THE SKIN SOURCEBOOK

THE
SKIN SOURCEBOOK

~ ~ ~ ~

by Alan S. Boyd, M.D.

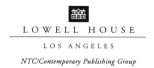

LOWELL HOUSE

LOS ANGELES

NTC/Contemporary Publishing Group

Library of Congress Cataloging-in-Publication Data

Boyd, Alan S.
    The skin sourcebook / by Alan S. boyd.
        p.   cm.
    Includes bibliographical references and index.
    ISBN 0-7373-0003-5
    1. Skin—Diseases—Popular works.   2. Skin—Care and hygiene–
    –Popular works.   I. Title.
    RL85.B69   1998
    616.5—dc21   98-51989
                                                              CIP

Published by Lowell House, a division of NTC/Contemporary Publishing
Group, Inc., 4255 West Touhy Avenue, Lincolnwood, Illinois 60646-
1975 U.S.A.

Design by Kate Mueller, Electric Dragon Productions

Printed and bound in the United States of America
International Standard Book Number: 0-7373-0003-5
10 9 8 7 6 5 4 3 2 1

CONTENTS

ACKNOWLEDGMENTS

The author would like to acknowledge the following people:

Jack and Joann Boyd—If I ever accomplished anything in my life, it was because of you two. I love you both.

My grandparents—Boy, did you raise some fantastic kids.

Susan Teel and Jeannie Forehand—Believe it or not, I am honored to be your brother.

The extended Scruggs family—You all raised a wonderful daughter.

Dwight Aston—Thank you for teaching me to work.

Lloyd Warner—It's nice to have a brother.

Jarret Forehand and Curt Williams—You were good guys. See you soon.

Wayne Reed—You're my hero, too.

Drs. Kenneth Neldner, Ron Rapini, and Lloyd King, Jr.—When no one else was willing to take a chance on me, you did. Thank you.

Paul McCord—Thanks, as always.

Stuart and Taylor—I cannot tell you two what it means to be your dad.

Binx—Worthless fleabag.

And most especially, to Lori—Without your love and support over the years, this project would have been neither begun nor worth doing. I love you.

PREFACE

This book is designed to provide you with an overview of different diseases of the skin, how they manifest themselves, their symptoms, and available therapies for their treatment.

The first section covers general skin care and therapy, since many patients have questions about routine skin maintenance (including sun protection) and cosmetic procedures to enhance their appearance.

Part II discusses several different types of dermatitis; most are explained at length.

Part III is dedicated to the topic of skin cancer. Since this is a particularly important subject for most people, both in terms of therapy and prevention, I believe it deserves a separate section. The three major types of skin cancer—basal cell carcinoma, squamous cell carcinoma, and malignant melanoma—are all discussed in depth, as well as are other, less common skin cancers.

In Part IV, I have compiled the most common skin conditions that afflict patients today. A complete listing of all known skin diseases is beyond the scope of a general guide for the consumer; however, therapies for various conditions are discussed in terms the layperson can understand. I have attempted to list as much as feasible all the possible treatments for a given condition.

The diseases are listed using the official nomenclature of clinical dermatology as well as the more common "unofficial" names. For instance, tinea corporis is the official name for a superficial fungal infection of the skin, but most persons know it better as ringworm. Similarly, shingles is known to dermatologists as herpes zoster. A nomenclature is provided to describe how areas of skin disease appear on the skin (for example, macule, papule, pustule, nodule, and so on). Use of these terms are not included in this text. Instead, I have chosen to designate the area of skin disease or involvement as a lesion.

The Appendices include a guide to medications used in dermatology, including commonly used drugs, their side effects, precautions for their administration, and estimated expense. A self-diagnosis appendix lists different diseases by how they might appear on your skin. It is not all inclusive, but it does cover the major disease categories and should help patients narrow down the possible conditions they may be experiencing. A list of skin disease organizations is also included. Those with a particular disorder may find it helpful to contact these groups for more information about new treatment advances, group meetings, lectures, and so on.

It is important to remember that this book is not a substitute for the care and guidance of a board-certified dermatologist. If you are concerned about a skin problem, consult a dermatologist.

PART I

SKIN CARE AND THERAPY

~ ~ ~ ~

MOISTURIZERS AND SOAPS

Types of Moisturizers

The production and use of moisturizers is a multimillion-dollar industry in the United States. These products are very important in dermatology; they are used to treat many different conditions such as eczema, psoriasis, and dry skin. None are capable, however, of putting moisture back into the skin. They are only able to *prevent* the loss of the body's natural moisture. Most products available on the store shelves are composed of some formulation of oil and water. Other ingredients are added as well, and occasionally these may cause problems.

The most moisturizing emollient available is petrolatum or Vaseline®, which provides a coating over the skin through which water cannot escape. Unfortunately, it is greasy and most people dislike the way it feels. In certain circumstances, however, it may be very useful. Ointments are usually very much like petrolatum, since most have an oily base. They are also very greasy and not always well accepted; some patients prefer to use them only at bedtime rather than during the day. Moisturizing creams contain more oil than water and, as a result, are also very effective. These may feel greasy but less so than petrolatum or ointments. Lotions have more water than oil; they are probably the most popular moisturizer. They are not as effective as ointments but are more likely to be used frequently since they are more pleasant. Humectants are a class of moisturizers which do not contain oil and may be classified as "oil free." These contain glycerin, propylene glycol, urea, glycolic acid, and lactic acid.

Many products contain ingredients added by manufacturers to enhance their products. These include fragrances, coloring agents, antimicrobials (to prevent bacterial contamination), and other chemicals to make the moisturizer more appealing. Some also include additional ingredients to increase the lotion's purchase appeal, such as vitamins, essential fatty acids, collagen, elastin, hyaluronic acid, and keratin. These may have some scientific basis and have catchy names, but they have not been proven to be of benefit.

Routine Moisturizers

There is certainly no shortage of moisturizers on the market. Table 1 lists several that are widely available and have few of the substances known to irritate the skin. As a rule, it is a good idea to avoid products containing lanolin, parabens,

Table 1 SUGGESTED MOISTURIZERS

Aquaphor® Ointment

Aveeno® Moisturizing Cream

Aveeno® Moisturizing Lotion

Beta Care® Lotion

Carmol® 10 Lotion

Colladerm® Lotion

Collastin® Oil-Free Moisturizer

DML® Forte Cream

DML® Forte Lotion

Eutra® Swiss Skin Creme

Jergens® All Purpose Face Lotion

Johnson's® Baby Oil

Lubriderm® Skin Conditioning Oil

Moisturel® Cream

Neutrogena® Body Oil

Pro-Cute® Cream

Purpose® Dry Skin Cream

Theraplex® Clearlotion

Theraplex® Hydrolotion

Vanicream® Moisturizing Skin Care Cream

quaternium-15, imidazolidinyl urea, and formaldehyde. These substances, while not irritating to everyone, may cause allergic reactions in some persons.

There is no way to moisturize the skin "too much," and those who need these products are encouraged to use them as often as possible. The best time to apply moisturizers is after a bath or shower while the skin is still moist. This seals in some of the water from bathing and leaves the skin lubricated.

Alpha Hydroxy Acids

Alpha hydroxy acids (AHAs) have been used since antiquity. Cleopatra is said to have used them for facial massage. These products have become very popular in the

Table 2   ALPHA HYDROXY ACIDS

AHA	Sugar Source
Glycolic acid	Sugar cane
Lactic acid	Milk
Tartaric acid	Grapes
Citric acid	Citrus fruits
Malic acid	Apples
Mandelic acid	Bitter almonds

past decade. They are all derived from different sugars (see Table 2) and are for-mulated as creams, lotions, cleansers, peeling agents, and facial masks. Their main effect seems to be altering the bonding between the skin cells. AHAs also affect the deeper layers of the skin, called the dermis, by increasing the fluid in the tissues. It is claimed that these products are capable of making the skin appear younger and healthier by decreasing skin wrinkling and pigmentation (age spots). The most pop-ular AHA is glycolic acid. This product is used extensively for chemical peeling and is the most common AHA added to various moisturizing creams and lotions (for ex-ample, Aqua Glycolic Lotion®, Shampoo®). Many cosmetic lines are now featuring moisturizers and makeup containing glycolic acid. Most formulations available over the counter have 8% glycolic acid. There is probably little danger from using these products, but their effectiveness is not completely proven; mild redness and sting-ing are the only known side effects. Combining the use of AHA-containing creams with tretinoin (Retin-A®, Renova®) is a popular method of trying to make the skin appear "younger."

Lotions containing lactic acid include Lac-Hydrin®, Amlactin®, Lactinol®, and Lactinol-E®. These are 10 to 12% creams and require a prescription for purchase. Lower-strength creams are available over the counter (Lacticare® and Lac Hydrin V®) but contain only 5% lactic acid. These creams and lotions are very effective at helping the skin retain its moisture. They are best used when the skin is damp and should be applied at least twice daily. There are few, if any, restrictions to their use; however, cuts and scrapes do not tolerate lactic acid–containing lotions well and will sting. Therefore, if the skin is dry and cracked, it is usually best to use a differ-ent product to allow healing before using these lotions. Lactic acid products have a slightly ammonialike smell, which some patients find objectionable. They are also relatively expensive.

Table 3   UREA-CONTAINING MOISTURIZERS

Aqua Care® Cream and Lotion (10%)

Aqua Lactin® Lotion (10%)

Atrac-tain® Cream (10%)

Atrac-tain® Lotion (5%)

Betamide® Lotion (25%)

Carmol® 10 Lotion (10%)

Carmol® 20 Cream (20%)

Carmol® 40 Cream (40%)

Eucerin® Plus Cream and Lotion (5%)

Gormel® Cream (20%)

Nutraplus® 10% Urea Cream

Nutraplus® 10% Urea Lotion

U-Lactin® (10%)

Ultramide® 25 Lotion (25%)

Ureacin® 10 Lotion (10%)

Ureacin® 20 Cream (20%)

Urea

Urea is a molecule that works much as do alpha hydroxy acids. When applied to the skin, it allows the cells to retain more water and gives the skin a lustrous look. Like lactic acid, it also tends to sting when it gets into a cut or abrasion. Urea gives moisturizers a slightly sticky feel but is otherwise very well tolerated. Most products are somewhat expensive; however, higher-concentration products may be very useful for thick, rough skin such as that found on the palms and soles (see Table 3). It is best to apply these moisturizers while the skin is wet. Some of the products on the market contain formalin, lanolin, and other substances which may be irritating to the skin, so read the product's ingredient list carefully before purchase.

Botanicals

Botanicals are plant products that are added to moisturizers in an effort to make the product seem "natural" or to capitalize on the popularity of herbal medicine. These

Table 4   DIFFERENT TYPES OF SOAPS

Type	Brand Name
Cleansing Creams and Lotions	Oil of Olay® Daily Facial Cleansing Lotion Ponds® Water Rinseable Cleanser Sea Breeze® Whipped Facial Cleanser
Moderately Moisturizing Soaps	Alpha Keri® Moisture-Rich Cleansing Bar Aveeno® Cleansing Bar for Normal to Oily Skin Caress® Bar Soap Eucerin® Cleansing Bar Faberge® Organics Bar Jergins® Gentle Touch Bar Lowila® Cake Soap
Mildly Moisturizing Soaps	Basis® Facial Cleanser Camay® Bar Soap Dove® Bar Soap Lubriderm® Body Bar Neutrogena® Cleansing Wash and Bar Oil of Olay® Foaming Face Wash Shield® Bar Soap
Drying	Acne Aid® Cleansing Bar Ivory® Moisturel® Sensitive Skin Cleanser Yardly® Oatmeal Soap
Acne Soaps	Aveeno® Cleansing Bar for Acne Buf Puf® Acne Cleansing Bar Drytex® Fostex® Medicated Cleansing Bar Oxy Clean® Medicated Bar Soap Pernox® Abraidant Scrub Cleanser Sulpho-Lac® Soap
Deodorant	Clearasil® Antibacterial Bar Coast® Johnson's® Foot Soap Lever 2000® Lifebuoy® Antibacterial Soap

Table 4 *continued*

Type	Brand Name
Deodorant continued	Liquid Dial® Antibacterial Soap
	Oxy Clean® Lathering Facial Scrub
	Palmolive® Gold
	Zest® Deodorant Soap

substances may give a moisturizer a different texture or aroma. The most popular additive is aloe vera. This substance has been shown to have some antibacterial properties when used in large quantities and is believed to have healing capabilities as well, although this has never been scientifically tested. Aloe vera is probably not harmful but may be mildly to moderately irritating to some patients. Other additives include almond oil, jojoba, licorice, seaweed, sesame oil, and wheat germ oil. These substances are not likely to cause irritation, but probably don't substantially enhance the skin.

Types of Soaps

Soaps are also a multimillion-dollar industry. Numerous brands are available and can be categorized according to how they were manufactured, how dry they leave the skin feeling, and the different functions they supposedly perform. Table 4 lists common soaps by these categories.

Soaps and washes with benzoyl peroxide are not included here since they are covered in the section on acne. Cleansing creams and lotions are the most useful for particularly dry or sensitive skin. They leave behind a layer of oil that helps to lubricate the skin much as moisturizers do, but they are only moderately effective at cleaning the skin surface. Mildly moisturizing soaps are probably the most useful for general use and are often recommended by dermatologists. They clean adequately and do not strip the skin of its natural oils. Soaps that dry the skin excessively are not inherently bad, particularly if a person tends to have oily skin. They may worsen conditions such as eczema (atopic dermatitis), however, and should not be used by those with sensitive skin. Deodorant soaps usually contain bacteria-killing substances. If a person is not allergic to these ingredients, their use should pose no problem. Unfortunately, patients with conditions caused by sensitive skin usually do not tolerate deodorant soaps.

There has been much focus in the past about the role that soaps should play in treating acne. Most of the acne soaps contain salicylic acid, precipitated sulfur, or benzoyl peroxide. These agents have a drying effect on the skin and cause some mild scaling and desquamation. They may be helpful in persons with mild acne, but for patients with more severe disease, these soaps are not likely to provide much relief. Some soaps contain abrasive scrubbers, usually ground-up fruit pits or polyethylene beads. These products are not inherently harmful and can indeed exfoliate some dead skin cells. However, they can be overused and may cause skin irritation. They should be used only about once or twice per week; daily use will probably not improve the acne and may worsen it.

SUN EXPOSURE

Light that strikes the earth is composed, in part, of ultraviolet light A (UVA) and B (UVB). Ultraviolet light C exists but is filtered out by the atmosphere and does not reach the earth's surface. UVB is responsible for most skin tanning and also for sunburn. UVA, on the other hand, is the ultraviolet light that provokes most of the sun-sensitivity disorders that are seen. Much more UVA strikes the earth than UVB, but UVB is capable of doing more damage to the skin.

Sunburn

Almost everyone is familiar with sunburn. People differ in their susceptibility to sunburn depending on skin type, the amount of protective pigment accumulated in the skin, recent medication intake, and clothing or sunscreen use. The peak times for sunburning are between 10:00 A.M. and 2:00 P.M. It is still possible to burn at other times, but maximum ultraviolet light exposure is during these four hours. Other factors include the amount of cloud cover (clouds, unless very thick, transmit almost all the ultraviolet light striking them), water or snow reflection, low humidity, high altitude and latitude (the closer to the equator, the greater the amount of ultraviolet light). Those who have been in the sun (or on suntanning beds) for extended periods and who have produced a substantial amount of pigment in the skin will be less likely to burn.

People who take certain medications may be more likely to burn, even with less exposure to the sun (see Table 5). These phototoxic drugs may encourage severe burns that may require hospitalization and have sometimes even resulted in death. Someone taking one or more of these medications is usually advised to remain out of the sun for several days after the last dose has been taken. If one must be in the sun, the use of a good sunscreen is imperative. Not everyone who takes these medications will become more sun sensitive, but there is no way to predict who will be affected.

A person's clothing makes a big difference in the amount of ultraviolet light that reaches the skin. For years, the traditional recommendation has been to wear a broad-brimmed hat, long sleeves, and long pants to minimize sun exposure. While this is good advice, there are other considerations as well. Lighter shades of clothing, particularly white, tend to transmit more ultraviolet rays. Therefore, darker colors are preferable. Unfortunately, they tend to be hot. Wet clothing also allows

Table 5   PHOTOTOXIC MEDICATIONS

Generic Name	Brand Name
Amiodarone	Cordarone®
Coal tars (and coal tar derivatives)	
Demeclocyline	Declomycin®
Doxycyline	Vibramycin®, Monodox®
Furosemide	Lasix®
Naldixic acid	NegGram®
Naproxen	Anaprox®, Naprosyn®
Phenothiazines	Compazine®, Mellaril®, Prolixin®, Serentil®, Stelazine®, Thorazine®
Piroxicam	Feldene®
Sulfonamides	Bactrim®, Septra®, Gantanol®, Gantrisin®, Pediazole®
Psoralens	
Methoxsalen	Oxsoralen®
Trioxsalen	Trisoralen®

more ultraviolet light through. The heavier the cloth, the less ultraviolet light transmitted. Synthetic fabrics such as rayon protect better than cotton, and clothing which is made from fabric with a "loose" weave is less desirable than tighter-woven fabric. Some companies, such as Sun Precautions, Inc. (425-303-8585), manufacture special lines of clothing with fabric that protects from ultraviolet light (Rayosan®). This clothing is most useful for persons exposed to a great deal of sun or who have previously developed a skin cancer. Almost all types of clothing (pants, shirts, jackets, hats, socks, and so on) can be purchased with sun protection in mind.

Treating Sunburn

It's important to remember that there are different types of sunburn. For persons with a mild degree of redness and discomfort, very little treatment may be needed. Use of a moisturizing lotion such as Aveeno® or Lubriderm® may be all that is required. Bath preparations, particularly colloidal oatmeal (Aveeno®), are also

Table 6 TREATMENT MEASURES FOR MODERATE SUNBURNS

1. Consume plenty of *nonalcoholic* fluids (water, Gatorade®, Kool-Aid®).
2. Take aspirin or ibuprofen on a regular basis until the discomfort subsides.
3. Stay in a shaded, cool room.
4. Take cool showers or baths with colloidal oatmeal (Aveeno®).
5. Apply corticosteroid *cream* to burned areas two or three times daily.
6. Apply moisturizing lotions liberally and often.

useful. Topical corticosteroid creams (preferable to ointments) may decrease the redness and inflammation. For a more serious burn, more aggressive measures are useful; these are outlined in Table 6.

Topical corticosteroid creams have numerous side effects if a strong preparation is used for too long. For a period of twenty-four to seventy-two hours, however, they may be used without worry. Even in children, a Class I corticosteroid cream may be safely used on the face for several days and may make the child much more comfortable. Sunburns peak at about eighteen hours. Those who realize that they have gotten a serious burn may be helped by a corticosteroid injection (triamcinolone [Kenalog®]) or a short course of oral prednisone (Deltasone®). People who moisturize their skin a great deal may be able to avoid a lot of peeling. Some gels are available containing a topical anesthetic and menthol (for example, Banana Boat®) that may be applied to sunburned skin; these relieve the stinging for a few days until the body can heal itself. Drinking lots of *nonalcoholic* beverages may also be beneficial. Drinks containing alcohol actually dehydrate the body and may make the problem worse.

Those who have received a particularly bad sunburn or who have burned while taking one of the photosensitizing medications listed in Table 5 should consider seeing a dermatologist. They may blister and experience headaches, nausea, vomiting, and chills. Corticosteroids taken orally or by injection may be helpful, as may aggressive replacement of fluids.

Tanning

A tan is the skin's response to an injury done by ultraviolet light. In order to tan, you have to stimulate the pigment-producing cells in the skin, and to do that, they must be exposed to the sun or some other light source. In other words, there is no way to obtain a safe tan. Having some pigment protection from the sun is beneficial if a person is about to be exposed to it, but ultimately it is safer to wear protective clothing and to use a good sunscreen. Unfortunately, a tan is considered "sexy," so many people don't heed this advice.

Tanning beds have also provided the opportunity to tan during the colder months. Commercial tanning beds are somewhat different from the ultraviolet light machines used in dermatologists' offices. First, they tend to put out almost solely UVA. They also vary widely in the amount of UVA that they emit. In other words, they are not uniformly calibrated–some machines put out a great amount of UVA and others much less. This makes it easier to burn. Additionally, the operators of tanning establishments are not always careful to inform customers about which medications interact dangerously with ultraviolet light. Unfortunately, most of the warnings dermatologists give about the dangers of too much light exposure seem to fall on deaf ears.

Tanning accelerators should also be avoided. These products may be purchased through mail-order houses and over the Internet. Some are relatively harmless; however, it is not known what chemicals may be in them. The most popular type has been tyrosine-containing creams and lotions which are applied to the skin several days before sun exposure. Theoretically, the tyrosine accumulates in the skin and when exposed to sunlight is converted by the body to melanin, the pigment contained in the skin. What little scientific testing has been done on these products has not shown them to live up to their claims. Another product, canthaxanthin, is potentially dangerous and should be avoided. This chemical has been shown to accumulate in the eyes of those who take it. While it has not been proven to affect vision, there is certainly a potential for problems. Some people become so susceptible to ultraviolet light when using these substances that they burn badly; deaths have even occurred. Taking or applying a drug and then purposefully exposing oneself to the sun (or worse, a tanning bed) is asking for trouble.

For many years, dihydroxyacetone (DHA) has been used to stain the skin a reddish-brown color to simulate a tan. Numerous products are available; some provide a more realistic "tan" than others. There is no way to know which product will work best for a given person. These products are harmless and if properly applied may give good results. Too much of the lotion or cream can produce a "streaked" appearance, however. Additionally, some persons do not appear "tan" but somewhat orange or yellow. It is wise to test a small area before widespread application. It will take about a month for the color to fade, and the palms may deeply stain. Remember, fake tans do nothing to prevent sunburn. They are not protective–persons exposed to extensive ultraviolet light exposure will burn.

Chronic Sun Exposure

Persons who have been in the sun for prolonged periods, either at work or at play, have what is termed "photoaged" skin. Their skin appears slightly yellowed, wrinkled, lax, dry, and leatherlike. The back of the neck frequently shows a diamond-like pattern of deep wrinkling (cutis rhomboidalis nuchae); on the front of the chest there may be small, superficial blood vessels with an overall appearance of reddened skin (poikiloderma of Civatte). Recent treatment of photoaged skin of the face and forehead includes several different therapies. Chemical peels (see the section on cosmetic concerns) are a popular method of treatment and are useful in removing precancerous lesions such as actinic keratoses. More popular is the use of tretinoin (Retin-A®, Renova®). Tretinoin is applied much as it is for acne but is used for much more prolonged periods (months to years). There is evidence that this medicine is helpful in reducing fine wrinkles and in eliminating dark spots (liver spots) called solar lentigos. Usually, medium strengths such as the 0.05% cream are used. With cutis rhomboidalis nuchae the wrinkling is generally too extensive to respond to tretinoin or peels. Poikiloderma of Civatte may be fairly disfiguring since it is present on the sides of the neck and upper trunk, but may be difficult to treat. Topical tretinoin may be helpful but the use of this drug in these sites may cause considerable irritation. Laser treatment for the fine blood vessels may be useful, but it is expensive and time consuming. Obviously, it is important to prevent any further damage with the regular use of a good sunscreen.

Sunscreens

One of the hottest-selling dermatological items of the past decade is sunscreen. There are currently over a hundred different brands available, and this is a multi-million-dollar industry. These products are useful not only to prevent sunburn; more importantly, they protect us from long-term damage from sun exposure such as skin cancer and wrinkling. Sunscreens are manufactured as creams, ointment, gels, lotions, sprays, sticks, and oils. Sunscreens are divided into two different types—chemical sunscreens and physical sunscreens. Chemical sunscreens are most common and popular. They contain different chemicals designed to block or scatter ultraviolet rays as they strike the skin (see Table 7).

Most commercial sunscreens contain more than one of these substances. The amount may depend on how soluble they are in the lotion or cream base. Most absorb UVB rays well but do a poor job with UVA. However, some absorb better in the UVA range.

Table 7 **ACTIVE INGREDIENTS OF CHEMICAL SUNSCREENS**

PABA and PABA-esters	Para-aminobenzoic acid (PABA)
	Octyl-dimethyl PABA (Padimate O)
	Amyl-dimethyl PABA (Padimate A)
	Glyceryl PABA
Benzophenones	Oxybenzone
	Sulisobenzone
	Dioxybenzone
Cinnamates	Cinoxate
	Octylmethoxycinnamate
	Octocrylene
	Ethylhexyl-p-methoxycinnamate
Salicylates	Homomethyl salicylate (Homosalate)
	Octyl salicylate
Anathranilate	Menthylanathranilate

Physical sunscreens are better for sun protection but they are not usually as cosmetically attractive and therefore are less widely used. These chemicals do not absorb ultraviolet light but rather reflect and scatter it. Table 8 lists physical sunscreening agents; these are most useful for persons with fair skin who have little or no protection from ultraviolet light.

An important aspect of any sunscreen is how well it stays on the skin. Early sunscreens worked well but had little staying power when the skin became wet with perspiration or water. Newer formulations, particularly those used for sports, are much better at staying on the skin. Some practically have to be washed off. To get the most out of your sunscreen, apply it to dry skin an hour before sun exposure. Even if the skin is wet, frequently apply sunscreen to continue getting the maximum benefits from it. In this instance, more is definitely better. It should be remembered that water is not the only thing that will diminish the amount of protective sunscreen on a person's skin. Wind and natural absorption of the chemical will also do this. There may also be a difference between fresh water and salt water with regard to how easily they wash off a sunscreen.

Table 8   ACTIVE INGREDIENTS OF PHYSICAL SUNSCREENS

Active Ingredient	Brand Name
Zinc oxide	RVPaque®
Titanium dioxide	Baby Garde® Sunblock Lotion
	Bain de Soleil® Sport Lotion
	Banana Boat® Sunscreen Lotion
	Coppertone® Faces Only Sunblock Lotion
	Johnson's® Baby Sunblock Lotion and Cream
	Sundown® Sunblock Ultra
	Total Eclipse® Lotion
Magnesium silicate (talc)	
Kaolin	
Ferric oxide	
Red petrolatum	RVPaba®
Magnesium oxide	

Sun Protection Factor (SPF)

Sunscreens come with a number called an "SPF," which stands for Sun Protection Factor. Most formulations are at least an 8, and some range up to 50 or more. The sun protection factor is a multiple of the number of hours a person can stay out in the sun while using a given sunscreen before he or she will have been exposed to the same amount of ultraviolet light in one hour of unprotected exposure. For instance, if a sunscreen has the label of 15, then with its use over a fifteen-hour period the skin will have only absorbed an hour's worth of ultraviolet light. Obviously, the higher the SPF the more protection that is theoretically provided. SPFs only apply to UVB-blocking agents, which make up the majority of the sunscreening ingredients found in sun protection products. It is important to remember that UVA, while not as capable of causing a sunburn, interacts the most with phototoxic drugs. It also penetrates deeper into the skin than does UVB and is suspected of being responsible for many of the signs of aging attributed to sun exposure. For this reason, it is a good idea to consider using sunscreens with either a physical blocking agent or that are specifically formulated to block UVA (for example, Shade®). It is important to remember that SPFs were developed by testing the sunscreens in a laboratory and not under "real-life" conditions. It is probably best, therefore, to con-

Table 9   PREFERRED SUNSCREEN FORMULATIONS

Bain de Soleil® Sport Lotion★

Banana Boat® Sunscreen Lotion SPF 34★

Cancer Garde® Ultra Protection Sunblock Lotion★

Bullfrog® Gel

Coppertone® All Day Protection Lotion

Coppertone® Moisturizing Sunblock Lotion

Hawaiian Tropic® Baby Faces Sunblock Lotion and Spray

Hawaiian Tropic® UVA Sunblock Lotion

Johnson's® Baby Sunblock Lotion and Cream★

Piz Buin® Lotion★

PreSun® products (SPF 15 and higher)

RVPaba® and RVPaque★

Shade® products

Sundown® products (SPF 15 and higher)★

Total Eclipse® Lotion★

★*Contains a physical sunscreening agent*

sider an SPF rating overly optimistic and not to count on it providing a full degree of protection. Keep in mind that sunscreens are only able to provide protection if they are utilized properly. Frequent and generous application is the key to their use. Some people may be allergic to sunscreen components; this may be to the sunscreening agents themselves or to the creams and lotions in which they are mixed.

How strong a sunscreen should a person use? There is probably not much benefit to using a sunscreen with an SPF over 20. Most persons don't spend a full day in the sun and if they do, hopefully they apply sunscreen more than once. A sunscreen with an SPF of 50 or more provides more protection than a person probably needs. It is more important to emphasize frequent application of the sunscreen and care in getting the product over *all* sun-exposed areas.

Which product to use? While it is probably more important that a sunscreen *be* used (it does no good sitting in a bottle), not all sunscreens are created equal. Most dermatologists recommend preparations with more than one sunscreening agent, preferably three or four, and be at least an SPF of 15 or more. Additionally, it is helpful if the product has a physical blocking agent such as titanium dioxide. Several sunscreens which meet these criteria are listed in Table 9.

Sunscreens are also available in sticks for use on the lips (Blistex®, Chapstick®, Coppertone®, Hawaiian Tropic®, Piz Buin®, Sundown®). Use of these may be very important if a person is susceptible to sun-induced fever blisters.

More and more people have taken to using a sunscreen every day in an attempt to prevent even the smallest amount of ultraviolet light exposure. This is probably a good idea. Most cosmetics now contain some type of sunscreen. Also, it has recently become popular for moisturizing lotions to contain sunscreen. For persons with fair skin, the practice of complete sun avoidance will go a long way toward preventing future skin problems.

The use of sunscreens for children has become widespread. Recent research has shown that children who experience significant sun exposure and/or sunburns, particularly prior to puberty, have an increased incidence of skin cancer, including melanoma. In other words, preventing serious sun exposure in children today helps prevent potentially life-threatening health consequences tomorrow. This applies to infants as well. Babies have little or no protection from the sun's ultraviolet rays; therefore, even if an infant is going to be in a carriage or in the shade, the liberal use of sunscreen is in order. A new product, Coppertone Kids 30®, has been formulated with a purple color. This is appealing to children and allows the parent to see where the sunscreen has been applied. The color will not stain clothing, hair, or skin.

Some sunscreens contain additional ingredients such as jojoba oil, aloe, and/or vitamin E. These reportedly help to soothe the skin or provide a missing nutritional ingredient. While such products are probably harmless, they have never been appropriately tested and their claimed benefits are unproven. Some persons are allergic to these ingredients, and a good rule of thumb would be to avoid them.

DRY SKIN (XEROSIS)

Xerosis affects more than half of people over age sixty-five. The skin becomes dry and slightly scaly and may itch. This promotes eczema (xerotic eczema). For some reason, the skin of older patients fails to retain the moisture that it once did. Application of water from external sources is not helpful in alleviating the problem, but holding the moisture in with emollients frequently is. The use of emollients, moisturizers, and soaps designed for atopic dermatitis and eczema is generally helpful. If the problem is particularly severe, the emollients listed in Table 10 are useful. Frequent application is the key to improvement.

Table 10   USEFUL LOTIONS FOR DRY SKIN (XEROSIS)

Emollient	Brand Name
Lactic Acid Containing	Amlactin® 12% (Rx)
	Epilyt®
	Lac-Hydrin® 12% (Rx)
	Lac-Hydrin® 5
	Lacticare® Lotion
Urea Containing	Aqua Care® Cream or Lotion
	Aqua Lacten® Lotion
	Atrac-tain® Lotion and Cream
	Betamide® Lotion
	Carmol® 10 Lotion and 20 and 40 Cream (Rx)
	Gormel® Cream
	Nutraplus® Cream or Lotion
	U-lactin® Cream
	Ultramide 25® Lotion

Topical Corticosteroids

The use of topical corticosteroids (or topical steroids) in dermatology is so widespread that a separate section about these products is in order. They are among the most popular medications because they are effective, easy to use, don't cause odor or discomfort, are compatible with other therapies, and, in the case of generic formulations, relatively inexpensive. Hydrocortisone was first marketed in the 1950s. Shortly thereafter a topical form of the drug was used for skin diseases such as eczema and psoriasis. Subsequently, triamcinolone ointment (Kenalog®) became available, and for the first time, physicians and patients had a powerful weapon in the fight against skin disease. Currently, there are close to fifty different brand-name topical steroids and scores of generic formulations.

Side Effects

While topical steroids are useful, they also have some side effects. Most of these are relatively minor and may be avoided with proper use of these medications. Almost all side effects result from either using a preparation which is too strong or using it under the wrong conditions. Some areas of the skin are able to absorb topical steroids better than others. Thin skin such as that of the eyelids and scrotum need only weak preparations since the absorption is so great. On the other hand, the palms and soles are very thick and usually require stronger steroids. It is important to use the appropriate preparation on the appropriate site. Skin also absorbs topical steroids better if the skin is very moist or well lubricated (such as after a bath) or if it is slightly broken down (as in eczema or psoriasis). It is also possible to greatly increase the amount of absorbed topical steroid by covering or occluding the skin with plastic wrap (Saran Wrap®). This is a popular method for increasing the effectiveness of midpotency topical steroids while avoiding some of the side effects of stronger medications.

The most common side effect is thinning of the skin. This makes the skin look pink or red since blood vessels are more visible and dilated (telangiectasias). It may take only a few weeks to develop thinned skin if a potent formulation is used on a sensitive site. This problem will resolve over several months if the topical steroid is stopped.

Very potent preparations tend to lose their effectiveness if used too often. This phenomenon is called tachyphylaxis and may occur after only a week's use. It is more common if the cream is being applied several times per day rather than just once. The topical steroid will become as effective as before if the drug is stopped for a week or so. It is, therefore, usually best to use topical steroids for only a few weeks at a time.

If these drugs are applied to the face and upper trunk, a mild case of acne or perioral dermatitis may begin. This side effect is somewhat difficult to control even if the topical steroid is discontinued; it is better prevented than treated.

Rarely, the use of a topical steroid may make a rash worse. This is seen as increased redness, scaling, and itching. Most often this is due to an allergy or irritation from one of the ingredients in the cream or ointment. Occasionally there is an allergy to the steroid itself.

The most dangerous side effect of topical steroid use is systemic absorption of the drug. This is not common, but may be seen in persons using large amounts of very potent preparations. If the problem is severe enough, it may give the patient symptoms identical to those on long-term oral or injectable steroids, including increased blood pressure, rounded facial features ("moon faces"), and increased blood sugar. Careful use of topical steroids allow them to yield the benefits for which they are intended without causing problems. Most scientific studies have shown that applying a steroid several times per day is no more effective than a single application. Once-per-day application cuts down the likelihood of side effects and decreases the cost of using these drugs.

Topical steroids are rated according to potency. Class I, or the superpotent formulations are about one thousand times stronger than 1% hydrocortisone. Most skin conditions can be treated using a midpotency topical steroid, although very potent or very weak formulations are most appropriate in some instances. Table 11 lists available topical steroids and their brand names, sizes, and approximate cost.

Forms of Topical Corticosteroids

The many different formulations of topical steroids are designed to treat different types of skin diseases as well as varying types of skin. Ointments are somewhat greasy and for that reason, many people do not like them. However, they not only moisturize the skin but also allow better absorption of the medication. These preparations are popular for rashes which are particularly dry and or scaly. Ointments are most appropriate for nighttime use, under occlusion with plastic film or gloves/socks or on hairless areas. They may occlude pores and might result in an acnelike rash if used on hairy sites.

Creams are the most popular forms of topical steroids. They are much more cosmetically acceptable than ointments and may be applied to almost any site.

Table 11 **TOPICAL CORTICOSTEROIDS**

Generic Name	Trade Name	Size	Cost
Class I			
Betamethasone dipropionate 0.05%	Diprolene® Ointment	15g, 50g	★★★★
	Diprolene® AF Cream	15g, 50g	★★★★
	Diprolene® Gel	15g, 50g	★★★★
	Diprolene® Lotion	30ml, 60ml	★★★★
	Generic Ointment	NA	★★★
	Generic Cream	NA	★★★
	Generic Lotion	NA	★★★
Clobatasol propionate 0.05%	Temovate® Ointment	15g, 30g, 45g	★★★★
	Temovate® Cream	15g, 30g, 45g	★★★★
	Temovate® E Cream	15g, 30g, 60g	★★★★
	Temovate® Gel	15g, 30g, 60g	★★★★
	Temovate® Lotion	25ml, 50ml	★★★★
	Cormax® Ointment	15g, 45g	★★★
	Cormax® Lotion	25ml	★★★
	Generic Ointment	NA	★★★
	Generic Cream	NA	★★★
	Generic Lotion	NA	★★★
Diflorasone diacetate 0.05%	Psorcon® Ointment	15g, 30g, 60g	★★★★
	Psorcon® Cream	15g, 30g, 60g	★★★★
Halobetasol propionate 0.05%	Ultravate® Ointment	15g, 50g	★★★★
	Ultravate® Cream	15g, 50g	★★★★
Class II			
Amcinonide 0.1%	Cyclocort® Ointment	15g, 30g, 60g	★★★★
Betamethasone dipropionate 0.05%	Diprolene® Cream AF	15g, 50g	★★★★
Betamethasone dipropionate 0.05%	Diprosone® Ointment	15g, 45g	★★★
Desoximetasone 0.25%	Topicort® Ointment	15g, 60g	★★★
	Topicort® Cream	15g, 60g, 4oz	★★★
Desoximetasone 0.05%	Topicort® Gel	15g, 60g	★★★
Diflorasone diacetate 0.05%	Florone® Ointment	15g, 30g, 60g	★★★
	Maxiflor® Ointment	15g, 30g, 60g	★★★

Generic Name	Trade Name	Size	Cost
Class II			
Fluocinonide 0.05%	Lidex® Ointment	15g, 30g, 60g, 120g	★★★★
	Lidex® Cream	15g, 30g, 60g, 120g	★★★★
	Lidex® Gel	15g, 30g, 60g	★★★★
	Dermacin® Creme	30g	★★
	Generic Ointment	NA	★★
	Generic Cream	NA	★★
	Generic Gel	NA	★★
Halcinonide 0.1%	Halog® Cream	15g, 30g, 60g, 240g	★★
Mometasone furoate 0.05%	Elocon® Ointment	15g, 45g	★★★★
Triamcinolone acetonide 0.1%	Aristicort® A Ointment	15g, 60g	★★★
Class III			
Amcinonide 0.1%	Cyclocort® Cream	15g, 30g, 60g	★★★★
Amcinonide 0.1%	Cyclocort® Lotion	20ml, 60ml	★★★★
Betamethasone valerate 0.1%	Valisone® Ointment	15g, 45g	★★★
	Generic Ointment	NA	★★
Desoximetasone 0.20%	Topicort® LP Cream	15g, 60g	★★★
	Topicort® Gel	15g, 60g	★★★
Diflorasone diacetate 0.05%	Florone® E Cream	15g, 30g, 60g	★★★
	Florone® Cream	15g, 30g, 60g	★★★
	Maxiflor® Cream	30g, 60g	★★★
Fluocinonide 0.05%	Lidex-E® Cream	15g, 30g, 60g, 120g	★★★★
	Lidex® Solution	20mg, 60ml	★★★★
	Generic E Cream	NA	★★
	Generic Solution	NA	★★
Fluticasone proprionate 0.05%	Cutivate® Ointment	15g, 30g, 60g	★★★
Halcinonide 0.1%	Halog® Ointment	15g, 30g, 60g, 240g	★★★
	Halog-E® Cream	30g, 60g	★★★
	Halog® Solution	20ml, 60ml	★★★
Mometasone furoate 0.05%	Elocon® Lotion	30ml, 60ml	★★★★
Triamcinolone acetonide 0.1%	Kenalog® Ointment	15g, 60g, 240g	★★★
	Generic	NA	★

continued

Table 11　*continued*

Generic Name	Trade Name	Size	Cost
Class IV			
Betamethasone valerate 0.1%	Valisone® Lotion	20g, 60ml	★★★
	Generic	NA	★★
Fluocinolone acetonide 0.025%	Synalar® Ointment	15g, 30g, 60g, 425g	★★★
Flurandrenolide 0.05%	Cordran® Ointment	15g, 30g, 60g, 225g	★★★
Halcinonide 0.025%	Halog® Cream	15g, 60g	★★★
Hydrocortisone butyrate 0.1%	Locoid® Ointment	15g, 45g	★★★
Hydrocortisone valerate 0.2%	Westcort® Ointment	15g, 45g, 60g	★★★
Mometasone furoate 0.05%	Elocon® Cream	15g, 45g	★★★★
Class V			
Betamethasone dipropionate 0.02%	Diprosone® Lotion	20ml, 60ml	★★
Betamethasone valerate 0.1%	Valisone® Cream	15g, 45g	★★★
	Generic	NA	★★
Clocortalone 0.1%	Cloderm® Cream	15g, 45g	★★
Fluocinolone acetonide 0.025%	Synalar® Cream	15g, 30g, 60g, 425g	★★★
Flurandrenolide 0.025%	Cordran® Ointment	30g, 60g, 225g	★★★
Flurandrenolide 0.05%	Cordran® Cream	15g, 30g, 60g, 225g	★★★
Fluticasone propionate 0.05%	Cutivate® Cream	15g, 30g, 60g	★★★
Hydrocortisone butyrate 0.1%	Locoid® Cream	15g, 45g, 60g	★★★
Hydrocortisone valerate 0.2%	Westcort® Cream	15g, 45g, 60g	★★★
Prednicarbate 0.1%	Dermatop® Cream	15g, 60g	★★★★
Triamcinolone acetonide 0.25%	Aristicort® Cream	15g, 60g, 2,520g	★★★
Triamcinolone acetonide 0.1%	Kenalog® Lotion	15ml, 60ml	★★
Class VI			
Aclometasone dipropionate 0.05%	Aclovate® Ointment	15g, 45g, 60g	★★★
	Aclovate® Cream	15g, 45g, 60g	★★★
Betamethasone valerate 0.1%	Valisone® Lotion	20ml, 60ml	★★★
	Beta-Val® Lotion	NA	★★
	Generic	NA	★★

Generic Name	Trade Name	Size	Cost
Class VI			
Desonide 0.05%	DesOwen® Ointment	15g, 60g	★★★
	DesOwen® Cream	15g, 60g, 90g	★★★
	DesOwen® Lotion	60ml, 120ml	★★★
	Tridesilon® Ointment	15g, 60g	★★
	Tridesilon® Cream	15g, 60g, 5lb	★★
Fluocinolone acetonide 0.01%	Synalar® Cream	15g, 30g, 60g, 425g	★★★
	Synalar® Lotion	20ml, 60ml	★★★
Flurandrenolide 0.05%	Cordran® Lotion	15ml, 60ml	★★★
Flurandrenolide 0.025%	Cordran® Cream	30g, 60g, 225g	★★★
Triamcinolone acetonide 0.025%	Kenalog® Lotion	60ml	★★
Class VII			
Decadron phosphate 0.1%	Generic Cream	15g, 30g	★
Hydrocortisone 2.5%	Eldecort® Cream 2.5%	15g, 30g	★
	Hytone® Ointment 2.5%	1oz	★★
	Hytone® Cream 2.5%®	1oz, 2oz	★★
	Hytone® Lotion 2.5%®	2oz	★★
	Nutracort® Lotion 2.5%	60ml, 120ml	★★
	Synacort® 2.5% Cream	30g	★★
Hydrocortisone 1.0%	Eldecort® Cream 1%	15g, 30g	★
	Hytone® Ointment 1%	30g, 120g	★★
	Hytone® Cream 1%	30g, 120g	★★
	Nutracort® Cream 1%	30g, 60g, 120g	★★
	Nutracort® Lotion 1%	60ml, 120ml	★★
	Penecort® Cream 1%	30g	★★
	Penecort® Lotion 1%	30ml, 60ml	★★
	Penecort® Solution 1%	30ml, 60ml	★★
	Synacort® 1% Cream	15g, 30g, 60g	★★
Hydrocortisone 0.5%	Cortaid®	15g, 30g	★
	Cortizone-5® Ointment	1oz	★
	Cortizone-5® Cream	1oz, 2oz	★
	Cortizone-10® Ointment	1oz, 2oz	★
	Cortizone-10® Cream	1oz, 2oz	★
	Cortizone-10® Liquid	1.5oz	★

continued

Table 11　*continued*

Generic Name	Trade Name	Size	Cost
Unusual Formulations			
Dexamethasone 0.04%	Decaspray®	25g	★★
Fluocinolone acetonide 0.01%	FS Shampoo®	4oz	★★
	Derma-Smooth® FS Oil	4oz	★★
Flurandrenolide	Cordran® Tape	12 patches, small roll, large roll	★★
Triamcinolone acetonide 0.1%	Kenalog® in Orabase	5g	
Triamcinolone acetonide 0.2%	Kenalog® Spray	23g, 63g	★★

★ = *inexpensive*, ★★★★ = *very expensive*

Some patients prefer certain brands of topical steroids because the base in which the drug is mixed is better suited to them. Lotions and liquids are popular for use on large surface areas. They are particularly useful for treating the scalp. Most liquids contain propylene glycol, which allows for easy spreading. Some lotions are slightly creamy and may leave a residue on the skin or in the hair. Gels are formulated in propylene glycol and isopropyl alcohol and have an alcohol-type smell. These are very useful for the scalp and other hair-bearing skin. Topical steroid sprays are not often used. They are somewhat expensive and wasteful. Some patients prefer them, however, since they are easy to use on the scalp. Kenalog® Spray has a small tube which attaches to a spray nozzle and allows the patient to squirt the medication directly through the hair to a specific area. Cordran Tape® is an occlusive tape which contains a topical steroid. It is not often used but is very helpful for treating small spots, especially in psoriasis. It allows the steroid to be applied in a concentrated manner and with some occlusion. Derma-Smoothe FS® is another rarely used steroid product, although it is very helpful for scalp conditions, particularly psoriasis. It is applied to a damp scalp for variable periods of time. Derma-Smoothe FS® is an oil that must be washed out. The best use of this product is by occluding it overnight with a shower cap or damp, warm towel. The only marketed steroid shampoo is FS Shampoo®. It is most useful for scalp conditions such as seborrheic dermatitis or mild psoriasis.

Vitamins and Minerals

Vitamins and minerals are compounds that function as the "supporting engine" for the body's metabolism. Actual deficiencies of vitamins and minerals in industrialized countries are rare, and people who eat a normal North American diet don't usually benefit by taking medicines containing vitamins and/or minerals. The rare patients who may be helped are usually either mentally ill or consuming an insufficient diet. People with metabolic diseases or eating disorders may also be vitamin deficient. Some older patients, or those with certain medical conditions (alcoholism, bowel obstruction, or chronic diarrhea) may have a borderline deficiency. These persons often benefit from taking a vitamin supplement.

One important thing to remember about vitamins and minerals is that applying them to your skin is usually of little value. The skin, hair, and nails are generally not capable of absorbing these compounds in their pure form. While the cosmetic industry has profited by advertising shampoos, moisturizers, and cosmetics as vitamin or mineral enriched, there is no evidence that these products are actually helpful. Taking these compounds by mouth is usually unnecessary and not likely to help a particular skin condition.

Vitamin C

This vitamin is found in fresh fruits and vegetables. Most persons need about 50 to 60 mg per day of this vitamin, which is adequately provided by a standard diet. Smokers tend to need a little more, about 100 mg per day. Supplementing the diet with additional vitamin C has not been shown to be helpful. Since this is a water-soluble vitamin, any excess is excreted in the urine. No scientific studies have ever shown that taking this supplement in large doses has an effect on any disease process. Taking several thousand milligrams daily may cause diarrhea and abdominal pain.

A deficiency of vitamin C leads to the medical condition known as scurvy. Today scurvy is only seen among persons eating a single food item (for example, canned soup) every day or who have a phobia about fruits and vegetables. Scurvy causes small scaly areas on the arms and legs, mild bleeding around hair follicles, bleeding and swelling of the gums, and loose teeth. Treatment with supplements of vitamin C for a few days will usually cure the problem.

There is some evidence that applying topical vitamin C will help "rejuvenate" the skin and make it appear younger. Cellex-C America® (1-800-235-5392) now markets this product as a lotion, cream, and gel. The theory is that the vitamin C inactivates the oxidizing influences to which the skin is subjected. As a result, it appears younger and healthier. Cellex-C is expensive and must be used daily. There does not appear to be any harm in the use of this product, although the evidence that it is genuinely useful is not particularly strong.

Vitamin B

Vitamin B is actually a combination of B vitamins. Thiamin (B_1), riboflavin (B_2), pyridoxine (B_6), and cobalamine (B_{12}) are the four compounds comprising this group. Deficiency of any of these is rare and usually found in alcoholics and persons on bizarre diets (food faddists). Riboflavin, pyridoxine, and cobalamine deficiencies lead to disorders of the mouth and mucous membranes. Swelling and soreness of the tongue, inflammation of the corners of the mouth, and irritation of the lips are seen in affected persons. Cobalamine deficiency may occur in strict vegetarians and persons who do not absorb food properly from the stomach and intestines, and it may also develop as a natural consequence of aging. A type of anemia called pernicious anemia is seen in cobalamine deficiency. Vitamin B deficiency is rare in healthy persons who are consuming a reasonable diet. Vegetables, fruits, and beans are good sources of these compounds. There are no topical formulations of B vitamins for use on the skin.

Vitamin D

Vitamin D is formed in the body in part by interaction with sunlight. Deficiencies are seen in persons who get no exposure to light, such as hermits and prisoners. This compound keeps the body's calcium at appropriate levels. The building blocks of vitamin D are found in dairy products and some vegetables. It appears to be very important in the health of certain organs, including the skin. Increased amounts of this vitamin make the skin proliferate less and are useful in diseases such as psoriasis. A derivative of vitamin D, calcipotriene (Dovonex®), has been approved by the FDA. Taking large doses of vitamin D is dangerous since this vitamin is not water soluble and toxic amounts may build up in the body.

Vitamin E

This vitamin is also known as alpha tocopherol and is believed to help the body by removing oxidized acids. Vitamin E is found in vegetable oils and wheat germ and deficiency is extremely rare. This vitamin has been touted as being capable of partially reversing the aging processes in the skin. It is available in numerous moisturizers, lotions, and vitamin supplements. However, there is no proof that it is helpful and it is not absorbed to any appreciable extent when applied to the skin.

Vitamin A

Vitamin A is probably the most publicized vitamin in dermatology. Derivatives of this chemical are called "retinoids." Retinoids are used frequently in the form of tretinoin (Retin-A®, Renova®, Avita®), isotretinoin (Accutane®), acitretin (Soriatane®), tozarotene (Tazorac®), and adalapene (Differin®). This vitamin promotes good vision, interacts with immune system cells, and causes the skin to develop normally. It is found primarily in animal products, such as liver and eggs. Deficiency of vitamin A is probably the most common of all the vitamin deficiencies. Since in many undeveloped countries there is a serious shortage of meat and animal products, children and adults may show signs of vitamin A deficiency. Affected patients have poor nighttime vision, dry mouth, loss of appetite, diarrhea, and ulcerations on the cornea.

In industrialized countries, it is much more common to see vitamin A toxicity from consuming too much of the vitamin. This usually occurs when a well-intentioned person tries to treat his or her acne or psoriasis with very large doses of vitamin A, or in children who accidentally swallow a number of pills. The signs and symptoms of excess vitamin A are similar to those experienced by persons taking the retinoid drugs isotretinoin and acitretin. Chapped lips, dry eyes, bone and muscle pain, headaches, and insomnia are common. Taking too much of this vitamin is a serious matter since it is stored in the body; overdose is capable of causing significant sickness and even death.

Other vitamins such as pantothenic acid, niacin, folic acid, and vitamin K are rarely the cause of deficiencies. They too have found their way into various cosmetics, creams, and lotions but have never been scientifically tested for effectiveness. One other vitamin, biotin, is recommended by some dermatologists as being useful for strengthening the hair and promoting hair growth.

Zinc

This mineral is considered a "trace element" in the body, meaning that a very small amount is necessary for normal functioning of certain cells. Zinc deficiency is the most common trace element deficiency. This metal is found in meats and shellfish. Most persons with a normal diet consume an appropriate amount of it. Persons with poor diets, impaired absorption from the gastrointestinal tract, alcoholism, or anorexia may have a marginal deficiency of zinc. They may develop a mild facial and scalp rash, inflammation at the corners of the mouth (perleche), hair loss, inflamed cuticles, and erosions in the groin. Zinc deficiency is diagnosed by measuring zinc blood levels and treated by giving a supplement. An uncommon disease called acro-dermatitis enteropathica affects infants who are not capable of absorbing zinc from their mothers' milk. These children have blisters and erosions in the groin and a bright red facial rash which weeps. Supplementing their diets with zinc usually solves the problem.

Cosmetic Dermatology

Cosmetic dermatology has been the fastest-growing area of skin care in the past ten years. While some of the procedures discussed here are performed purely for the sake of aesthetics, many are also used to correct certain physical defects, including scars (from acne or burns), birth defects, pigmentation problems, skin damage from sun exposure, and varicose veins, to name a few. Some physicians' practices are now dedicated solely to this aspect of dermatology; there were few, if any, such practices fifteen years ago. This field is expansive and entire books have been dedicated to cosmetic dermatology. This section will review some of the most popular procedures and therapies. Those wishing for more in-depth information on treatments of a cosmetic nature should refer to the Bibliography as well as to dermatologists and plastic surgeons in their communities who specialize in cosmetology.

Chemical Peels

Chemical peels have become popular in the past ten years and many physicians and medical paraprofessionals are performing them. There is a variety of different types of peels (see Table 12). In theory, they are very straightforward and easy to perform, but in practice they are tricky and full of potential complications. Peels are useful for a variety of skin conditions including acne, scarring, sun damage, melasma (darkening of the facial skin), pigmentation abnormalities, and others.

Chemical peels are classified as superficial, medium, and deep depending on the depth of effect on the skin's layers. The deeper the peel the greater the amount of skin affected and the more time will be required for the treated area to repair itself. It is this "stripping" of the skin's layers and their replacement by new, healthier skin which results in the beneficial effects of a chemical peel. Different types of peels are indicated for different types of skin conditions and there are patients for whom chemical peels should not be performed. Patients prone to fever blisters such as herpes labialis or other herpes infections, with psychiatric or personality disorders, with a tendency to scar or form keloids, who have recently used isotretinoin (Accutane®), have had radiation therapy, or who are unable to avoid ultraviolet light should not have a chemical peel.

Table 12 TYPES OF CHEMICAL PEELS

Degree	Type of Chemical Peel
Superficial	Alpha hydroxy acids (glycolic acid) 30–70%
	Carbon dioxide, solid
	Jessner's solution
	Liquid nitrogen
	Resourcin paste
	Trichloroacetic acid 10–25%
Medium	Phenol, full strength
	Trichloroacetic acid 35–50%
Deep	Baker Gordon phenol formula

Alpha Hydroxy Acid

This family of chemicals derives from the breakdown of acids which occur in sugar (glycolic acid), milk (lactic acid), apples (malic acid), grapes (tartaric acid), and citrus fruit (citric acid). While all may theoretically be utilized for chemical peels, only glycolic acid is used with any frequency. How these acids induce a peel is not clear. They are minimally destructive to the superficial layers of the skin and cause a mild peeling several days after application. Glycolic acid is usually used in 50 to 70% concentrations in physicians' offices. Several over-the-counter products are available with lesser concentrations and some spas and beauty shops do "mini-peels" with concentrations in the 20% range. Patients may have glycolic acid peels done with gradually increasing strengths until a full 70% treatment is performed.

Glycolic acid peels are usually done for acne, mild skin discoloration (age spots), and long-standing sun damage with precancerous changes. Patients feel that their skin is "refreshed" and that they have an improved appearance. Some people incorporate these peels into their routine cosmetic regimen by having them done regularly (every two to three months), especially before holiday entertaining. Glycolic acid may be applied to most skin surfaces but is usually reserved for the face and forehead. The neck is treatable but complications are more frequent at this site, so it is generally avoided. Other sensitive skin areas are rarely treated.

Most physicians performing these peels have a regimen they ask their patients to follow for two to four weeks prior to the chemical peel. This includes use of tretinoin (Retin-A®), glycolic acid–containing creams and lotions, and sunscreens. The individual treatment regimens vary. These prepare the skin to better accept the peel and give improved results. Just before the chemical peel is performed, the skin is thoroughly cleaned. Acetone, chlorhexidine (Hibiclens®), alcohol, or Jessner's solution are used to rid the skin of any debris and loose skin scales. The glycolic acid is applied with cotton-tipped applicators in smooth strokes. Small paint-brushes or gauze pads may also be used. Care is taken to avoid contact with the eyes, and the glycolic acid is applied differently depending on the area of facial skin being treated. The procedure is timed so that the glycolic acid does not remain on the skin for longer than necessary. There is mild to moderate discomfort with this type of chemical peel depending on a patient's tolerance, the prepeel regimen used, and how long the glycolic acid is allowed to remain in contact with the skin. The acid is removed by neutralizing it with water or a solution of sodium bicarbonate or washing it off with soap and water.

After the treatment has been performed patients will usually experience redness, peeling, and some mild pain. If they have reacted fairly strongly to the acid, a topical corticosteroid may be prescribed, but usually a topical antibiotic ointment (Bactroban®, Polysporin®) will be used as will an emollient ointment or cream. Avoidance of sun exposure is strongly encouraged and sunscreen use is mandatory for the weeks and months following the peel. The peeling and redness usually subside after a week or two.

Glycolic acid peels are not without potential risks. Since they are superficial, however, these are usually minimal. Scarring is occasionally seen but generally only occurs in patients who have had the glycolic acid on too long or are excessively intolerant to it. Increased or decreased pigmentation is also seen and is a particular risk factor for dark-skinned individuals. Infection is also possible but very infrequent.

Trichloroacetic Acid and Jessner's Solution

Tricholoroacetic acid (TCA) is one of the most popular peeling agents, since it can be used for both a superficial and medium-depth peel. This chemical is commonly used on persons with significant sun damage and precancerous changes. While TCA peels involve a significant degree of cost and discomfort, these must be weighed against the other therapies used for patients with similar diseases. When analyzed over time, the other treatment modalities are likely to be just as expensive if not more so, equally uncomfortable, and much more inconvenient with regard to office visits, pharmacy visits, and so on. TCA peels therefore are frequently more economical than other therapies for precancerous changes. They are also helpful for most of the conditions for which glycolic acid peels are used except active acne. TCA is occasionally used in combination with other medications and procedures including 5-fluorouracil (Efudex®), tretinoin, phenol, dermabrasion, dry ice, and Jessner's solution. The degree of peeling and depth of skin penetration depend on the concentration of TCA used and how long it is allowed to remain on the skin. Most skin surfaces may be treated but TCA is most commonly applied to the face and forehead. TCA is used almost exclusively by physicians since it is more complex and potentially problematic than glycolic acid.

The preparation of the skin prior to the peel is similar to that for glycolic acid peels. Application of TCA is done using 10 to 25% solutions for superficial peels and 35 to 50% for medium-depth peels. Higher concentrations are occasionally used but only with great caution, since at those strengths TCA may become dangerous. The chemical is applied in the same manner as glycolic acid. The eyes are sometimes protected with cotton or plastic covers to prevent contact with the TCA. The acid is applied carefully and evenly. Eventually the skin becomes somewhat white or "frosted." The patient will usually complain of burning discomfort and a handheld fan is sometimes used to help "cool" the face. Gauze pads soaked in ice water may then be applied to the skin to neutralize the acid and diminish the discomfort.

When the peel is finished, the skin is usually moderately swollen or puffy, red, and hot. The patient is in some discomfort but not excessively so. A coat of antibiotic ointment is usually applied and the patient is allowed to go home. If the skin is very swollen and irritated a shot of a short-acting corticosteroid (Celestone®) may be given. Some physicians apply a layer of moisturizing wound dressing and a "mask" of gauze to hold it in place. This is allowed to remain on the face for about twenty-four hours and then removed. If the patient is expected to be in significant pain or have difficulty resting, pain pills and/or sleeping pills may be used. The postoperative wound care is similar to that for glycolic acid peels. Depending on the concentration of the TCA used, it takes about ten days for the skin to heal. Vigilant use of sunscreens is mandatory.

Complications are similar to those of glycolic acid peels but there is a greater risk of activation of fever blisters (herpes labialis) and scarring, especially with higher concentrations or longer contact times. Increased or decreased skin pigmentation is more of a problem than with glycolic acid peels. Constant sunscreen use and ultraviolet light avoidance are helpful in avoiding this complication. Finally, infection can be a problem, particularly if antibiotic ointments are not applied.

Jessner's solution is named for the physician who developed this mixture. It contains resorcinol, salicylic acid, lactic acid, and alcohol. It may be used by itself for peeling and is probably most similar to glycolic acid. It is commonly used in combination with TCA to "soften" the skin layers and allow the TCA to work more effectively. It is often uncomfortable and sedation and/or pain medication may be used. The Jessner's solution is applied with cotton-tipped applicators after the face has been appropriately cleaned. The TCA is then applied over it and the peel stopped by the application of soaked gauze pads. These patients usually experience more postpeel pain or burning and take longer to heal, usually two weeks or more. Since this is a medium-depth peel, the results are usually much more noticeable; the skin appears pinker, healthier, and smoother. The risks and precautions are essentially the same as for other peels.

Phenol

The phenol peel is the deepest of the customary chemical peels and is not performed very frequently. This type of peel is most useful for scarring and deep wrinkling such as crow's feet and furrows around the lips. It may be useful for persons with severe sun damage and precancerous changes, but TCA is usually preferred. "Ice pick" scarring from acne may also respond to phenol peels. Dark-skinned people are not good candidates for phenol peels since there may be serious alterations in their pigmentation. Patients taking birth control pills, estrogens, or progesterone should stop since the skin may be more prone to develop increased pigmentation after the peel. Treatment is restricted to the face and forehead since complications are commonplace when the neck or chest is treated. Patients are sedated and given pain medication beforehand and most areas to be treated are numbed with anesthetic injections, and the face is cleaned as with other peels.

The phenol solution deeply penetrates the skin and causes significant damage and irritation. Additionally, the phenol is absorbed to a mild degree and may cause irregular heart rhythms. For that reason, the patient is usually evaluated with a heart monitor during the procedure. The phenol is applied carefully with cotton-tipped applicators. Application causes the upper layers of the skin to dissolve and a "frost" is seen after a few minutes. The phenol is eventually neutralized in the skin and loses its potency.

Phenol peels cause significant burning and pain. Application of cool compresses is helpful but virtually all patients need some form of pain medication and sedation. Frequent follow-up visits in the weeks after the peel are usually the rule. Application of antibiotic ointment is mandatory since serious infections may otherwise result. Sunscreen use is required and the patient is usually pink and mildly swollen for several weeks or months after the peel. The most worrisome complication is scarring. Persons with a past history of herpes labialis are usually given prophylactic acyclovir (Zovirax®) or valcyclovir (Valtrex®) to prevent this complication.

Phenol peels may be spectacularly effective with dramatic results. However, they are complex, complicated procedures.

Other Peels

Resourcin paste has been used for facial peeling for over a century. It is more commonly used in Europe than in North America but is helpful for patients with acne and sun-damaged skin. The patient is tested with a spot of the medication before it is applied to the face. If there are no problems, the resourcin is applied to the face and forehead for three consecutive days for about thirty minutes. The patient usually experiences some mild stinging and pain. If the discomfort is excessive, pain medication may be used or the resorcinol paste removed early. There is mild redness, swelling, and peeling for a week to ten days after the last application. Care of the skin is similar to the other types of peels. Side effects and complications are few.

Dry ice (carbon dioxide) and liquid nitrogen peels are similar. They are used for the same indications as glycolic acid peels; namely, sun damage and acne, but are no longer very popular. The carbon dioxide is applied to the skin for a brief period of time and causes peeling. Some physicians prefer to crush the carbon dioxide into smaller fragments, collect them in a gauze bag, and soak them for five to ten seconds in acetone before application. This is called a "dry ice slush" and is one of the older methods for in-office acne therapy. Liquid nitrogen is lightly applied with a spray gun to the skin until a mild frosting occurs. It may also be applied using cotton-tipped applicators. Both liquid nitrogen and carbon dioxide are somewhat painful and result in a mild to moderate peeling in about five to seven days.

Topical tretinoin is a skin irritant which results in mild scaling. In many patients, this property may be exploited to induce a mild, superficial peel. This mild peeling improves acne, sun damage, and precancerous lesions and blotchy pigmentation. In certain patients it may be much more desirable than a TCA or glycolic acid peel.

Collagen Injection

Injecting substances into the skin has been popular since the early part of the twentieth century. Initially, oils and silicone were used with moderate success, but bad reactions arose in some patients. In the past fifteen years, collagen from animal sources has been used with good outcomes. The two most popular collagens, Zyderm® or Zyplast® and Fibrel®, are made from cow and pig collagen, respectively. Collagen is the tissue found in deeper layers of the skin which give it substance and toughness. These products are usually used for scars (particularly "ice pick" scars from acne), facial defects, wrinkles, and cosmetic enhancement of features such as the lips. Since these are foreign proteins, an allergic reaction to them is possible. During production the material is treated to minimize this possibility, but some degree of risk remains. To guard against such an occurrence, patients must be tested before undergoing therapeutic injections. A small amount of collagen is injected under the skin on the forearm and evaluated after several days and again after four weeks. If there is no reaction, there is little likelihood that the patient will react negatively to the therapeutic injections. The collagen is injected under the skin to fill the defective areas. The areas may be "overfilled" to allow for some shrinkage of the material.

Aside from discomfort and a possible allergic reaction, the side effects are mild bruising and infection. Expense must be considered as well. Most collagen injections must be repeated every six to twelve months, depending on the site treated. It has also been suggested that there is an association between these injections and developing collagen vascular diseases (lupus erythematosus, rheumatoid arthritis, dermatomyositis, and so on); however, this has been subsequently disproved. Collagen injections have probably peaked in popularity but remain a very viable technique for scar revision in some patients.

A new technique, termed autologous collagen injection, has been developed using a patient's own collagen, thereby minimizing the possibility of an allergic reaction. The collagen is harvested by withdrawing fat from an area such as the thigh, then extracting all the fat from the material. What remains is largely collagen; this is injected as with cow and pig collagen. The area is usually massaged to smooth out the injected material. Complications are few, aside from pain and swelling. The degree of correction and its duration appear comparable to collagen from animal sources.

Sclerotherapy

Sclerotherapy is a procedure which involves injecting substances into superficial veins to induce their disappearance. Initially this was performed on larger veins on the legs (varicose veins), but it has become popular for treatment of very superficial veins (spider veins). Varicose veins are moderate to large blood vessels, most commonly found on the legs, which have become enlarged and engorged and are often painful. They may be associated with mild dermatitis in the overlying skin. They form when the valves inside the veins become nonfunctional and blood begins to pool in vessels of the skin and superficial fat. Spider veins form in a similar manner. To some extent this tendency is inherited but is enhanced by pregnancy, weight gain, and prolonged standing.

Sclerosing solutions cause irritation to the lining of the vessels walls, inducing their collapse and destruction. These vessels are destroyed, forcing the blood flow to veins with normal function. There are several substances used for sclerotherapy including polidocanol (Aethoxysklerol®), sodium morrhuate (Scleromate®), and strong salt solutions called hypertonic saline. The procedure causes some pain. Patients are usually given tight-fitting clothing (compression garments) to wear, which keep the injured blood vessels adherent to one another.

Complications include phlebitis (inflammation of the veins), infection, and skin ulcer formation. Increased pigmentation over the area of the vein is seen in more than 10 percent of patients. Patients with diabetes, bleeding disorders, or who are prone to develop phlebitis are not candidates for this procedure.

Use of sclerosing solutions may not be as popular in the future since a new laser (Sclerolaser® [Candela Corporation]) may be capable of performing the same procedure more quickly with less discomfort.

Liposuction

This procedure has become extremely popular in the past decade, due to new advancements in its performance. Liposuction is generally performed for removal of unwanted fat from the trunk, buttocks, and thighs but may also be used for fatty deposits in the neck and jowls. Additionally, liposuction may improve the patient's appearance and allow for improved mobility in some rare conditions where fat is inappropriately deposited.

Liposuction is almost always performed in outpatient surgery units or in the hospital itself. Some physicians, usually plastic surgeons or those specializing in liposuction, have their offices equipped for such procedures, but this is a rarity. Candidates for this procedure must have realistic expectations about liposuction and not have any significant health problems such as uncontrolled heart disease, kidney failure, excessively high blood pressure, or bleeding problems. Photographs are almost always taken before and after the procedure. Routine blood work is also performed. The procedure is done under anesthesia since it is painful. This may be a shot of painkiller or full general anesthesia. However, a newer type of anesthesia called "tumescent liposuction" has been developed in which a solution containing an anesthetic is infused into the fat and allowed to remain for half an hour.

The skin is anesthetized with an injection and small incisions into the skin are made. Metal cannulas which are attached to a suction machine are inserted into the fat. As the cannulas are moved back and forth, the fat is disrupted and suctioned away. Perhaps the most important part of liposuction occurs after the procedure is finished. Compression garments are applied and the patient must wear them constantly for the next week or so. Liposuction patients are instructed to "take it easy"; they may do light exercise or return to work after a few days, depending on how they feel. There is mild to moderate bruising but this subsides in several weeks, and antibiotics may be given to prevent infection. The newest form of liposuction is called "ultrasonic" liposuction and involves less blood loss. It is more expensive, but the recovery time is quicker. It is currently available in only a few centers around the United States.

Endodermologie

This is a new method of treating cellulite. Endodermologie was developed in Europe and has become popular in the United States in the past several years. While it is still somewhat controversial, it is believed to work by "breaking up" the pockets of cellulite in the skin so that its contour is much smoother and more pleasing to the eye. A handheld device picks up the skin and rolls it between two rollers before dropping it back down again. Endodermologie is noninvasive and painless, but requires fifteen to twenty sessions of about thirty minutes each. It is expensive (approximately $100 per session) but is obviously less costly than laser surgery or liposuction. This treatment method has shown some beneficial effects and is particularly useful in patients who have recently undergone liposuction.

Dermabrasion

Dermabrasion is an older cosmetic technique and was widely used in the 1960s and 1970s. With recent concern about HIV, hepatitis, and other blood-borne pathogens, the popularity of dermabrasion has fallen. Additionally, chemical peels are a useful substitute in many patients. There is an extensive list of potential indications for this procedure, but its principal use has been for patients with facial scarring due to acne. It may also be used for tattoo removal, rhinophyma, seborrheic keratoses, actinic keratoses, and other benign tumors.

Dermabrasion uses an instrument not unlike an electric drill and a wire metal brush. The brush is run at high speeds to remove the superficial portion of the skin. The skin is numbed beforehand with an injection of lidocaine. A topical refrigerant such as freon or ethyl chloride is sprayed on the skin, and while the skin is "hard" the dermabrader is activated and the brush used to "sand" away the appropriate areas. This is, of course, an oversimplification, since this technique is difficult to learn and requires considerable skill and expertise. Some patients are not good candidates and are excluded from therapy. Pre- and postoperative treatments are similar to that for chemical peels. Postoperative recovery takes several weeks and patients who have had dermabrasion may look frightening until they heal. Perhaps the most worrisome concern is that this procedure involves significant, though not dangerous, bleeding and splattering of the patient's blood.

Hair Transplantation

Hair transplantation was pioneered almost forty years ago. It was based on the knowledge that hairs from one part of the body tend to grow and behave in a constant pattern even if they are moved to another anatomic site. When men (and women) suffer from "male pattern baldness" they tend to lose hair along the frontal hairline and on the top of their scalps (see the section on hair loss). The lower portion of the scalp above the neck and behind the ears tends to retain hair. Consequently, hair from that area can be removed along with surrounding tissue and transplanted onto the front of the scalp. Almost anyone may undergo a hair transplant if he is in good health. Routine evaluation includes checking for anemia and the ability of the blood to clot.

The areas to be transplanted are numbed with lidocaine injections and marked with ink to facilitate plug placement. Hair plugs are removed from the back of the scalp using a power tool called a power punch. Reciprocal holes are placed on the frontal scalp. They are slightly smaller than the hair plugs. Placement of the plugs is usually done in stages so that the frontal hairline looks natural. Postoperative instructions are given to prevent the plugs from falling out or being pulled out. One of the new techniques in hair transplantation has been the use of very small grafts (minigrafts and micrografts), even to the point of transplanting single hairs. This allows the hairline to appear much more natural. This is obviously more labor intensive and more expensive. The disadvantages of hair transplantation are few, infection and postoperative bleeding are occasionally seen but are rare. Poor technique and improper placement of the plugs may result in an unacceptable cosmetic appearance. Finally, cost of a hair transplant is from $5,000 to $6,000 or more depending on the technique used and the number of plugs placed. Use of antibalding medications such as minoxidil and finasteride (Propecia®) over a period of years may be equally expensive, making a hair transplant more cost effective.

The newest technique for balding is the scalp reduction procedure. In this surgery the area of balding is essentially "cut out" and the edges of the hair-bearing scalp sewn together. There are a number of different techniques used, depending on the areas of involvement. These may be quite effective and do not require as much operative time as hair transplants. Infection and bleeding are potential problems, but are usually easily managed or prevented. The most disappointing aspect of the surgery is a mild stretching back of the closure that some patients experience. This does not usually approximate the original area of hair loss, however. The scalp often responds to trauma (such as a transplant) by the hair shafts in a certain area dropping out after several months. This is not permanent and the hair will regrow, but it is very discouraging to patients who have gone to so much trouble and expense to acquire a full head of hair.

Laser Surgery

What was once considered science fiction a few years ago is now reality with the use of lasers. The word *laser* stands for Light Amplification by Stimulated Emission of Radiation. These machines align light waves in a single line, which increases their potency and ability to perform certain functions. There are approximately ten different types of lasers in clinical use, and certain types have more than one manufacturer. They are categorized based on the color of the light beam they emit, the frequency of that wavelength, and the way they function. They may vary in the size of the light beam they emit, the amount of time they come into contact with the skin, and the amount of energy they possess.

The original lasers were used to remove lesions, usually by destroying them. The carbon dioxide (CO_2) laser was and still is the most popular laser for this purpose. Warts, benign tumors, precancerous changes, and skin cancers can be treated with the CO_2 laser, but as with many other destructive methods of therapy, it is a painful procedure and may result in scarring. Most CO_2 lasers are used to excise or cut the tissue or to vaporize an area or lesion. The excision of a lesion using a carbon dioxide laser generally leaves a cosmetically undesirable wound with a visible scar but this laser has a great advantage in that it almost immediately seals the blood vessels being cut. As a result, blood loss is minimal and for those with bleeding difficulties, this may be an ideal way to remove a lesion. The vaporize mode results in destruction of the lesion being treated, though the resulting scar may not be attractive. A newer model, the ultrapulsed carbon dioxide laser, is gentler on treated tissues and may cause much less scarring. This laser may be used in situations where chemical peels have been successful, namely, precancerous changes, scarring, stretch marks, and superficial skin cancers. The area is anesthetized, and the patient must care for the treated site like they would for a routine excision or wound. The carbon dioxide laser is the least expensive of the lasers and the most widely available.

Lasers have been at the center of a great expansion of treatment options for vascular tumors such as port wine stains, spider veins, varicose veins, and hemangiomas. While these are mostly cosmetic, children with very large port wine stains or hemangiomas may suffer significant psychological damage as well as physical danger if their lesions are not treated. Previously, treatment options were few and unappealing. The argon laser, copper vapor laser, ruby laser, pulsed dye laser, and Neodynium:YAG laser all play a role in the removal of certain types of vascular lesions. Scarring is a problem in certain situations, but overall the treatments are much better than ten years ago. Disadvantages include discomfort (worse with some lasers than with others) and the need for multiple treatments; a large hemangioma may require ten or more therapy sessions. Unfortunately, the greatest drawback seems to be cost. These lasers may cost over $100,000. Additionally, the source that generates the wavelength (for example, copper, argon, dye) must periodically be replaced and is usually very expensive. Some costs may be reimbursable by insurance companies, but this is usually not the case.

The final use for lasers is the removal of tattoos. These include not only professional tattoos applied in "tattoo parlors" but also amateur tattoos and "traumatic" tattoos. Traumatic tattoos result from gunpowder explosions, asphalt abrasions, or being stabbed with a leaded pencil. Lasers which work on tattoos include ruby, alexandrite and Neodynium:YAG lasers. Multiple treatments may be required and reimbursement by insurance companies is rare, so someone wishing to have a tattoo removed must usually pay out of pocket. Degree of discomfort varies, and posttherapy care for the site is required but is usually minimal. Tattoos which are composed of different pigments may require treatment by different lasers. Multiple treatment sessions are also usually required, making this a potentially extended and expensive therapy.

There has been some use of lasers in the treatment of moles and other pigmented lesions. For routine moles, this will not likely become a standard therapy but for some conditions in which pigment is found deeply in the skin and is cosmetically deforming (Nevus of Ota, Nevus of Ito, Becker's nevus, lentigos, melasma, and so on) laser therapy offers a realistic chance for improvement. The ruby, Neodynium:YAG, copper, pulsed dye, and alexandrite lasers are the most useful. Treatments, posttherapy follow-up, wound care, and expense are essentially the same as for treatment of tattoos and vascular tumors. There is great hope that someday these tools may be useful for persons with congenital moles, particularly those with very large lesions in whom the risk of melanoma is increased. They may allow for removal of numerous melanocytes within in the skin and diminish the chance that they will become malignant.

PART II

DERMATITIS

~ ~ ~ ~

Atopic Dermatitis and Eczema

Atopic Dermatitis

This disease is one of the most common skin conditions. Atopic dermatitis (AD) also goes by the term *eczema*. This disorder is associated with *atopy*—the tendency to develop allergic rhinitis (allergy, hay fever), asthma, and atopic dermatitis. Atopic dermatitis develops mostly in children but adult onset is possible. Two to five percent of all children are affected with AD to one degree or another. They often have relatives with atopy. Slightly more boys are affected than girls, and there seems to be more disease in children of Asian descent. There is evidence that the incidence of AD is increasing. This may be due to pollution, food additives and chemical preservatives, decreased breast-feeding, and awareness by physicians and the public about AD. Most evidence points to a genetic component to the disease. Children inherit a tendency to develop AD from their parents. If both parents are or were affected, the likelihood that the child will also have it approaches 80 percent. Atopic dermatitis is also closely linked with the immune system. Sophisticated tests have been developed which demonstrate that the immune cells in AD patients are different and react differently than in persons without AD. Some of these abnormalities may be of no significance, but they may provide the basis for new medication testing.

Causes and Symptoms of Atopic Dermatitis

The list of things which incite this disease is long and getting longer. One of the most recent discoveries has been that mites living in house dust (house-dust mites) seem to provoke the disease. These insects don't cause the disease, but in susceptible persons they may elicit and/or aggravate dermatitis. Dust mites live on the scales from human skin and apparently prefer that from persons with AD. Therefore, treatment of AD includes cleaning the area where the patient lives and using specialized air conditioning and furnace filters. Some say diet can provoke AD; however, the association between certain foods and AD has probably been exaggerated. Still, some persons have learned that certain foods worsen their disease and they should avoid them. Breast-feeding children seems to help prevent or diminish the severity of AD, and these children at high risk to develop atopic dermatitis (parents or siblings with AD) should be breast-fed to diminish the risk. Mothers who are breast-feeding can adopt certain dietary practices such as following a "hypoaller-genic" diet to help their children avoid AD.

Other causes of the disease include illnesses such as ear infections, colds, and strep throat, wool or other irritating fabrics, stress, cold weather, and irritating soaps or lotions. The itch of AD seems to worsen at night and may prevent restful sleep. Some patients continue to scratch their skin even when completely asleep. Evidence of nighttime scratching such as blood on the sheets and bedclothes is common. Patients are divided into three groups depending on their age: infantile, childhood/adolescent, and adult atopic dermatitis. The symptoms and findings are much the same regardless of the category, but there is some evidence that younger children will "grow out" of their disease over time.

The most characteristic and continuous feature of atopic dermatitis is the itch. It is sometimes difficult to tell if there is an itchy rash initially or if the itch occurs first and the patient scratches themselves into a rash. The classically affected areas include the folds of the arms and legs, back of the neck, back of the hands, tops of the feet, and wrists, especially in children. There are exceptions; the rare patient will demonstrate involvement over the entire body (erythroderma). These patients are very sick and are usually hospitalized to administer intravenous fluids and aggressive skin care.

The initial rash is red, mildly scaly or with small blisters, swollen, and in some cases, scratched or rubbed raw. With infection of the skin, crusting may be seen. If broad areas are involved and especially if the skin is infected nearby, lymph nodes will become swollen and tender. After constant scratching, the skin becomes dark and thickened with very prominent ridges, a process known as *lichenification.* This may be seen anywhere but is most prominent on the arms and legs. The skin also typically has a quality of fine dryness known as *xerosis.* Xerosis is seen in numerous other disorders but is a central theme in atopic dermatitis. These patients tend to have skin which is inclined to be dry and to itch. Other symptoms include:

1. Dennie-Morgan folds, a small fold of redundant skin on the lower eyelid. This is seen in patients with other forms of atopy such as asthma and may be present in healthy patients as well. A nasal crease is commonly found in these patients. This occurs toward the end of the nose where the nasal bone stops and soft tissues begin. It is believed to arise from constant pushing of the hand or arm on the tip of the nose in persons with allergies such as hay fever.

2. The palms in persons with AD may show many more lines or grooves than in unaffected persons. This condition is called "hyperlinear" palms, and is especially common in a subset of patients with AD who also have

ichthyosis vulgaris or a "fish-scale" eruption of dry skin on the legs and arms. Some AD patients have a great deal of hand involvement, and hyperlinear palms are more common in them as well. Persons with AD have an increased incidence of ichthyosis vulgaris and it is likely that those with hyperlinear palms simply belong to that subset of persons with ichthyosis vulgaris.

3. Geographic tongue is a condition in which the tongue's surface loses its roughness in various spots so that it resembles a relief map. It is most commonly seen in atopic dermatitis but may also be present in psoriasis and other diseases.

4. Persons with AD have an increased incidence of cataracts. This was previously believed to be due to the disease alone, but it is now thought that indiscriminate use of corticosteroids by mouth or potent formulations used around the eyes contribute to cataract formation.

5. Keratosis pilaris is a skin-colored or slightly orange eruption on the backs of the arms and legs commonly associated with AD. It consists of mildly raised spiny lesions. Patients usually find the eruption annoying. Keratosis pilaris may also be seen in persons without AD but with other signs of atopy.

6. White dermatographism may be seen in some patients. This consists of a tendency for the skin to blanch when stroked vigorously by a finger or blunt object; it is related to an abnormality in the skin's blood vessels.

7. Many affected persons have cold hands that tend to be somewhat white in color.

8. Patients with atopic dermatitis may also experience less common symptoms such as nausea, vomiting, diarrhea, itching around the anus and within the mouth, mouth ulcers, and an increased sensitivity to insect bites.

9. Finally, there are a number of rare genetic diseases in which atopic dermatitis is a prominent factor. Patients typically have other, life-threatening problems, such as deficiencies of the immune system.

Since atopic dermatitis can involve a large amount of the skin's surface area and represents an abnormal reaction of the immune system, it is not unusual that several different diseases and/or complications often affect these patients. One of the most spectacular and dangerous is termed Kaposi's varicelliform eruption (eczema herpeticum). In this disease, a person, usually one with moderately severe AD, becomes infected with Herpes simplex virus (HSV) or the chicken pox virus (varicella-zoster virus; VZV). Other viruses can also cause this disease. Initially, the symptoms are typical, but they become more widespread, more symptomatic, larger, and ulcerate more frequently. Most patients with Kaposi's varicelliform eruption are very ill and must be hospitalized; deaths have even been reported. Fortunately, acyclovir (Zovirax®) is now available and is given intravenously in very large doses.

Other viral infections of the skin such as warts and molluscum contagiosum (see *molluscum contagiosum*) are common and usually more difficult to treat in AD. Occasionally, these lesions will be restricted to areas of involved skin.

The skin of affected persons is usually colonized by bacteria and fungi that are not present, or not present to the same degree, as in healthy persons. This results from the increased amount of fissuring, cracking, and skin breakdown in these patients. *Staphylococcus aureus* is usually found both on healthy and involved skin. Since antibiotics are commonly given to patients with AD, there is the possibility that the *S. aureus* on the skin of a person with AD may be resistant to the usual medications used for such infections. If most of the breaks in the skin are relatively superficial and heal without problems, there is little possibility of scarring. However, when deep skin infections arise or the skin is very abraded, scarring may occur. More common is the presence of increased and decreased pigment in the skin. This is termed hyper- or hypopigmentation and is often believed by the patient to represent "scarring." It is most problematic for blacks and Hispanics. While this will subside with time, it may be emotionally upsetting. Finally, there is some evidence that AD may play a role in the development of Hodgkin's disease and other types of lymphoma.

Psychological Aspects of Atopic Dermatitis
There has been considerable research on the emotional and psychological aspects of atopic dermatitis. Previously, it was believed that "nerves" or emotions were the cause of the disease. While this is no longer thought to be true, there is a certain psychiatric profile that fits many of these patients. Persons with atopic dermatitis tend to be nervous, sensitive, tense, hyperactive, and intolerant. They tend to be easily depressed, which may spring from suppressing feelings of resentment about their disease. Child patients may become manipulative of their parents or caretakers to get what they want. Often combating the psychological problems associated with this disease is as frustrating and time consuming as dealing with the skin symptoms themselves. There is no question that stressful situations and experiences worsen, precipitate, and aggravate atopic dermatitis. Many physicians successfully treat this disease using medications for relief of anxiety and depression.

Treatment of Atopic Dermatitis

LUBRICATION   Treatment of atopic dermatitis centers around keeping the skin well moisturized and free of irritating factors. Patients are often simply told to use a moisturizer, but this is not enough information to be helpful. There are a great number of lubricants available but they are not equivalent. Many contain antimicrobials such as formaldehyde or formaldehyde releasers, fragrances, stabilizers, antioxidants, lanolin and coloring agents. The following sidebar is a handout used for persons with AD. It addresses the need for proper moisturizing with a good lubricant. Several suggested brands are listed. Unfortunately, these are more expensive than some of the generic or brand-name emollients available, but they are much less likely to irritate the skin or worsen the disease. Lubricants often contain catchy ingredients such as vitamins, minerals, collagen, aloe vera, elastin, hyaluronic acid, and so on. It is best to avoid these substances, since they are unable to pass into the skin or be absorbed by it, generally add to the cost of the moisturizer, and may make the formulation irritating or cause allergies.

The need for frequent and liberal moisturizing of the skin in those with atopic dermatitis cannot be overemphasized. The skin of these patients has a tendency to both itch and become dry (causing further itching). If the dryness is alleviated, this will go a long way to keeping the disease in check. Moisturizing may have to be done six to eight times per day and is best accomplished when the skin is slightly damp (as after a bath or shower). Petroleum-based products such as Vasoline® or white petrolatum are useful but are unpleasant to use since they are greasy. Additionally, they may occlude follicles and result in folliculitis. Petrolatum Mousse (Lancome®) is a useful petroleum product that causes less mess. When the disease is flaring and particularly when there are discrete outbreaks on the arms or legs, application of wet compresses is useful (see the section on wet dressings).

BATHING   Bathing is important, since bathtime habits can worsen the disease. Some physicians suggest that bathing be eliminated altogether or restricted to one to two times per week. While this is effective for some patients, it presents difficulties for others. A short shower or bath (five minutes) with lukewarm water once per day will allow for personal hygiene and not aggravate the skin. Hot water and prolonged contact with warm water dry out the skin and worsen the disease. Certain soaps, such as deodorant soaps (Dial®, Safeguard®) may be very drying to the skin. Superfatted soaps are the least drying and are recommended for general use. Some soap substitutes are applied and removed without use of water (Cetaphil®, Aquanil®). While these are not harmful, they offer little advantage over careful use of superfatted soaps and water. Soaps with additives such as sulfur, abrasives, vegetable and nut oils, fragrances, vitamins, and aloe vera should generally be avoided

Eczema and Atopic Dermatitis

You have been diagnosed by your dermatologist as having atopic dermatitis or eczema. The skin in patients with atopic dermatitis or eczema is easily irritated, frequently itchy, commonly dry; it is often associated with asthma and allergies (hay fever). Atopic dermatitis is usually considered to be synonymous with eczema. This handout is designed to help you better care for your skin and to minimize any complications of the underlying disease or its treatment.

General Considerations

In general, the less irritation and trauma that affects your skin, the better. You will find that the more care you take of your skin the less likely it will be to itch, break open, blister, turn red, or get infected. Do not put anything on topically that you have not okayed with your doctor. This includes topical antibiotics, astringents, perfumes, and so on. Many of these can be bought without a prescription (over the counter; OTC) and may potentially complicate or negate the therapy your physician has designed for you. It is also a good idea to make sure that the doctor has a complete list of all the medications you regularly take, including birth control pills and nonprescription medicines.

Bathing

Contact with water washes away the natural oils in a person's skin. These natural oils play a substantial role in keeping skin soft, well protected, and appropriately lubricated. They are the most natural and most effective lubricants available. Hot water results in a loss of these natural oils and worsens dry skin. Therefore, baths or showers should be as brief and infrequent as possible. Five to seven minutes in the shower or tub is a good rule of thumb.

Soaps can play a substantial role in aggravating atopic dermatitis through their ability to irritate the skin. Soaps that are excessively harsh (Ivory®, Lifebuoy®) or contain additives such as deodorants (Safeguard®, Zest®, Lever 2000®), perfumes, or lanolin (Palmolive®) are frequently a source of problems. Gentle, bland soaps such as Cetaphil®, Aveeno®, Dove®, Oilatum®, Neutrogena®, or Lowila® are best. A tar soap, Polytar®, can also be soothing. The same is true of shampoos. Neutrogena® and baby shampoos are recommended.

Bath oils are helpful but it is best to avoid the inexpensive, heavily perfumed ones. Keri oil® and Aveeno® are both soothing and will help the skin retain moisture. Bath oils containing tar sometimes make the skin less irritated. Most drug stores have several tar solutions such as Zetar®, Balnetar®, or Tar Doak®; these are available without a prescription but may not be on the store shelves. Pharmacists sometimes keep these items behind the counter or can order them for you. The addition of one-half teaspoon of chlorine bleach to bathwater is soothing as well .

After your bath or shower, dry with a heavy absorbent cotton towel. Do not rub the skin. Patting dry is the best method, but don't overdo it; two to four pats should be enough for any one region of the body. If you are going to apply a cream or ointment prescribed for you by your physician, this is the best time to do so, while the skin is still full of moisture. Application of your moisturizing lotion or cream should follow. Apply prescribed medications or moisturizers in the same direction as hair growth.

Skin Lubrication

One of the most important aspects of skin care in patients with atopic dermatitis centers around the need to keep the skin well moisturized at all times. Low humidity, frequent washing, and contact with certain chemicals and astringents will dry the skin and present real problems. You should apply your emollient as frequently and liberally as possible. It is important to avoid the use of lubricating lotions that contain parabens, lanolin (or wool wax), and fragrances. We usually recommend the use of Moisturel Lotion or Cream®, DML Lotion or Forte Cream®, DML Forte Cream®, Eucerin®, Eucerin Plus®, Aveeno Lotion or Cream®, Vanicream®, Eutra Swiss Skin Cream®, Keri Light Lotion®, Theraplex Clearlotion or Hydrolotion®, or Neutrogena Facial Moisturizer®. Petroleum jelly or Vaseline® is an acceptable moisturizer (but not Vaseline Intensive Care Lotion®) and may be preferred by some patients. If you wash your hands frequently, you may find it helpful to keep a pump bottle of your favorite emollient nearby for use following hand drying. You should apply your lotion to your entire body after bathing; this is best accomplished *immediately* following towel drying. Oily or greasy formulations are best used at bedtime.

Avoidance

There are many chemicals and substances encountered each day that might cause your atopic dermatitis or eczema to worsen. You will do yourself a favor if you avoid these substances as much as possible. This usually means wearing gloves if you will be touching chemicals (as in mixing paint) or will have your hands in water for prolonged periods (as in washing dishes).

Foods

Many physicians and patients believe that certain foods worsen atopic dermatitis or eczema. In children, foods to consider avoiding are milk, milk products (cheese, ice cream, and so on), citrus fruits and juices, eggs, and fish. Adults might try avoiding pork, eggs, mushrooms, tomatoes, corn, chocolate, caffeine, and nuts. Alcohol and fermented beverages may also play a role in this disease.

Miscellaneous

Clothing may irritate your skin, especially wools and synthetic fabrics. We recommend that, if possible, 100 percent cotton clothing be used. Loose-fitting clothes and light weaves are also helpful.

Many patients like to use a humidifier or vaporizer at night to help moisturize their skin. While there have never been any scientific studies that have shown this to be of benefit, it doesn't seem to be harmful and does help some patients.

Stress can frequently worsen atopic dermatitis. Minimizing stress through exercise, proper rest, and appropriate diet may help prevent skin problems.

There is some evidence that fish oil and evening primrose oil (both available at health food stores) help people with atopic dermatitis. While expensive, these substances are unlikely to be harmful and may be worth trying. Timed-release vitamin C (1,000 mg) has also been used with some success.

Sarna® and Aveeno Anti-Itch Cream®, over the counter anti-itch creams, are usually very helpful and can be purchased without a prescription. These are safe for long-term use and can be applied liberally and as often as desired.

Table 13 BATH ADDITIVES

Brand Name	Active Ingredients
Alpha Keri®	mineral oil and lanolin
Aveeno®	colloidal oatmeal
Aveeno Bath Oil®	colloidal oatmeal and mineral oil
Balnetar Bath Oil®	coal tar
Doak Oil®	coal tar, mineral oil, and lanolin
Jeri-Bath®	mineral oil and lanolin
Lubriderm®	mineral oil
Neutrogena Body Oil®	sesame oil
Nivea Bath Silk®	mineral oil and lanolin
Nutraderm®	mineral oil
Nutra Soothe®	colloidal oatmeal and mineral oil
Polytar Bath®	coal tar
RoBathol®	cottonseed oil
Zetar Emulsion®	coal tar

since they have an increased tendency to irritate the skin and worsen the disease. Numerous oils and bath additives are available (see Table 13). Lubricating bath oils and oatmeal-based bath products are very soothing for dry and inflamed skin. Tar bath oils are helpful but many patients dislike them. Toweling down after a bath or shower should be done with a 100 percent cotton towel. Patting the skin dry is preferable to rubbing. While the skin is still moist and damp is the best time to apply moisturizers. If the patient has active disease, a thin layer of corticosteroid cream followed by a thicker overlying coat of lubricant is an excellent means of therapy.

TOPICAL ANTI-ITCH MEDICATIONS   These medicines have a role in the treatment of AD. Sarna® lotion and Aveeno Anti-Itch® cream contain menthol and help control the itch. They are available over the counter and are useful for patients with limited disease. They may be used as often as needed. Compounded medications containing menthol and phenol are also helpful but are expensive.

CLOTHING AND LIFESTYLE   The way a person dresses may have to be modified to accommodate the disease. One hundred percent cotton clothing should be used as much as possible. Synthetic fabrics are occasionally irritating, and wool should be strictly avoided. Homes and work areas should be kept moderately humidified. The dry air of wintertime combined with the drying effect of most heating systems will worsen the disease.

Use of a cool-vapor humidifier or vaporizer is encouraged, particularly in children's rooms. Some of these machines allow medications to be added but this is not necessary with AD and may be harmful. Turning the heater off in the wintertime as much as is comfortable may also be useful. Since the house dust mite seems to play a significant role in atopic dermatitis, keeping living and work environments as dust free as possible may make a remarkable difference. Frequent vacuuming and dusting, particularly in children's rooms, can be helpful. Some patients believe that their atopic dermatitis is worsened by fabric softeners or certain brands of laundry detergent. Since fabric softeners are not essential for clean clothes, their use is discouraged. Dreft® and Hypoallergenic All® are good detergents for routine laundry use. Keeping clothes in the rinse cycle twice is useful in eliminating any soap residue.

CORTICOSTEROIDS One of the mainstays of treating atopic dermatitis is corticosteroids. For disease which is not extensive or complicated, topical preparations are ideal. They relieve the itching, stinging, redness, and swelling of affected skin. These products are best used for short periods (several days to several weeks) and then used less frequently. Most are designed to be applied once or twice per day but dermatologists often suggest their application more frequently for the first few days to help bring the disease under better control. Topical corticosteroids are manufactured as creams, ointments, lotions, gels, solutions, and sprays. They may also be the main ingredient in shampoos and oils. Different preparations are useful for different body sites and for different ages. Children and babies may absorb significant amounts of topically applied corticosteroids, so use of low-potency preparations is appropriate. For older patients and treatment areas with thicker skin, more potent preparations are used.

Ointments are greasy and oily but most useful for absorption into the skin. Creams are the most popular formulation since they are more cosmetically acceptable. Lotions are helpful for larger surface areas and for babies and children. Solutions are usually propylene glycol based and are best for large surface areas and hair-bearing regions. Unfortunately, they may sting if they are used on an area with a fissure or crack. Gels are also alcohol based and can be a problem on open wounds or cracked skin, but are very useful for hair-bearing areas such as the scalp and groins. Sprays are rarely used but are useful for high-intensity application to an area such as the scalp or a large plaque over the trunk.

If topical corticosteroids are applied too frequently, they begin to lose their potency, so it is important not to overuse them. Most patients with atopic dermatitis do not need to use these medications daily but appreciate having them around when a patch arises or their disease flares. Mixing some creams at one-quarter strength with a moisturizer is a useful way to apply a lubricant and topical corticosteroid. This is a popular means of therapy but may be costly for extended use. Applying a thin layer of the cream to the affected area and then occluding the skin with plastic wrap (Saran Wrap®) can be helpful. This is useful for disease on the arms and legs but difficult to do on the trunk. The plastic wrap may be left in place for several hours or overnight. If ointments are used or the wrap is left on too long, folliculitis may develop. There are numerous means of using these effective medications, but it is important to remember that they may have serious long-term effects and that they need to be used carefully.

Corticosteroids are also useful when taken by mouth, intramuscular injection, or intravenously. This can be a lifesaving therapy but it has numerous drawbacks. The most popular oral medication is prednisone or prednisolone, although methylprednisolone (SoluMedrol®) is also used. These drugs are usually given on a tapering dose over a seven- to fourteen-day period. The most common initial dose is about 30 to 60 mg per day for adults.

One of the most popular methods of initial treatment, particularly for persons with severe or recalcitrant disease, is an intramuscular injection of triamcinolone (Kenalog®) or dexamethasone (Decadron®). Triamcinolone stays in the body with gradually decreasing blood levels for about three weeks, so in effect it provides its own tapering dose. Doses are usually 20 to 60 mg. Dexamethasone is also useful but there seem to be more treatment failures when this drug is given. Triamcinolone takes about eighteen hours to begin providing relief from the itching and redness so dermatologists may give the patient a 6 mg dose (1 cc) of Celestone® (betamethasone phosphate/betamethasone acetate) in the same injection. This drug begins to work in about six hours; its effects are gone by eighteen hours.

Intravenous medications are usually reserved for hospitalized patients. Hydrocortisone and methylprednisolone are the most commonly used corticosteroids. These drugs have numerous drawbacks and they are not intended for regular use. It is not clear how often they can be safely given but any more often than every three months is considered risky. Overuse or abuse of these drugs may lead to increased blood pressure, elevated blood sugar, weight gain, increased body hair, and personality or mental changes.

The use of these preparations in children is somewhat controversial. An injection or intravenous administration of these drugs is unusual and undertaken only in dire circumstances. The use of oral prednisolone for three to five days, however, may provide the patient (and the family) some relief. Use of this drug allows the involved areas to heal since they are no longer scratched, and lets the patient sleep better at night. Unfortunately, some patients and parents become addicted to the use of these corticosteroid preparations and "doctor-shop" until they find a physician who will prescribe or administer them.

ANTIBIOTICS Many patients have an increased amount of bacteria, particularly *Staphylococcus aureus*, on their skin. Additionally, when there is a flare, the abraded and scratched areas become secondarily infected. For that reason, antibiotics are frequently given to patients with AD. One of the most popular is erythromycin because it is effective not only against *S. aureus* but also because it has some anti-inflammatory effects as well. Unfortunately, some people are resistant to this drug. Other antibiotics are also used with various degrees of success. Topical mupirocin is helpful for individual lesions which have become infected.

DIET Much has been made of dietary therapy for atopic dermatitis. It is unquestionably effective in certain patients, but a failure in others. Foods which a patient knows will worsen his or her disease should obviously be avoided. Patients are usually much better at discerning these foods than are physicians. A diary in which periods of calm and worsening of the AD and the activities and food intake surrounding them is helpful. This allows patients and physicians to evaluate what is happening just before the disease flares and make appropriate behavioral changes. Some foods which have been associated with flares include colas, chocolate, coffee, tea, eggs, milk, pork, mushrooms, tomatoes, fish, shellfish, nuts, citrus drinks (orange juice, grapefruit juice, and so on), corn, and fermented beverages. It is best to eliminate these one at a time from the diet for ten to fourteen days. If improvement is not seen, the food is reinstituted and another is eliminated until they have all been tried. Elemental diets from which the most common allergy-inducing ingredients have been eliminated are available; however, they are time consuming to prepare and are not very satisfying. As mentioned previously, there is evidence that mothers with "at-risk" pregnancies or who are breast-feeding may prevent or reduce atopic dermatitis by avoiding "high-allergen" foods.

Several dietary oils including evening primrose oil (EPO), fatty acid supplements, and fish oil have been touted as effective in treating AD. These may be purchased over the counter at food and nutrition stores. There is some evidence that EPO may be helpful; it is marketed in Great Britain for patients with atopic dermatitis, but it is not very popular in the United States. Fatty acid supplements such as EPO or fish oil have been shown to be no more effective than placebos. Gamma-linoleic acid may be of some help in persons with atopic dermatitis, but it is unlikely to be effective enough to replace conventional therapies.

ANTIHISTAMINES Antihistamines are widely used in atopic dermatitis. They offer relief from itching and often cause mild to moderate drowsiness, allowing patients to get much-needed sleep. These medications are particularly useful in persons who unknowingly or unconsciously scratch their skin. Antihistamines are usually divided into sedating and nonsedating categories. Sedating antihistamines include diphenhydramine (Benadryl®), promethazine (Phenergan®), doxepin (Sinequan®), hydroxyzine (Atarax®), chlorpheniramine (Rescon®), brompheneramine (Bromphed®), triprolidine (Actifed®), and cyproheptadine (Periactin®). The most common side effect with these medications is drowsiness, which may be intolerable or dangerous. Taking the medication only at bedtime avoids this problem, but there may be a lingering effect in the morning. Additionally, these medications, though making the patient fall asleep easier, alter the sleep patterns and may leave the patient feeling less than refreshed. Stomach upset and nervousness are also occasionally seen. Many antihistimines are dangerous if ingested in large quantities by children. These drugs are usually available generically and some are formulated in suspension. Chlorpromazine (Thorazine®) is a powerful antipsychotic with some antihistamine properties and may occasionally be used in patients with severe disease in whom breaking the itch-scratch cycle has become imperative. It promotes sleep and allows the patient to rest.

The nonsedating antihistamines include terfenadine (Seldane®), astemizole (Hismanal®), cetirizine (Zyrtec®), and loratidine (Claritin®). A few patients become drowsy when taking these medications, but overall they are well tolerated. They are available only in pill form (except for cetirizine) and are expensive. These drugs also may interact with different antibiotics and must be cautiously given.

A final category of antihistamines include the so called "H$_2$" blockers, which are given to diminish stomach acid production; these include cimetidine (Tagamet®), ranitidine (Zantac®), and famotidine (Pepcid®). These are probably more useful for hives and other skin disorders. Their ability to control itching appears limited; however, for certain patients they may be extremely useful. They are well tolerated with few side effects, and some are available generically or over the counter.

There are two topical antihistamine formulations containing diphenhydramine and doxepin (Zonalon®). Topical diphenhydramine is effective in certain patients but is usually not strong enough for significant AD. Additionally, it may make the disease worse by irritating the skin. Topical doxepin is useful in certain patients. It is effective in AD and may be helpful for patients with limited disease. It is very expensive, however, may occasionally be absorbed enough to induce drowsiness, and is capable of causing contact dermatitis. For patients with disease manageable with topical doxepin, the use of a moderate-strength topical corticosteroid is generally more cost efficient.

TAR PRODUCTS Topical tars may be very helpful for persons with atopic dermatitis. These medications are covered more extensively in the section on psoriasis. The most commonly used tar formulations include liquor carbonis detergens (LCD). Tar bath oils and topical creams are the most useful. If a patient's disease is flaring or very sensitive, tars may be too irritating. However, physicians commonly urge patients to use these products since they are believed to be safer for long-term use than are topical corticosteroids. A helpful product for persons with limited disease is the compounding of LCD (usually 10 to 15%) with triamcinolone ointment 0.1%, which may be generically purchased. Tar shampoos are also useful for persons with scalp involvement.

LIGHT TREATMENTS Light therapy (phototherapy), much like that prescribed for persons with psoriasis, is one of the most effective and best-tolerated forms of treatment for AD. In most patients, it is reasonably safe (when given properly), effective, and cost efficient. Its downside is that it is somewhat expensive and inconvenient. Certain cities and medical institutions have specialized phototherapy centers. Ultraviolet light B (UVB) is the most popular form of treatment; many dermatologists have these light units in their offices. Recently, combining UVB with ultraviolet light A (UVA) has become popular. PUVA (*Psoralens* and *UVA* light) is very effective in AD but is usually reserved for patients with more severe disease (see the section on psoriasis). Physicians may recommend that persons with limited disease spend thirty to sixty minutes daily in the sunlight. Obviously, this must not be overdone. It is important to emphasize that the use of a tanning bed is *not* equivalent to standardized, well-monitored, and properly dosed light treatment. While it is true that some patients benefit from the use of a tanning bed, some improperly treat their disease and worsen their symptoms. There is a subset of patients with AD whose disease is irritated by exposure to any and all forms of light therapy. These patients have what is termed *photosensitive eczema* and usually become skilled at sunscreen use and light avoidance. The use of light treatment in AD has become much more sophisticated in the past five years.

SYSTEMIC IMMUNOSUPPRESSANTS Cyclosporine (Sandimmune®) is a medication used by transplant patients to prevent organ rejection. It has been in use in the United States for about fifteen years. Recently, cyclosporine has been found to have profound effects on many skin diseases such as psoriasis, alopecia areata, and atopic dermatitis. It has been tested in a large number of studies in AD and found to be very helpful. Itching is relieved within a few days, and in about two weeks the patient's skin is greatly improved. There is some evidence that treatment with cyclosporine beyond two weeks is not helpful. Patients tend to relapse to some extent after stopping the medication. However, some patients, despite a return of their disease, are improved overall and require fewer conventional treatments. Patients with severe disease may be tapered to a very small dose or given a full dose every several days.

Cyclosporine is intended only for the most severe cases; it may harm the kidneys and cause high blood pressure. Some medications such as erythromycin and antifungal agents may not be taken with cyclosporine, and the drug is very expensive. A topical formulation may be mixed up by the pharmacist, but this has not proven to be particularly helpful. In the future, cyclosporine-containing creams and lotions may be developed. A new formulation of cyclosporine (Neoral®) has come on the market and allows the drug to be better absorbed from the gastrointestinal tract. It has not been tested on persons with atopic dermatitis as yet, but may allow for lower dosing of the drug.

INTERFERON Interferon is a protein made by white blood cells which is being used and evaluated for numerous diseases. Interferon-gamma (Actimmune®) has been found useful in some patients with AD. It is given as a shot several times per week and is dosed based on the patient's weight. Response tends to be rapid but so does relapse after the drug is discontinued. Interferons cause flulike symptoms. This complication may be avoided by pretreatment with acetaminophen. Most treatment trials have been in adults, but some children have benefited from IFN-gamma as well. Interferon alfa (Intron A®) has been used as well but has been disappointing. The interferons are an unusual class of medications and are intended for use only with severe cases. No oral or topical formulations exist.

RADIATION Radiation therapy was previously used in patients with atopic dermatitis. It was very effective but had a number of unacceptable long-term side effects. As a result, this treatment modality has fallen out of favor. However, a form of "light x-ray" known as Grenz rays is useful and safe when properly administered. The word *Grenz* comes from the German word meaning "border." The wavelength of these ultraviolet rays are found on the border between that of light and x-rays. Treatment is usually given once per week for three weeks. Individual sites are treated, so this therapy is not useful for patients with widespread disease. Grenz-ray therapy become less popular about fifteen years ago due to concerns over the safety of "radiation treatments." However, it has since become clear that for certain patients this may be a helpful and safe means of controlling their disease.

PSYCHOLOGICAL INTERVENTION Patients with a significant degree of anxiety and depression may benefit from administration of psychiatric medications, counseling, and/or psychotherapy. While this is not a typical scenario, many dermatologists have noted improvement in patients who begin these therapies. The use of antianxiety medication such as diazepam (Valium®) or alprazolam (Xanax®), however, is not recommended. While these medications may be useful in the short term, they often do more harm than good if chronically used.

HOSPITALIZATION There is a subset of patients for whom almost all therapies are unhelpful or untenable. These patients are commonly hospitalized for several days or weeks for more intensive therapy. They are usually given a good diet, intravenous antibiotics, and corticosteroids and may be started on light treatments. Aggressive use of antihistamines is also usually instituted, since this allows the patient to sleep and helps prevent scratching. Wet soaks and lubricant application up to eight times daily are also common. While this is an expensive means of treatment, in some instances it is the only therapy which will allow control of the disease. Hopefully, upon discharge the patient's AD will be manageable with more conservative treatment measures.

Other Treatments

There are numerous anecdotal reports of helpful medications and treatments for atopic dermatitis. Chinese herbal therapies have long been claimed to be beneficial in treating AD. Recent scientific studies seem to back up these claims. However, the exact ingredients in these herbs is not clear and there is some concern that liver damage may occur. Additionally, they reportedly have a very bad taste. Timed-release vitamin C (about 1,000 mg) has been reported as helpful. Ichthammol in zinc oxide is effective (similar to topical tar) but is not very cosmetically acceptable. Biotin, which may be purchased at health and nutrition stores, is touted as beneficial in childhood disease and is given as 300 µg per day. Propanolol, a medication used for control of high blood pressure, also helps reduce itching in some patients. It may worsen asthma, however. Naloxone is used for narcotic overdose but in patients with atopic dermatitis it may reduce itching. Oral sodium cromolyn is used to control asthma and has been tried with some success in atopic dermatitis. It seems to work best in persons whose disease is worsened by certain foods or allergens. It is easy to take and well tolerated, but expensive.

Eczema

The word *eczema* literally means "to boil over," which is what ancient physicians thought the skin was doing when it broke out. There are a number of different clinical conditions in which the skin behaves much as in atopic dermatitis but the affected areas and overall course is different. Many are named for the anatomic site of involvement.

Nummular Eczema

Nummular eczema is named for the configuration of the patches of involved skin. This word means "coin shaped" and the individual spots are circular or round. They range in size from that of a pencil eraser to a half dollar. They are usually mildly red or pink but often have a somewhat orange color. Crusting and scaling is seen. If present for prolonged periods and continually scratched, individual lesions will become dark and thickly scaled. Nummular eczema principally affects the extremities (particularly the legs) but may also involve the trunk. The head and neck are usually spared. The major complaint is moderate to severe itching. This disease affects primarily two groups—patients in their late fifties and early sixties and adolescent girls. There does not appear to be a connection to atopy, but the disease is associated with dry skin and the events which precipitate atopic dermatitis. It tends to be worse in the winter, probably due to decreased humidity. There is also a significant association with psychological stress.

Treatment is similar to that for AD. Topical steroids and tars, oral antibiotics, and corticosteroid injections are useful. Injection of corticosteroid suspensions into individual lesions may be very effective, but are not appropriate for persons with widespread disease. Light therapy may be helpful, and liberal and frequent moisturizing is required. Precipitated sulfur added to triamcinolone ointment 0.1% is beneficial in certain patients. The itch of nummular eczema can interfere greatly with sleep, so antihistamines may be useful.

Hand Eczema

See the section on hand dermatitis.

Pompholyx

Pompholyx is a term for a type of eczema affecting the hands and feet. Small bumps and blisters are seen along the sides of the digits and extending back onto the palms and soles. The tops of the feet and back of the hands are also involved. The itch may be maddening and may be accompanied by a burning sensation. There is a weak link with atopy in these patients, and most complain that their palms and soles sweat a lot. Pompholyx is most common in women beginning in their late twenties. Some patients are nickel sensitive and are unknowingly ingesting quantities of nickel in their diets, which causes their pompholyx to flare. An even more unusual subset includes patients with what has been termed an "id" reaction. These persons have a fungal infection elsewhere, such as athlete's foot or ringworm of the scalp. Diets low in nickel and treatment of the fungal infection may help these patients considerably.

Treatment is similar to other forms of eczema. Corticosteroids orally or by injection are useful for initial control of the disease; however, topical preparations are the mainstays of therapy. Use of a very potent topical corticosteroid early in an outbreak may help thwart worsening of the disease. Wearing latex or white cotton gloves over the corticosteroid for several hours (usually overnight) is helpful. Avoidance of irritating substances such as cleaners and solvents will help, as will liberal moisturizing (six to eight times per day). Ultraviolet light therapy, including PUVA treatments, are useful in severe cases. Pompholyx may respond beautifully to grenz-ray treatments. Topical tar preparations are helpful in some patients but generally don't help as much as with atopic dermatitis or nummular dermatitis. In persons whose feet sweat a lot, frequent sock changes with 100 percent cotton crew-type white socks are useful. This may require taking one or more pairs to school or the workplace. Skin which has become very weepy and inflamed responds well to wet compresses. Soaking in tar-based bath oils is also useful. Three to four capfuls can be put in a basin of tepid water and the hands and/or feet soaked for thirty minutes.

Xerotic Eczema

Xerotic eczema goes by a number of different names including "winter itch," "asteatotic eczema," and "eczema craquele." This disorder occurs mostly on the legs, but it is also seen on the arms and trunk. The skin is very dry and usually demonstrates a fine cracking; it resembles cracked porcelain. It is most common in older patients and in the wintertime when the air is dry and central heat is being used. Itching is moderate but infection may occur after prolonged scratching. Treatment centers around restoring moisture to the skin with appropriate bathing habits as in atopic dermatitis. Topical corticosteroids are helpful for the redness and itch, but the disease may be put into remission and eliminated with an avoidance of hot water, use of a mild soap, and moisturizing four to six times per day. Moisturizers containing urea and lactic acid are very useful for xerotic eczema, but if the skin is cracked and fissured they may sting. Bath oils, including those containing tar, are helpful.

Juvenile Plantar Dermatosis

Juvenile plantar dermatosis is an unusual but not uncommon form of eczema. This skin eruption occurs on the feet and soles of preadolescent children. It is red and scaly and usually involves the tops of the feet, particularly the toes, with little involvement of the toe web spaces. Itching is the predominant complaint; most patients believe their feet sweat a great deal. Parents usually worry that a child has athlete's foot or some type of contact allergy, but fungal infections such as athlete's foot are rare in children prior to puberty. Treatment consists of wet compresses if the eruption is very weepy, oral antibiotics, and topical steroids. If the soles are involved, walking may be difficult.

Eyelid Dermatitis

Eyelid dermatitis is an extremely common form of eczema and one which affects women almost exclusively, since they are likely to use nail polish, makeup, hair spray, and other cosmetics. The skin may show mild redness and irritation, but is more likely to display flaking and shedding. Eyelid dermatitis may be better classified as a contact dermatitis. In most instances, the offending agent has been transferred to the eyelids by the hands. Fingernail polish is a classic example. Eyeglasses or contact lens solutions may also be responsible. It is usually possible to eradicate the problem if the patient is willing to meticulously avoid all cosmetics, perfumes, fingernail products, hair-care products, and so on. This is rarely practical; most persons choose to simply treat the problem. Use of a good, bland moisturizing cream and a low-potency topical steroid are usually enough to keep the problem under control. Very potent corticosteroids applied to the tissue surrounding the eye may result in absorption into the eye itself and worsening of glaucoma, and should be avoided. If this eruption continues without resolution, patch testing for specific causes of this dermatitis should be considered.

Nipple Eczema

This condition involves the nipples and surrounding tissue of the breast. It may be seen in men but is much more common in women. There is usually redness, cracked skin, weeping, and mild to moderate itching, often on both nipples. It commonly afflicts nursing mothers and may hinder their attempts to breast-feed their children. Most worrisome is that it may mimic a form of cancer called Paget's disease. This cancer is usually the result of an underlying breast malignancy; therefore, many women have their nipple eczema biopsied to exclude the possibility of this neoplasm. Treatment consists of medium-potency topical corticosteroids and moisturizing creams. Discontinuing breast-feeding is usually recommended.

CONTACT DERMATITIS

The field of contact dermatitis has blossomed in the past several years as awareness has grown of what a significant role our environment plays in our lives. The number and variety of chemicals we use in everyday living has increased considerably in the past quarter century. While these may make living easier, some persons will react, sometimes violently, to the presence of these elements. When these substances come into contact with the skin or are ingested, they may cause a variety of reactions. There are basically three subtypes of contact dermatitis—allergic contact dermatitis, irritant contact dermatitis, and contact urticaria.

Allergic Contact Dermatitis

Allergic contact dermatitis (ACD) occurs when chemicals come in contact with the skin of persons who are allergic to them. The classic example is that of poison ivy or poison oak. These eruptions occur within a day or two of contact and usually itch or burn. There is mild to severe redness and blistering is common. As the rash fades the blisters dry up, forming crusts and scale. Residual pigmentation may remain. The eruption tends to resemble the shape of the culprit. For example, if ACD is due to poison ivy or oak, streaks where the plant brushed the skin will appear. If due to nickel allergy, the eruption may be round from the nickel in the wristwatch or snaps on the pants. Allergic reactions to hair dyes are usually streaked since the water and dye may run down the back of the neck. If the allergen is in the air, the exposed skin will be involved. The hands are commonly affected in persons exposed to chemicals at work (industrial chemicals). Allergic contact dermatitis differs from irritant contact dermatitis in that with the former the initial contact with the offending chemical may elicit no rash, it takes very little of the chemical to cause an eruption, and only certain persons are susceptible to this reaction. The patient's immune system is involved in the production of the eruption of allergic contact dermatitis, whereas it is not with irritant contact dermatitis.

Diagnosis
Diagnosis of contact dermatitis often proves confusing. Correct identification is often time consuming. Dermatologists and allergists rely on what is called "patch testing" to determine what, if any, chemicals are causing problems for the patient.

In this procedure, small metal wells about the size of a pencil eraser are filled with an appropriate amount of a chemical and are taped in place on the back of the person being tested. This test is usually performed with multiple wells and multiple chemicals so that a single test will yield as much information as possible. The wells allow the substances to come into contact with the patient's skin and cause contact dermatitis if the person is genuinely allergic to them. The wells are kept dry (no bathing or showering) and allowed to remain in place for seventy-two hours, at which time they are removed and the dermatologist evaluates the sites. Those sites which have reacted are usually red, are mildly swollen, and may itch. A strong reaction may involve the formation of a small blister. The reactions are graded on a scale of 0 (normal skin) to 4 (blister formation). Dermatologists experienced with patch testing often use 80 to 100 of these wells to maximize their testing efforts. A commercial patch test kit (T.R.U.E. TEST®) is available and tests for twenty-four chemicals. A common and less expensive means of testing is to apply the suspect substance to the fold of the arm twice daily for up to a week and observe any reaction that occurs.

The number of chemicals capable of causing ACD is extensive and is increasing. There is no practical way to avoid contact with all the chemicals that may cause ACD. Most all foods, medicines, cosmetics, toiletries, and consumer products have chemicals that might potentially provoke ACD. Table 14 provides a partial listing of some of the more common substances and chemicals.

Formaldehyde and formaldehyde-releasing agents are becoming known for the widespread disease they cause. Formaldehyde is a commonly used industrial chemical and exposure in everyday living is extensive. Formaldehyde-releasing agents are chemicals which slowly release formaldehyde and provide an antiseptic effect for cosmetics and lotions. Contact allergy to nickel is probably the most common ACD in North America. Low-nickel diets and medications used to "bind up" nickel in the gastrointestinal tract (disulfiuram) are used for persons with this allergy. Latex allergy has become a significant problem in the past ten years with the widespread use of gloves by health-care professionals. Use of vinyl gloves is suggested for these patients.

Treatment

The treatment of ACD is much simpler to envision than effect. In theory, simple avoidance should prevent any further problems with the eruption. However, chemicals in widespread use allow many opportunities for contact. Additionally, many products do not list what ingredients they contain. The dermatologist counsels the patient about what they are allergic to and the best means of avoiding the allergen. Sometimes this involves changing occupations or even moving to another city or state. There are lists and handouts available for persons with allergies to the more

Table 14   SUBSTANCES KNOWN TO CAUSE ALLERGIC CONTACT DERMATITIS

Substance	Where It Is Found
Acrylics	synthetic resins
	artificial nails
	plastics
Chromates	inks and paints
	leather processing
	cement
Epoxy Resins	
Ethylenediamine	Mycolog® cream
	certain antihistamines
	aminophylline
	merthiolate
Formaldehyde and Formalin	cosmetics
	shampoos
	nail polish
	soaps
	fabrics
	embalming fluid
	paper products
	glues
Formaldehyde-Releasing Agents	
Quaternium-15	moisturizers
	cosmetics
	shampoos
Imidazolidinyl urea	moisturizers
	cosmetics
Diazolidinyl urea	cosmetics
Bronopol	moisturizers
	cosmetics
	shampoos
Fragrances	colognes
	cosmetics
	perfumes
Lanolin	moisturizers
	cosmetics

continued

Table 14 *continued*

Substance	Where It Is Found
Latex	condoms
	gloves
Neomycin	topical antibiotics (Neosporin®)
	cosmetics
	deodorants
Nickel	diet
	metal objects
	insecticides and fungicides
Paraphenylenediamine	hair dyes
	leather processing
Plants	poison ivy
	poison oak
	poison sumac
	Japanese lacquer tree (lacquer dermatitis)
	cashew
	mango
	philodendron
	chrysanthemum
	dieffenbachia
	alstroemeria (Peruvian lily)
	ragweed pollen
	sesame seeds and sesame oils
Rubber	
mercaptobenzothiazole	rubber products
tetraethylthiuram disulfide	rubber products
	certain medications
Vegetables	celery
	cucumber
	parsley
	turnip
	asparagus
	garlic
	onion
	tomato
	mushroom

common chemicals which describe helpful things to avoid and items which may be substituted for their use. However, for some patients this is not enough. Topical corticosteroids, particularly potent preparations, are very effective in removing the redness and itching that commonly accompanies ACD. If patients have widespread disease, oral prednisone (Deltasone®) or an injection of triamcinolone (Kenalog®) is more humane. While this may help the acute symptoms substantially, it cannot be relied on for extended therapy. Topical use of astringents such as Domeboro® will help dry up the eruption and diminish the itch. Colloidal oatmeal preparations (Aveeno®) are useful. Oral antihistamines such as diphenhydramine (Benadryl®) or hydroxyzine (Atarax®) are helpful for itching. *Tolerance*, a term meaning persons with ACD who have been gradually exposed to increasing amounts of the offending chemical, can become "tolerant" of the allergen, is theoretically possible; however, its practical application is difficult since it requires specialized training, is expensive, and is considered an experimental therapy.

Barrier creams help prevent contact with the offending agent. These are most popular for use on the hands, particularly in persons whose profession or avocation puts them at risk. These may be used before working around poison ivy or poison oak as well as solvents, grease, glue, and oils in the workplace. These products include Work Shield®, Dermaffin Cream®, Dermofilm Spray®, Ivy Shield®, Multi-Shield®, and Travabon®.

Photoallergic Contact Dermatitis

A subset of ACD is photoallergic contact dermatitis. In this disease, a patient comes into contact with a substance such as certain medications, sunscreens, fragrances, and plants that is activated by exposure to sunlight. Other forms of light such as those from sunning lamps and tanning beds may also provoke this disease. Testing for sensitivity to one of these medications involves applying some of the substance and then giving the patient light (usually ultraviolet light A) in gradually increasing doses to the affected skin. This is called photopatch testing and is usually done in specialized dermatology treatment centers.

Systemic Contact Dermatitis

An unusual reaction in persons allergic to one or more chemicals is called systemic contact dermatitis. This occurs when a patient ingests or is injected with an allergen to which they have developed an allergic contact dermatitis. The skin eruptions range from dermatitis on the hands and sides of the fingers to an extensive red itchy eruption all over the body. Sometimes a flare of the dermatitis at the original site of contact will occur. Numerous chemicals have been described as causing this phenomenon including antibiotics, sulfa drugs, oral antidiabetes medications, salicylates, and some B vitamins.

Irritant Contact Dermatitis

Irritant contact dermatitis (ICD) differs from ACD in that the immune system is not involved, so previous contact with the offending chemical is not required. In other words, the irritation begins almost immediately. Skin which is intact, well hydrated, thick, and otherwise healthy is less likely to develop problems with ICD. Similarly, different chemicals have different properties which make them more likely to irritate the skin. The skin changes are almost identical to those of ACD and include redness, itching, skin breakdown, and burning. Distinguishing between ACD and ICD may be difficult or impossible; it is often done by the use of patch testing. The list of substances which may induce ICD is also long and growing. Alkalis and acids are probably the most common. Chemicals with these properties dissolve the overlying layers of the skin to a certain degree and allow for penetration into the deeper aspects of the tissues. Many acids and alkalis are contacted on the job (solvents, cutting fluids, fiberglass, dusts, and so on). Sometimes contact with these chemicals is in the setting of an industrial accident and emergency therapy is required. Airborne irritants such as dusts and gases also cause ICD. Examples include tear gas or mace (chloroacetophenone), dusts from woods and nuts, and tobacco dust. Photoirritant dermatitis may arise in persons who come into contact with offending substances or who ingest medications which make them susceptible to this reaction (see Table 15). The features are essentially identical to those of photoallergic contact dermatitis. Photopatch testing may prove useful.

Treatment of ICD is similar to that for ACD. Avoiding contact with these substances is essential. Again, this may involve a change in profession, particularly in those persons exposed at work. Initial therapy includes topical or oral corticosteroids and wet compresses (Domeboro®). Secondary infection may also be a problem and antibiotics may be required. Since so much of the susceptibility of ICD is due to environment (humidity, temperature, and so on), these factors must be controlled as best as possible. Protection of the skin to allow healing is mandatory and use of liberal and frequent moisturizing is required. Thick nonirritating creams such as Moisturel Cream® and Aveeno Cream® or ointments such as white petrolatum should be applied four to six times per day. The skin must repair itself and seven to ten days may be needed for the skin to become intact again.

Contact Urticaria

This phenomenon occurs when a substance, often a food, comes into contact with the skin and induces hives or urticaria. The skin reaction is essentially identical to hives from other causes and includes some mild swelling and redness with blanching in the center of the lesion. Other findings which may be seen include gastroin-

Table 15   CHEMICALS WHICH CAUSE PHOTOIRRITANT CONTACT DERMATITIS

Medications	griseofulvin (Gris-PEG®)
	tetracyclines (Sumycin®)
	sulfanilamide (AVC Cream®)
	vinblastine (Velban®)
	5-fluorouracil (Efudex®)
	dacarbazine (DTIC-Dome®)
	chlorpromazine (Thorazene®)
	amiodarone (Cordarone®)
	thiazide diuretics
	piroxicam (Feldene®)
	naproxen (Naprosyn®, Aleve®)
	tolbutamide
	Psoralens®
Fragrances	
Plants	limes
	figs
	parsnip
	celery
Tars	crude coal tar
	liquor carbonis detergens

testinal upset, shortness of breath, generalized itching, swelling of the throat, headache, and wheezing. The most common substances to cause contact urticaria are foods such as apples, potatoes, eggs, milk, shellfish, strawberries, spices, carrots, and raw meats (all types). Moths and caterpillars, antibiotics, fragrances, rubber (latex), topical anesthetics, antipsychotic medications, preservatives, and solvents may also provoke this reaction. Virtually any allergen which may provoke a reaction of one type or another is capable of inciting contact urticaria. Testing is usually done with the suspect substance and is performed in the physician's office, since the reaction is usually immediate. Treatment is essentially the same as for contact dermatitis and urticaria in general. Avoidance is the best method but may not be easily accomplished. Topical corticosteroids are useful as is topical doxepin (Zonalon®). Antihistamines such as doxepin (Sinequan®), hydroxyzine, and diphenhydramine are helpful but many patients prefer nonsedating compounds such as astemizole (Hismanal®) or terfenadine (Seldane®).

HAND DERMATITIS

Hand dermatitis affects 5 to 15 percent of the populace depending on how it is defined. It is more common in women than in men, probably because women are more likely to come into contact with water and cleaning fluids which are a common cause of this disorder. Several different diseases make up this complex including contact dermatitis (from cleaners, solvents, and chemicals), infection, eczema (pompholyx, nummular eczema), psoriasis, and keratolysis exfoliativa. Each disease must be addressed differently because the underlying cause is different. Making a distinction between the different categories of hand dermatitis is occasionally easy but can be very difficult. The cuticles and folds of skin around the nail may be swollen and irritated and produce pus. The nails may also be thinned, ridged, and deformed if the hand dermatitis has been present for a long time. Because a person uses the hands intimately in day-to-day living, it is not surprising that skin diseases in this area are particularly disabling. Some of the disorders which will be discussed here are covered in other areas of the book; the reader is encouraged to consult those sections.

Contact Dermatitis–Induced Hand Dermatitis

This may be divided into two categories of contact—substances to which the patient is allergic and contact with those that are simply irritating. The most common cause of hand dermatitis is irritation from prolonged contact with water and harsh chemical cleaners or soaps. Foods to which the patient is allergic such as tomatoes, shellfish, fish, cheese, radishes, parsnips, carrots, garlic, or onions may also provoke this disease. This condition is also known as "housewife's hands." Allergic contact dermatitis of the hands is also very common in persons who work around different chemicals on the job. (Some of these are discussed in the section on contact dermatitis.) Persons with chemical-induced hand dermatitis often find their symptoms improving on the weekends or when off work during holidays or vacations. Some people are allergic to chemicals from hobbies or pastimes they pursue. Deciding which substances are the problem is best done using patch testing (see section on contact dermatitis). Avoidance of the offending substances is the best means of solving the problem, but this may be impossible or impractical, especially if work related. The use of gloves and other barriers may be sufficient to solve the problem.

In some patients, the dermatitis does not result from an allergy but rather the harshness of a cleaner or solvent they are using. Constant exposure to water, particularly hot water, will worsen the problem. Patch-testing these patients will not provide an answer. Avoidance of hot water, the use of latex gloves, and decreased exposure to chemicals is suggested.

The skin of patients with this type of hand dermatitis is usually red, chapped, scaly, and cracked. Blisters are not common, and itching is more of a problem with allergic contact dermatitis than with the irritant variety. Patients may experience pain and soreness. The backs of the hands are more affected than the palms. The sides of the fingers may be spared. If the problem has been present for a long time, infection may occur.

Infection

Bacterial or fungal infection of the hand itself does not often cause hand dermatitis. However, in certain patients a bacterial or fungal infection elsewhere may induce hand dermatitis; this looks very much like that caused by eczema. These conditions are called "trichophytids" if caused by a fungal infection and "bacterids" if caused by bacterial infections. With fungal infections, the most commonly involved site is the feet. Athlete's foot or infection of the toenails is a common scenario. Bacterial infections may theoretically be at any site. Treatment of the underlying fungal or bacterial infection will result in disappearance of the hand dermatitis. In this situation, small blisters develop along the sides of the fingers with redness and scaling on the palms. Itching is usually the major symptom. This is a relatively uncommon form of hand dermatitis; some dermatologists no longer believe that it actually exists.

Pompholyx

Pompholyx is an older name for hand dermatitis or hand eczema. This is one of the most common, if not the most common, form of the disease. Pompholyx presents as small blisters along the sides of the fingers and on the palms. The feet may be involved as well, but to a lesser extent. The blisters are about the size of a pinhead but may enlarge to the size of a pea or larger. The problem is much more common in women than in men, particularly those in their twenties and thirties. Flares occur in the spring and summer and last for several weeks. Itching is the main symptom, and may be maddening. Many patients have a history of asthma, allergies, or eczema either personally or in their families. A large number of patients also have a history of excessive sweating on the palms and soles. Some persons have allergies to substances such as nickel, cobalt, and other metals. In this case, the person is ingesting quantities of nickel through the diet. Stress usually makes pompholyx worse but does not cause the disease. Some patients can relate their flares to a recent illness. As the disease progresses and the skin is traumatized by scratching, it becomes thickened (lichenified) with scaling and crust formation. Secondary infection may take place but serious infections are uncommon. The disease may appear to "spread" up the hand and wrist. Breakouts in locations typical for eczematous dermatitis such as the folds of the arm and behind the knee may also occur. The nails may show some mild involvement such as small "pits," much like those seen in the nails of persons with psoriasis. A type of hand dermatitis termed *hyperkeratotic palmar eczema* may begin as pompholyx. This variant shows red palms with very thick scaly skin. Itching is common and the person may become incapacitated from the skin's crusting and cracking.

Psoriasis

Hand psoriasis is difficult to manage and usually must be approached differently from other types of hand dermatitis. Routine psoriasis will occasionally occur as small patches on the hands and feet. However, certain patients will have widespread involvement. The patches are red and scaling. Nails are involved with pitting and other deformities. If the skin displays pustules, a similar eruption may occur on the palms and soles. Psoriasis of the hands and feet usually is uncomfortable with some modest itching.

Keratolysis Exfoliativa

This is an unusual type of hand eruption which primarily occurs in adolescents and young adults. The skin over the palms and soles develops small white spots which gradually break down and form scaling skin. There are few, if any, symptoms and little evidence of inflammation. Some patients have a history of increased sweating in these areas.

Treatment

To some extent the treatment for each of these types of hand dermatitis is different and the therapy regimen must be constructed uniquely for individual patients. However, some common ground does exist; the therapy is similar to that for atopic dermatitis.

Avoidance

One of the most important things for patients with hand dermatitis to do is to avoid circumstances which make the problem worse. Wearing gloves on the job or when working in the home is important. Some persons have allergies to latex, in which case vinyl gloves should be used. These may be purchased through a surgical supply store. Extensive contact with water, particularly hot water, should be avoided. The more protection and "pampering" a patient's hands receive, the better. Protecting the hands from the weather is also important, but wool gloves usually worsen the problem. Leather gloves are the most useful. Strong soaps, detergents, solvents, acids, greases, and other irritating chemicals should be avoided.

Lubrication

Moisturizing the hands is extremely important. The use of a topical corticosteroid cream or ointment will help, but these products do not provide enough lubrication to adequately fill this role. There are numerous moisturizing creams and lotions on the market but many may contain lanolin (wool wax), antimicrobials, perfumes, coloring agents, and various forms of formaldehyde. These may make some patients' skin disease worse. Some useful brands of lotions and creams are listed in the handout in the moisturizers and soap section. Using cheaper generic moisturizers may save money but can contain irritating substances that may worsen hand dermatitis. Remember, the thicker the moisturizer the better the result. Moisturizers do not actually resupply the skin with fluids. Rather, they provide a barrier which stops the loss of moisture. Some persons prefer to use petroleum-based products for lubrication. These are excellent, because they allow almost no moisture from the skin to escape, and they promote healing. Vaseline® and white petrolatum are the two most popular emollients used. Unfortunately, they are greasy; many patients don't like their thick texture. It is better to apply a less optimal emollient than have a fantastic one gathering dust. It is important, therefore, to find an acceptable product and use it regularly. Pump bottles at home or at work are great since they encourage frequent usage. Wearing gloves at night is helpful. White cotton gloves are popular; they allow the hands to breathe and are cool. Moisturizers and other medications should be put on the skin and the cotton gloves then pulled on. Vinyl or latex gloves are even better. They are put on after the emollients are applied. If only a few fingers are affected, the fingertips of the gloves may be cut out and used for occlusion. Some people don't like wearing gloves while they sleep. In these instances, the use of gloves for several hours in the evening may suffice. Obviously, the more time they are used the better the skin will respond. The most important thing to remember about moisturizers for hand dermatitis is that it is impossible to moisturize the skin too much. Frequent and continual application of moisturizers is essential.

Corticosteroids

Cortisones are frequently used, as described in the section on atopic dermatitis. Most persons will improve considerably after a shot of triamcinolone (Kenalog®) or a short course of prednisone (Deltasone®) tablets. However, these medications cannot be used for long-term treatment of hand or foot dermatitis. Similarly, topical corticosteroids are useful but require special precautions if used over a prolonged period. Since the skin in these areas is usually quite thick (it may be even thicker if the surface has been chronically scratched or rubbed), less potent topical steroids usually have little effect. Creams and ointments are most useful, since lotions and solutions tend to be irritating to skin if cracking or blistering is present. These medicines are initially applied several times a day with an eye toward decreasing the frequency of application. If a very potent topical corticosteroid is applied too frequently, the skin will become "immune" to the medication and it will become less effective. Thinning of the skin may also occur with chronic overuse. In this case, "less is more." Some persons control their disease by applying the medications every other day or just on weekends. A very useful way to use topical corticosteroids is at bedtime with moisturizer application. The corticosteroid is applied over the affected areas only. A thick layer of emollient (preferably a thick cream formulation) is then added over it and gloves are put on. This keeps the corticosteroid cream or ointment in contact with the skin for a longer period and occludes it with the gloves and the moisturizer. Injecting steroid suspensions into the affected skin may also be very helpful. This is painful, however, and practical only when there are a limited number of involved areas.

Antibiotics

Antibiotics are frequently used in persons with hand and foot dermatitis. Cracked and blistered skin easily becomes infected. This infection makes the skin more uncomfortable and worsens the disease. Antibiotics are most useful for acute flares. In persons with chronic stable disease, these medications are not as effective. The most commonly prescribed drugs include erythromycin (PCE®), azithromycin (Zithromax®), amoxicillin-clavulanate (Augmentin®), cephalexin (Keflex®), cefadroxil (Duricef®), and cloxacillin/dicloxacillin (Dycil®).

Wet Dressings

Wet dressings are useful for dermatitis of the hands as well as elsewhere. These solutions tend to work best if the skin is very inflamed and irritated with oozing and crusting. They relieve itching and allow the skin to "dry up" with less redness and scaling. The solutions are also capable of killing certain bacteria and thereby provide some antiseptic treatment as well. These products may be purchased over the counter. The most popular is aluminum acetate, packaged as tablets or powder and sold as Blueboro® or Domeboro.® It is nonstaining, easily used, and odorless. Silver nitrate and potassium permanganate are equally useful but stain the skin and clothes. A 5% solution of acetic acid (white vinegar) may also be used and is less expensive. The solutions are made according to the package instructions, usually in a 1:40 dilution. Strips of cloth are soaked in the solution. Gauze, bedsheets, pillowcases, and handkerchiefs make the best dressings. The solution should be gently squeezed from the cloth so that it remains very wet but does not drip. The dressings are applied to the skin in a wrapping fashion and kept in place for about fifteen minutes. Some drying should occur. After fifteen minutes the dressing should be removed, rinsed, and reapplied. This should be done for one-half to two hours several times daily. Soaking the skin directly in the wet dressing solution is not particularly helpful. Dressings may be washed between applications. After the soaks have been completed, application of a corticosteroid creme, not an ointment, to affected skin is beneficial.

Light Therapy

Ultraviolet light treatment (as for atopic dermatitis or psoriasis) is useful for patients with hand dermatitis. Special units designed for use on the hands and feet are available, but most dermatologists do not have them in their offices. It may be necessary to have this treatment in a specialized light therapy center. PUVA and UVB therapy is given in essentially the same manner as for other skin ailments. Precautions and side effects are also similar. These forms of therapy may be quite helpful for long-term control.

Grenz Ray

Grenz-ray therapy is one of the most effective and convenient means of treating hand dermatitis. This treatment modality was very popular in the past but has been linked with the adverse long-term effects of radiation therapy and has declined in popularity. Today, this therapy is difficult to obtain for most patients. Treatments are given weekly for three consecutive weeks. This may be repeated approximately every nine months or so; however, many patients do not need additional treatments.

Topical Tars

Some persons respond well to topical application of tar products. Tar lotions and creams may be purchased over the counter or may be formulated with a prescription. Those mixed up by the pharmacist may be more expensive but may contain different medications, including topical corticosteroid creams, which may be more effective and soothing. If the skin is very irritated and inflamed, application of tar may worsen the condition. Soaking in tar solutions as described in the section on eczema is useful. Tar creams applied at night with occlusion by gloves may be useful.

Antihistamines

Antihistamines may be useful for persons with hand dermatitis. For more information on their use, see the section on atopic dermatitis. Topical antihistamine creams such as diphenhydramine (Benadryl®) or doxepin (Zonalon®) may be of some help. Unfortunately, these medications may worsen the dermatitis and are expensive.

Psychological Medications

A certain subset of patients with hand dermatitis have a component of depression and/or anxiety which is driving their disease. Until these symptoms are addressed and dealt with, adequate control of the disease will be difficult to achieve. These persons may benefit greatly from use of antidepressants such as fluoxetine (Prozac®), nefazadone (Serzone®), or sertraline (Zoloft®). Antianxiety agents such as buspirone (Buspar®), alprazolam (Xanax®), and lorazepam (Ativan®) may also be helpful. These medications have significant side effects and the potential for abuse. Consequently, they should not be used in all situations.

Immunosuppressants

Systemic immunosuppressants such as azathioprine (Immuran®), cyclophosphamide (Cytoxan®), and cyclosporin (Sandimmune®) are rarely used in persons with hand dermatitis. These drugs should be only a "last-ditch" therapy since they have the potential for severe side effects and must be given with great care and caution.

Seborrheic Dermatitis

Seborrheic dermatitis is one of the most common skin conditions, affecting 2 to 5 percent of the population. It is seen in all age groups from infants to the elderly and in all races; men are more often affected than women. Poorly functioning immune systems, such as with AIDS, put persons at risk of developing seborrheic dermatitis. The cause of this condition is not clear but may be related to bacteria such as *Staphylococcus aureus* and *Propionibacterium acnes* or yeasts such as *Candida albicans* or *Pityrosporum*. As a result, some treatments for this disease are directed at these organisms. While seborrheic dermatitis occurs in the areas where people have the most oil glands, it still is not clear if there is something about the oil, or sebum, that these people produce or the means by which the skin clears it. This skin condition is worsened by stress and is commonly seen in persons with Parkinson's disease and different types of neurological disorders. The features of seborrheic dermatitis overlap to some degree with psoriasis and eczema. When a clear distinction between the two is not possible, the term *sebopsoriasis* is occasionally used.

The appearance of seborrheic dermatitis may depend on the patient's age. In adults and adolescents, a mild redness and scaling around the sides of the nose, in the eyebrows, on the scalp, and behind the ears is most common. Inside the ears and on the front of the chest are other sites of involvement. The scale may be thickened and somewhat "greasy." In severe cases there may be oozing and crusting. Some patches are a slightly yellow to orange color. Itching, if present, is usually mild. Patients may complain of stubborn "dandruff." In extensive disease, the groin, underarms, and sides of the neck are involved. Total body involvement (erythroderma) may be seen with particularly severe cases. In infants, the scalp may be affected (cradle cap). The scales can be thick and adhere to the skin. Diagnosis is usually not difficult but a skin biopsy may be helpful in some situations, particularly if a distinction from psoriasis needs to be made.

Treatment

The most common therapy is application of topical corticosteroids. Corticosteroid pills or injections are usually needed. Low- to midpotency preparations are usually sufficient. Creams work well but lotions, gels, or solutions also help. Ointments or greasy creams and lotions may make the problem worse. Corticosteroid-containing shampoos or scalp oils may be helpful. In the past several years, the use of anti-*Pityrosporum* agents such as ketoconazole (Nizoral®), selenium sulfide (Selsun®, Exsel®), and zinc pyrithione (DermaZinc®) have been shown to be useful. Ketoconazole cream is not only effective but may be used safely for prolonged periods. This drug is also present in shampoo form and has become one of the mainstays of scalp treatment. It is best to allow shampoos for seborrheic dermatitis to remain on the scalp for five to ten minutes before rinsing. Ketoconazole shampoo may be used daily; it is expensive, however, and requires a prescription. It may be used for children but has to be applied carefully to avoid the eyes. Alternating every other day with a cheaper shampoo is popular. Lathering up the body and scrubbing with this shampoo may also be helpful. Selenium sulfide shampoo and zinc pyrithione shampoo (Head & Shoulders Dandruff Shampoo®) are also useful and may be purchased without a prescription. Other antifungal medications such as itraconazole (Sporanox®) and econazole (Spectazole®) may also be effective. Tar shampoos, as used for psoriasis, also work and are available without a prescription. If scalp crusting is particularly bad, as with cradle cap, salicylic acid compounded in olive oil may help loosen the debris. Children are very susceptible to salicylic acid, however, and since some may be absorbed by the skin, this should be used only under a physician's supervision. Metronidazole cream (Metrocream®) is useful in some patients. Gentle removal of crusts from inside the ear may be done with a cotton-tipped applicator.

PART III

SKIN CANCER

~ ~ ~ ~

Awareness of skin cancer has increased over the past decade with the ballooning number of patients diagnosed with malignant melanoma and the realization that disease is related to the amount of exposure to ultraviolet light.

Skin cancer is not just one disease. There are a number of different malignancies that may occur in the skin and are believed to be related to overexposure to the sun or ultraviolet light. Some are more dangerous than others. Additionally, in many cases before a skin cancer arises a "precancer" occurs. These precancers are not dangerous and if appropriately treated will cause no further problem. While the risk of skin cancer seems to be most closely related to sun exposure, other risk factors including x-ray treatments (as for acne and thyroid disease), smoking history, certain genetic diseases, other carcinogen and chemical exposures, and the presence of viral infection (particularly human papillomavirus [HPV]) are also involved.

Before discussing the different types of skin cancer, it is important to realize that different people handle ultraviolet light differently. Table 16 notes how different skin types react to ultraviolet light.

Table 16 DIFFERENT SKIN TYPES AND THEIR REACTIONS TO UV LIGHT

Skin Type	Tan	Burn	Hair	Skin Color	Skin Reaction
I	Never	Always	Red/Blond	White	Freckle easily
II	Rarely	Usually	Red/Blond	White	Freckle easily
III	Usually	Sometimes	Blond/Brown	White	Tan lightly
IV	Almost always	Rarely	Brown/Black	Light brown	Tan well
V	Always	Rarely	Brown/Black	Brown	Will darken
VI	Always	Never	Black	Brown/Black	Tan difficult to see

Actinic Keratosis

Actinic keratoses are precancers that may ultimately form skin cancer (usually squamous cell carcinoma or basal cell carcinoma). Actinic keratoses (AKs) are among the most common lesions found on the skin. Not surprisingly, they tend to be found among older patients and on sun-exposed sites. However, they are being found in increasing numbers among younger persons as well. Most patients have just a few lesions but it is possible to have hundreds. Persons who tolerate the sun poorly (types I and II) or who have had significant sun exposure tend to have a great many AKs. Patients with poor immune systems such as kidney transplant patients also develop numerous AKs. The worry with actinic keratoses is that if they are not removed they may "turn the corner" and become skin cancer. This is considered a small risk for persons with just a few lesions, but for those with many the risk proportionally increases.

Actinic keratoses are small red to gray raised spots with scaling and crusting. They may often be felt better than seen. In some areas, such as the backs of the hands, they can become very thick. They may itch or sting mildly but usually are without any symptoms at all. When present on the lower lip (actinic cheilitis), they occur as mild scaling which may feel slightly thickened.

Treatment

The easiest treatment is to spray AKs with liquid nitrogen. This will cause them to become slightly inflamed, swollen, and possibly even blistered depending on how many times the liquid nitrogen is applied. After the lesions fall off in a week or so, the underlying skin will be new and healthy. This is a quick and effective treatment for most lesions. Thick actinic keratoses, particularly over the hands and arms, may be difficult to remove with this method because they may be too thick for the liquid nitrogen to fully freeze. Having patients with many lesions return monthly is a good way to stay on top of the situation and get rid of the lesions before they become too big.

The next most popular therapy is topical chemotherapy. 5-fluorouracil cream (Efudex®, Fluoroplex®) has been used for years to remove AKs. This medicine is available in several different strengths and is applied to the skin once or twice daily for several weeks. It must be used with a sunscreen if applied during the day, since interaction with the sun can make the skin very sensitive. It may also be applied along with tretinoin cream (Retin-A®) to enhance its effects. As time passes, the AKs will become red and inflamed and may crust over. The "normal" skin may also become reddened and painful but usually will not break down. A great number of invisible AKs often "light up" when using this drug. This has the benefit of not only removing lesions that were not visible previously but also showing the patient the degree of damage that exists on their skin. Usually after ten days to two weeks of twice-daily treatment of the face, there is considerable discomfort and the patient should stop using the 5-fluorouracil. Topical corticosteroids (triamcinolone [Kenalog®]) may be applied to particularly uncomfortable areas for temporary relief.

Over the next one to three weeks, the skin will gradually heal and the tissues will appear healthier and more vibrant. In effect, the patient has just undergone a facial peel and he or she may look spectacular. Unfortunately, this treatment may be very uncomfortable and it is often difficult, if not impossible, to convince a patient to undergo another round of therapy. The "tougher" skin of the arms and forearms will usually tolerate this treatment much better and without the inflammation and discomfort experienced on the face and forehead. Treatment for these areas may be done for three to six weeks if needed. The actinic keratoses from this part of the body are generally much thicker and more difficult to remove in a short time period. Some patients opt for a treatment course once a year just to remove all the lesions that have accumulated in the previous twelve months. Treatment during the cooler months is often preferred since there is usually less stinging and burning.

Recently, a better-tolerated regimen has become popular for facial application. Using the 5-fluorouracil twice daily for two consecutive days of the week seems to be just as effective as the method described above. This is done for several months or even longer. There is less inflammation or discomfort.

Facial peels using alpha-hydroxy acids are a popular means of removing AKs. These peels may be done to different depths, depending on their strength, and leave the skin feeling refreshed and regenerated. Home use of creams containing alpha-hydroxy acid may continue the beneficial effects. This method of treatment is somewhat expensive, but very popular; it is discussed further in the section on cosmetic dermatology.

Long-term use of tretinoin is believed to be useful in some patients with minimal disease. This medication is used as for acne but must be applied over a long time period. It is believed to prevent the development of AKs.

Finally, application of topical substances such as trichloroacetic or bichloroacetic acids to individual AKs may be used for their removal. This is an older method of treatment but is effective and usually well tolerated. It has been shown that use of sunscreen is helpful in preventing actinic keratoses and persons with

Table 17   PRECANCEROUS KERATOSES

Keratosis Type	Inciting Factors
Actinic keratosis	Ultraviolet exposure
Arsenical keratosis	Arsenic exposure
Tar keratosis	Use of or exposure to hydrocarbons (tar)
Thermal keratosis	Chronic heat exposure
Radiation keratosis	X-ray exposure
Scar keratosis	Long-standing scars

these lesions are encouraged to begin a pattern of long-term sunscreen use, not only for episodic sun exposure but for daily application as well.

There is a long list of other precancerous keratoses outlined in Table 17. These are considerably more rare but are still capable of forming skin cancers, usually squamous cell carcinomas, in affected patients.

Basal Cell Carcinoma

Basal cell carcinomas (BCCs) are the most common human malignancy and the most common skin cancer (more than 300,000 per year). The incidence of this cancer is increasing. It may occur in darker-skinned populations but is much more common in Caucasians, particularly persons with long-term sun exposure and/or lighter skin types. Most patients are forty years of age or older but BCCs in the twenties or thirties are not uncommon. In younger age groups, women seem to be more commonly affected, perhaps because of frequent sun tanning or use of tanning beds. Other risk factors are exposure to arsenic or x-rays and certain inherited conditions, such as basal cell nevus syndrome. Long-standing ulcers of the legs (stasis ulcers) may also develop these tumors.

Basal cell carcinomas typically occur as painless, skin-colored to slightly red bumps on the head and neck. They can contain dilated blood vessels and occasionally have a "pearly" look. A certain type of BCC, called a superficial basal cell carcinoma, occurs on the trunk. This tumor is usually flat, reddened, and mildly scaly. It may have been mistakenly thought to be a small patch of eczema. Pigmented basal cell carcinomas have pigment-producing cells (melanocytes) within them and may appear very dark. They have been mistaken in the past for melanomas and can cause considerable concern. Some BCCs, called sclerosing basal cell carcinomas, appear scarlike. These are very aggressive tumors which may invade deeply and may be destructive to surrounding tissues or organs.

Basal cell nevus syndrome is an inherited condition. Persons begin to develop BCCs in adolescence and may have hundreds of these tumors. They also have some abnormalities of their bones (typically the ribs), cysts in their jawbones, and pits in their palms. These patients are difficult to treat, since they frequently produce tumors as fast as they can be removed. Scarring is a problem. It is important to remember that basal cell cancers are not life threatening and do not behave as other "cancers" do. They metastasize only under the rarest of circumstances (usually when neglected for many years). The major problem with BCCs is that they may grow so large as to involve or invade organs such as the eyes. With reasonably early removal, there is nothing to fear from these lesions.

Treatment

The usual method of treatment for basal cell carcinomas begins with a biopsy. A small portion of the tumor is removed and evaluated by a pathologist. This will allow the dermatologist to determine what type of BCC is present and the best method of treatment. The oldest form of therapy is termed *electrodessication and curettage* (ED&C). With this treatment, the area is numbed with local anesthetic and the majority of the tumor is scraped away. The wound is then gone over with an electric needle, charring the tumor bed, and the debris again scraped away. This may be done several times. Since most BCCs are soft and fall apart easily, finding how far the tumor has spread in the skin is relatively simple. The wound is then allowed to heal with a bandage and application of an antibiotic ointment. Scarring does occur and if the tumor is large the scar may be cosmetically unacceptable. For some tumor types, such as a sclerosing BCC, this method of treatment will not work since the tumor cannot be completely scraped away. ED&C is relatively easy to do and is effective for many tumors. It is also inexpensive and does not inconvenience the patient. The downside of this treatment method is that in a substantial number of cases the entire tumor is not removed and it recurs.

Treatment of recurrent BCCs with ED&C is often not successful and other methods are then preferred. Probably the most popular therapy is simple excision. The area is numbed with local anesthetic, the tumor is scraped away to determine its dimensions, and the entire area is then cut out. Stitches are used to sew the edges together and the wound usually heals without further problems. Large wounds which have been created by excision removal, particularly on the central part of the face, may not allow for simple closure. Under these circumstances, the surgeon may decide to do a "flap" in which surrounding normal skin is brought in to help cover the defect, or a "graft" in which skin from another part of the body (behind the ear is a popular site) is applied to the wound and stitched in. Removal of BCCs in this method is more complicated, expensive, and uncomfortable but usually decreases the chance that the tumor will recur. The removed tissue is then evaluated by a pathologist to check for complete removal of the cancer.

Radiation treatment of BCCs is not as common as it once was, although it is still a very effective means of treatment. It is most often used when the patient is elderly (and therefore less likely to develop another BCC from the radiation treatment itself) or infirm and perhaps unable to tolerate any type of surgical procedure. The results of x-ray treatment may be very good and it should probably be considered more often than it is. Previously, many dermatologists had small x-ray units in their offices. However, with the current negative public image of radiation treatments, this method of therapy has dropped considerably in popularity.

Cryosurgery refers to the use of liquid nitrogen for tumor removal. This is an older treatment method but may be very appropriate for certain tumors. It is practiced differently than simple application of liquid nitrogen as for precancerous changes. The freeze is deeper and more prolonged. "Cryoprobes" are inserted into the skin to measure the temperature and when that reading is reached, the frozen tissue is allowed to gradually thaw over a several-minute period. This method of treatment may be quite effective but may not yield the best cosmetic result. As a consequence it has declined in popularity over the years.

One of the most effective and popular treatments for basal cell carcinomas is Mohs chemosurgery. This technique was developed by Dr. Frederick Mohs at the University of Wisconsin. It entails surgically excising the cancer and, while the patient is still in the office, evaluating the edges of the specimen to determine if any tumor remains. This allows the surgeons to remove the least amount of tissue; this results in a better cosmetic outcome. After the skin area has been shown to be cancer free, the wound is closed as with other excisions. Not every BCC requires Mohs surgery. The most common indications for the use of this technique include very aggressive tumors (sclerosing), recurrent BCCs which have not responded to other treatment methods, tumors in compromising sites (eyelids, corner of the eye, rim of the nose, lip, and so on), and lesions arising in unusual circumstances such as following radiation treatment. Mohs chemosurgery is time consuming and expensive, but offers the best chance for many persons to be completely rid of a tumor since recurrence rates are much lower than with other methods of treatment. This surgical technique has also been successfully used on squamous cell carcinomas and other skin malignancies. Its use in malignant melanoma is somewhat controversial.

In persons who are prone to develop many BCCs, such as patients with basal cell nevus syndrome or those who have had organ transplantation, there is some evidence that administering isotretinoin (Accutane®) may slow the development of such lesions. The drug is usually given in slightly lower doses than for acne. Unfortunately, once the drug is stopped, the tendency to develop more cancers returns. Other chemotherapeutic agents have been noted to halt or slow the progress of developing BCCs as well.

Topical acids and chemotherapy drugs (for example, 5-fluorouracil) are not helpful in treating BCCs since they do not treat far enough into the skin to remove the tumor.

Squamous Cell Carcinoma

Squamous cell carcinoma (SCC) is the second most common malignancy of the skin. Essentially the same things that make a person susceptible to developing a BCC apply also to SCCs. The most common risk factor is sun exposure. Around 100,000 persons in the United States develop an SCC each year. The typical patient is someone with long-standing sun damage or who is light complected and unable to tolerate the sun well. The skin usually appears weather-beaten, wrinkled, and discolored, with numerous actinic keratoses. Persons living closer to the equator have an increased number of SCCs. Men are more commonly affected than women, probably because they have a greater amount of sun exposure. Squamous cell carcinomas are on the increase and tend to occur after age forty. Other environmental factors including wind exposure, decreasing ozone layers, and hot weather may play a role in provoking SCC. A subtype of SCC called verrucous carcinoma is associated with human papillomavirus infection (HPV). Persons who have had kidney, liver, or heart transplantations are also much more susceptible to developing an SCC.

Squamous cell carcinomas are typically raised, crusty, or warty lesions which are mildly pink to red. They may be very large and if present for prolonged periods may erode into an eye or ear. SCCs may also appear as ulcerations and nodules. Verrucous carcinomas appear as large warty growths on the bottoms of the feet (epithelioma cunniculatum), large tumors on the genitalia (Buschke-Loewenstein tumor), and as a slowly enlarging whitish-gray growth in the mouth on older patients (oral verrucous carcinoma). Squamous cell carcinomas may also occur in scars and radiation-treated skin.

Oral SCCs appear as a whitish to reddish growth on the floor of the mouth, the sides of the tongue, and the back of the soft palate. These are usually related to smoking or tobacco chewing. These cancers are not painful but have an increased risk for spreading outside the mouth. The same is true of SCC of the lower lip. This type of cancer is linked to tobacco use (smoking or chewing), long-standing sun exposure, and alcohol consumption. About a quarter of these tumors will eventually metastasize to lymph nodes in the neck. As a result, all suspicious lesions or ulcerations in susceptible persons should be biopsied and if found to be a cancer, removed with due speed. Diagnosis of SCCs is done the same way as for BCCs. Treatment is similar.

The great worry for squamous cell carcinomas is that they will metastasize. While the likelihood of this happening is small, it is still greater than for basal cell carcinomas. Tumors which have been present and slowly growing for many years seem to be the most prone to metastatic spread. Additionally, SCCs arising from arsenic, x-ray, heat, and chemical exposure are more aggressive. Therefore, more cancers of this sort are treated with surgical excision or Mohs surgery than are BCCs. Squamous cell carcinomas arising on the lip or in the mouth may be removed by head and neck surgeons and the surrounding tissues explored for any evidence of spread. In short, the presence of an SCC is not considered an emergency, but it is certainly a situation that deserves attention in a forthright manner.

Malignant Melanoma

Melanoma, or malignant melanoma as it is usually called, is the skin cancer that is most worrisome to patients and dermatologists. Of the several different types of skin cancer, this is the most likely to metastasize and to ultimately kill the patient. These tumors arise from the pigmenting cells of the skin, called melanocytes, and sometimes appear as a mole.

In the past few years, dermatologists have witnessed considerable growth in the number of patients they see with melanoma. In fact, the number of cases of this disease is increasing faster than any other cancer. In 1997, an estimated 40,300 cases of melanoma will be diagnosed and 7,300 deaths will occur. There is credible evidence that the reported incidence of these cancers is badly underestimated and that the actual number exceeds 100,000. In the 1940s, the chance that a person would develop a melanoma was about 1 in 1,000. By the year 2000, those odds will be down to about 1 in 75.

Melanoma is the most common malignancy in women aged twenty-five to twenty-nine and the seventh most common cancer overall in the United States. Clearly, something has changed and has given us this epidemic of melanoma. What is different now? First of all, a number of dermatologists do not believe that melanoma is more prevalent today than previously. Rather, the public and physicians are better about spotting melanomas and that accounts for more of them being diagnosed. Additionally, considerable research has been done on this disease and the criteria for making the diagnosis microscopically has changed.

While there is some merit to these contentions, there surely are other factors not accounted for. In the past thirty years, the amount of people's exposure to light both from the sun and artificial sources has increased. The evidence that melanoma arises in people who spend too much time in the sun has long been proposed and evidence in favor of this hypothesis continues to accumulate. Some of this is self-induced or occupational, but some may also be caused by the thinning of the ozone layer. Again, this is a controversial subject but there is compelling evidence that the ozone layer above the earth is changing and may account for more damaging rays reaching the skin of its inhabitants. Finally, people today are living longer and with a greater number of immune-suppressing conditions than before. A person's immune system plays a key role in how they respond to cancer. This applies not just to melanoma but also to other malignancies. Patients who fifteen to forty years ago would have died of kidney failure, hepatitis, heart disease, or leukemia are now

Table 18 RISK FACTORS FOR DEVELOPING A MELANOMA

New mole or one that is changing

Presence of dysplastic moles

Family history of melanoma or dysplastic moles

Personal history of previous melanoma

Presence of a congenital mole

Presence of many (more than fifty) moles

Presence of many large moles (larger than a pencil eraser)

Caucasian

A suppressed immune system

Presence of freckles

Sensitivity to the sun

Poor ability to tan

Red or blond hair; green or blue eyes

Excessive sun exposure

given therapy that may make them more susceptible to developing melanoma. People with unusual-looking moles (called dysplastic) are more susceptible to developing melanoma. Finally, melanoma, like other types of cancer, tends to run in families. If a patient or a member of his or her family has had a melanoma, the other members are also at greater risk. Table 18 lists the risk factors for developing a melanoma.

There are more than a dozen types of melanoma but the most common are called superficial spreading melanoma, acral lentiginous melanoma, nodular melanoma, lentigo maligna, and lentigo maligna melanoma. They are categorized by what the lesion looks like to the dermatologist and the dermatopathologist (a physician who evaluates skin biopsies under the microscope). The melanocytes that give rise to melanomas are most commonly thought of as occurring in the skin but they can also be seen in the lining of the eyes, in the covering of the brain, and in the gastrointestinal system. Therefore, a melanoma can occur in any one of these locations. If a patient's melanoma is already widely metastatic to other parts of the body, as not uncommonly happens, the physician must begin a search for the initial site of malignancy. The most common place for melanomas to start is the skin, but other organ systems obviously must be evaluated as well.

Diagnosis

Melanomas show up on the body most commonly as a mole which has "gone bad." Moles usually don't have any symptoms and don't grow very much after they arise. Some of the early signs of a melanoma can be remembered by the anachronym "ABCD":

A—asymmetry; one side of the mole doesn't mirror the other side

B—border; it should be smooth and not ragged or blurred

C—color; the color should all be the same and not different shades of black, gray, red, or white

D—diameter; melanomas are not usually less than 6 mm in diameter (about the same size as a pencil eraser)

Early warning signs of malignancy include frequent bleeding, pain, or other symptoms, scaling or scabbing, and a rapid increase in growth.

Diagnosing a melanoma involves taking a sample of the cancer and having it examined under the microscope. Melanomas are graded based on how deeply they invade the skin. They do not have to invade very far before they become deadly. A person's prognosis is largely based on this depth of invasion. Invasion is usually measured with two different scales. The older one, called a Clark's level, renders a Roman number I to V, depending on the depth. The greater the number the deeper the invasion and the poorer the prognosis. A newer and more accurate method of evaluation is the Breslow level. This also measures the depth of invasion by cancerous melanoma cells but an actual numerical measurement (in millimeters) is generated. In some melanomas (lentigo maligna), all the malignant cells are confined to the uppermost portion of the skin called the epidermis and no invasion takes place. These patients virtually never die of their disease if the tumor is completely removed. On the other hand, people with very thick melanomas (over 2 mm in depth) have a high death rate. Evaluation of patients with a newly diagnosed melanoma may include chest x-rays, blood work, and Cat scans to check for metastatic disease.

Unfortunately, melanomas commonly metastasize. They do so primarily through the lymphatic system, which transports tissue fluid. Melanomas spread to lymph nodes, skin, brain, lung, liver, and bone. If the melanoma cells involve only the lymph nodes, only about a third of patients will survive. If the cancer has spread to other organ systems, there is little hope. The average life span of patients with metastatic disease is six months.

Treatment

Treating melanomas has historically been very frustrating, since these tumors are not only largely preventable but largely curable provided they are diagnosed and treated in a timely fashion. Fortunately, the survival rate for this cancer is increasing. Fifty years ago, only half of patients survived five years; today, the figure is over 90 percent.

The standard therapy has always been and continues to be surgical removal of the tumor. Melanomas are most effectively removed along with a border of normal skin. In the past, patients have been subjected to excisions of their cancers with unnecessarily wide margins of normal tissue, resulting in very mutilating surgeries. Research in the past decade, however, has shown that such wide-margin approaches are not only not necessary, they frequently aren't helpful. Patients with "thin" melanomas have such a good prognosis that after the biopsy minimal or no follow-up surgery is warranted. On the other hand, patients with "thick" melanomas have such poor prognoses that even a very wide excision may be of no benefit. Patients with melanomas of intermediate thickness seem to benefit the most from wide excision of their tumors and additional treatment. Theoretically, any residual cancer cells that have remained behind and are not removed might result in a recurrent tumor. Consequently, many physicians choose to excise around an area even where it appears that all the lesion has been removed. This point is somewhat controversial and many dermatologists and cutaneous surgeons believe that you only have to remove the visible tumor. There is scientific evidence to support both claims. Most dermatologists have adopted a modified "better safe than sorry" approach in dealing with this controversy.

One debatable point in managing patients with melanoma is the evaluation of a patient's lymph nodes. Melanoma spreads through the lymphatic vessel system, much more so than through the blood. As a result, lymph nodes are usually the first place to which melanoma spreads and dermatologists and surgeons may recommend that melanoma patients consider what is called an elective lymph node dissection (ELND). This involves the surgical removal of clinically normal lymph nodes which drain the tissue where the melanoma had arisen. These lymph nodes will then be evaluated to determine if the melanoma has spread. Patients with thin or thick melanomas may not benefit from this procedure, but those in between may derive some advantage. A variation on this procedure is injecting dye or radioactive material in the region of the melanoma and then tracing the substances' movement to the draining lymph nodes. The nodes taking up the dye or radioactive material are then removed and evaluated microscopically. This provides a better chance of locating the draining lymph nodes and accurately evaluating the possibility of spread.

Chemotherapy has traditionally been of little use in melanomas. The most commonly used drug is called dacarbazine (DTIC-Dome®); it is helpful in a small percentage of cases. The likelihood of cure is virtually nil but some patients will receive a lengthening of their life. Most chemotherapy for melanoma is given according to a "protocol." Protocols are usually available only at major medical centers where a group of physicians has recruited patients, all of whom are given the same types and doses of medication. Their outcome is then evaluated as a group. Typical medications found in these protocols include chemotherapy agents. Interferon (Intron-A®) has been shown to help lengthen the life span of persons with larger melanomas and is also currently in use.

There are a number of experimental therapies being evaluated for treating melanoma (again, most of these are protocols). Interleukin 2, antibodies, and immune system stimulants are being tested with some success. It remains to be determined how helpful these are. A vaccine may someday be available.

Follow-up consists mostly of frequent physician visits. Many dermatologists want a chest x-ray intermittently to check for metastases. They will also carefully evaluate the site of the tumor and look for evidence of lymph node spread.

Miscellaneous Skin Cancers

Keratoacanthoma

Keratoacanthomas (KAs) are somewhat controversial in that some dermatologists consider them to be benign growths, whereas others believe that they represent a form of squamous cell carcinoma. These are common lesions and arise in areas of sun damage such as the head and neck. In women, they occur on the lower legs, the arms, and the hands. They can also be found in the oral cavity. Most patients are older and many are or have been smokers. The risk factors for developing a KA are essentially the same as for an SCC. Infection by human papillomavirus (HPV) may be a factor. KAs usually arise as single lesions, but in some cases, hundreds of tumors occur. They begin as small flesh to red colored nodules and may enlarge to the size of a small marble. In the center of the nodule is a plug of compressed tissue which may fall out as the KA ages. They grow rapidly, attaining their full size within a few weeks. Over the next several months, they gradually regress and eventually leave a small depressed scar. There is some evidence that if KAs are not removed or destroyed they will metastasize and harm the patient in the same manner as an SCC. While this may be true, it seems likely that in such situations the tumor was not a KA to begin with but rather an SCC.

Treatment of KAs is also somewhat controversial. Some dermatologists do not believe that they require treatment, since they are benign and self-limited. With some patients, particularly those with underlying health conditions who may not tolerate extensive treatment, appropriate management of these tumors may be to simply leave them alone and allow them to resolve on their own. However, the cosmetic result from allowing a KA to resolve in this manner is usually poor and not acceptable to most persons. Electrodessication and curettage has been a popular means of treatment but results in scarring. Excision is probably the most common therapy. Mohs chemosurgery is another option. Since these tumors arise in older patients, many of whom have health problems, nonsurgical therapies are often preferred. Reasonable options include radiation treatment and cryosurgery. Injecting solutions containing methotrexate (Rheumatrex®) or 5-fluorouracil into the KA are other successful methods of treatment. These have the advantage of being quick, relatively easy, less expensive, and well tolerated. They are uncomfortable, however, and since multiple injections may have to be given, they are not always convenient. In patients with numerous KAs, giving methotrexate orally may be useful. Isotretinoin given as for BCCs and SCCs may also be helpful in such patients.

Bowen's Disease

Bowen's disease is also called "squamous cell carcinoma in situ," meaning that the cancerous cells don't actually invade the deeper parts of the skin. In almost all circumstances, the tumor arises in persons with long-standing sun damage. It is typically seen on the face, hands, arms, and legs. Some patients also develop Bowen's disease in nonexposed areas such as the groin. There may also be involvement of the mucous membranes of the mouth or genitalia. Infection with human papillomavirus and past exposure to arsenic can cause this disease.

Unfortunately, the appearance of Bowen's disease does not usually suggest a skin cancer. Most lesions are reddish brown, scaly, and no bigger than a nickel. They may ooze and crust and as such often look like nummular eczema. Consequently, they are often misdiagnosed and treated with topical corticosteroids or antifungal creams. If these lesions are left alone long enough, they will eventually break through and invade the deeper skin. They then behave like typical SCCs. Treatment is usually with surgical excision. The cancerous cells of Bowen's disease extend down into hair follicles. Since ED&C and topical fluorouracil do not remove the cells of hair follicles, tumor recurrence is common. The use of Moh's chemosurgery is popular when this tumor arises in areas which require extra care such as the genitalia and mucous membranes.

Merkel Cell Carcinoma

Merkel cell carcinoma is a somewhat rare cancer that occurs on the head and neck of elderly patients. Tumors are reddish to brown or blue and may ulcerate. These are very dangerous and aggressive lesions with poor survival rates if they have metastasized. Treatment consists of surgical excision. If the cells have metastasized to lymph nodes or other organs such as the lungs, there is little hope for a complete cure. Chemotherapy is used for such cases but with minimal success.

Dermatofibrosarcoma Protuberans

The name of this tumor is very similar to that of a dermatofibroma; this is a benign tumor that occurs on the legs and arms of young people. A dermatofibrosarcoma protuberans (DFSP), however, is a malignant tumor which arises on the trunk, particularly around the shoulders. This is not a common condition but it is not rare, either. Men are more commonly affected than are women and DFSPs are more frequently seen in blacks. Tumors are marble sized or larger and are usually red to plum colored. They are considered low-grade malignancies since they do not commonly cause death. DFSPs have a tendency to recur if not completely removed, so surgeons usually excise widely around them. They do have the capacity to metastasize, but this is uncommon.

Atypical Fibroxanthoma

Atypical fibroxanthoma (AFX) is a malignancy almost solely restricted to elderly patients with significant sun damage. It occurs on the head and neck as a small pink to red nodule. AFXs often ulcerate but have no symptoms. They appear very much like SCCs and BCCs but behave differently. They have a good overall prognosis provided that they are adequately excised. Recurrence may be a problem but metastatic spread is uncommon.

Paget's Disease

This malignancy comes in two different forms. The most common is found on the nipple and is associated with underlying breast cancer. The tumor cells from the breast travel by sweat ducts and begin to involve the overlying skin. The second type of Paget's disease is a malignancy of sweat glands or internal organs such as the cervix that invades the skin and is present away from the breast, usually in the groins. Both types of cancer begin as small scaling patches which gradually enlarge. They may be yellow to red in color and some oozing is occasionally found. A "velvety" feel is described in some cases. Itching and discomfort are also a problem. If left alone long enough, Paget's disease of the breast may eventually become thickened and dimple in as the underlying cancer enlarges. Nipple eczema may have virtually identical features to Paget's disease and so dermatologists almost always biopsy these patches to make the diagnosis. Treatment consists of surgical excision. Obviously the overall prognosis depends on what, if any, tumor is found underlying the skin changes.

PART IV

DISEASES AND CONDITIONS AFFECTING THE SKIN

~ ~ ~ ~

Acne and Acne Rosacea

Acne Vulgaris

Acne (acne vulgaris) is a disease most people experience at some point in their lives. While not everyone has a full-blown case, most persons have an occasional pimple. Although it is a benign disease, there can be significant psychological consequences. Long-term scarring may also be a problem. Some types of acne are very severe with symptoms such as fever and chills. These are discussed at the end of this section.

Acne begins around the time of adolescence. In some patients, the development of a few pimples is the earliest sign of puberty. Initially, most lesions are comedones or "blackheads," with more inflammatory lesions arising later. Most cases peak in severity during the teen years and subside during the twenties and thirties. This is not absolute by any means, however. Many patients are still suffering from acne as they approach their forties. There seems to be an inherited pattern to this disease; parents with a past history of acne often have children with acne.

There have been an endless number of "old wive's tales" regarding acne. This may stem from the fact that it is not clear exactly what causes this disease. The underlying problem seems to be a faulty means by which the follicles extrude the oil that they produce. The follicle becomes plugged by "sticky" cells, with inflammation building up behind the obstruction. There can be bacterial infection by the organism *Propionibacterium acnes* and an increased production of oil by glands associated with hair follicles. Rupture of the follicle into the surrounding skin causes inflammation and pain. Scarring may occur. Male and female sex hormones also play a role. Finally, stress may worsen acne. It's likely that these various factors combine to produce acne. The contribution of diet has been extensively evaluated with no evidence that food plays a significant role in worsening or improving acne. Despite these scientific studies, most patients can list foods or beverages that they find worsen their disease.

Acne principally involves the face, back, and chest. The initial lesions are comedones, which are dilated follicles (pores) that have accumulated a clear to dark plug (blackhead). Inflammatory acne is composed of red, raised bumps, some of which are topped by a pustule. These bumps range from the size of a pinhead to that of a marble. Persons with large deep-seated cysts have what is termed *nodulocystic* acne. This is a severe form of acne and leads to increased scarring. "Icepick" scarring is seen over the cheeks. Some scarring on the chest and back may be very thick and broad (hypertrophic scarring). Scarring from routine acne is usually mild if present at all. Pimples are usually painless, but nodulocystic acne may be very uncomfortable.

The first step in taking care of acne is taking care of your skin in general. Keep the skin clean and try not to traumatize it. Picking or "popping" acne pimples risks infection of the skin and scarring. This does not cause acne to spread, but a deep-seated skin infection may occur. The skin is not dirty and grime does not play a role in initiating acne. Consequently, excessive washing will be of no benefit and may worsen the disease. Gentle cleansing with soap and water once or twice a day is sufficient.

Acne Medications
Over-the-counter agents (Clearasil®, Rezamid®, RA Lotion®) often contain resorcinol and other agents to dry the skin and promote peeling. These may be helpful for mild acne, but are of little use in patients with significant disease. Other proprietary products contain "pseudomedicinal" materials loosely based on prescription drugs such as vitamin A derivatives. These have not been proven to work and may worsen acne by inflaming it. Mixing medications (applying them at the same time) may inflame the skin or diminish the effectiveness of one of the drugs. Astringents are of no proven benefit. Generally it is best to apply only soap, water, and the medications your dermatologist has prescribed or suggested for you.

Benzoyl Peroxides
Benzoyl peroxides (BPO) are popular since they may be purchased without a prescription (see Table 19). These drugs kill bacteria and promote a mild degree of exfoliation. For the most part, they are safe, but some persons react adversely to benzoyl peroxide and develop inflamed skin. These compounds also bleach out clothing, pillowcases, and sheets. BPO is available as bar soap, liquid wash, cream, lotion, and gel in 2.5 to 10% strengths. The soaps and washes are helpful for large surface areas such as the chest and back. The creams and gels are applied to the skin and washed off some hours later. Most evidence shows that higher-potency preparations are no more effective than are lower ones, and are much more likely to irritate the skin. Benzoyl peroxide is useful for mild to moderate acne but not for severe disease. Some preparations contain erythromycin (Benzamycin®) or sulfur (Sulfoxyl®).

Table 19 BENZOYL PEROXIDE PREPARATIONS

Brand Name	Form
Acne-Aid®	cream
Benzac AC®★	gel, wash
Benzashave®★	shaving lotion
Brevoxyl®★	gel
Clearasil 10%®	lotion
Clearasil Maximum Strength®	cream
Desquame E®★	gel
Fostex BPO®	gel, cream
Neutrogena Acne Mask®	mask
Noxzema Acne 12®	lotion
Oxy 5, 10®	cream
Pan Oxyl®	gel, bar soap
Persa-Gel®★	gel
Vanoxide®★	lotion

★Available by prescription only

Topical Antibiotics

Topical antibiotics such as erythromycin, clindamycin, sulfa drugs, meclocycline, and tetracycline are used to eradicate the *Propionibacterium acnes*; this is believed to contibute to acne. These drugs are available in gel, cream, lotion, pledget, and liquid (alcohol-based) form (see Table 20). They are not available without a prescription. Topical antibiotics can benefit some patients with mild to moderate disease. They are convenient, and aside from some occasional mild irritation, are without side effects. Rarely, the application of one of the tetracycline formulations will cause a person to be sensitive to the sun. Most of these products are available generically and are effective. A formulation of erythromycin and zinc is also available (Theramycin Z®).

Azelaic Acid (Azalex®)

This is a new product that is applied to the skin once or twice daily. It is believed to work by killing *Propionibacterium acnes*, but the exact mechanism of action is

Table 20 TOPICAL ANTIBIOTIC PREPARATIONS (PRESCRIPTION ONLY)

Brand Name	Form	Antibiotic
Akne-Mycin®	ointment, solution	erythromycin
ATS®	solution, gelery	thromycin
Cleocin T®	solution, gel, pads	clindamycin
Erycette®	pads	erythromycin
Erygel®	gel	erythromycin
Erymax®	solution	erythromycin
Klaron®	lotion	sulfacetamide
Meclan®	cream	meclocycline
Metrogel®	gel, cream	metronidazole
Staticin®	solution	erythromycin
Sulfacet-R®	lotion	sulfur
Topicycline®	solution	tetracycline
T-Stat®	solution, pads	erythromycin

unclear. Aside from some mild skin irritation, the drug appears to be safe and effective. As with most topical medications, it is intended for patients with mild to moderate disease. It may cause lightening of the skin in persons with pigmented skin, and it is expensive.

Physical Therapies

These include x-ray, ultraviolet light, liquid nitrogen or frozen CO_2 (dry ice), surgery, and corticosteroid injections. X-ray treatments were very popular forty years ago and helped control acne in some patients with severe disease. Unfortunately, these patients have had an increased incidence of thyroid and other head and neck tumors and this mode of therapy is no longer used. Most acne will improve following prolonged exposure to the sun or a mild sunburn. This likely has to do with sunlight's antiseptic properties. While ultraviolet light therapy is still sometimes used, this is an uncommon mode of treatment. The use of a tanning bed will not likely be of benefit and the light may interact adversely with other medications (for example, tetracyclines) being taken for the patient's acne. Spraying liquid nitrogen very lightly on the skin will cause a mild exfoliation and some improvement in mild acne, especially for acne cysts. Some dermatologists mix acetone with dry ice to form a slush and gently rub the mixture over affected skin. The results are the same as with liquid nitrogen. Acne surgery consists of expressing the contents of open comedones (blackheads) with an instrument called a comedone extractor. While this is usually effective, occasionally the comedone contents are extruded into the skin and produce inflammation. Injecting corticosteroid solutions into inflamed acne cysts is a very effective means of quickly controlling the disease. Corticosteroids reduce the inflammation, pain, and swelling associated with large acne cysts and improve the cosmetic appearance. They are useful when a particular lesion is either uncomfortable or very visible. This therapy is painful and cannot be used for long-term control. Injection of too much or too concentrated a solution may result in a sunken-in appearance in the overlying skin.

Oral Antibiotics

Perhaps the most popular treatment option is oral antibiotics. These have been a mainstay of acne therapy for many years. They are reasonably effective, safe, and easy to use. There is some evidence, however, that use of these drugs in patients taking oral contraceptives may cause the birth control pills to fail.

Several different antibiotics are prescribed for acne. The tetracycline family (tetracycline [Achromycin®, Sumycin®], doxycycline [Doryx®, Monodox®, Vibramycin®)], minocycline [Dynacin®, Minocin®, Vectrin®]) is probably the most popular group of antibiotics. Some of these drugs have to be taken on an empty stomach and may make the skin more sensitive to the sun. Erythromycin (E-Mycin®, Ery C®, Ery-Tab®, E.E.S.®, Ery-Ped® suspension, Erythrocin®, PCE®) is another good medication but is generally not as effective as the tetracyclines. It also may cause stomach upset and/or diarrhea in some patients. Penicillin-type drugs (beta-lactams) such as ampicillin, amoxicillin, cephalexin, dicloxicillin, and so on are effective but less so than other antibiotics. Sulfa drugs such as trimethoprim/sulfamethoxasole (Bactrim®, Cotrim®, Septra®) are another option. All of these drugs and classes of drugs are very effective in some patients and ineffective in others. It is mostly a matter of chance what will work for a given person, so switching from one drug to another is a common occurrence. Patients cannot indefinitely remain on these or any other antibiotics. Some dermatologists do blood work periodically, particularly if their patients are taking tetracyclines. One unusual side effect of antibiotic therapy is called gram negative folliculitis. Patients develop red bumps with pustules around hair follicles. This may appear to be a worsening of the acne but does not respond to routine acne therapy. Antibiotics effective against gram negative bacteria and retinoids are used to control this outbreak.

Retinoids

In the past, vitamin A was used to treat acne. It was given in large doses and had significant side effects. It is rarely used today. Vitamin A derivatives called retinoids, however, have become the mainstay of most acne therapy. Tretinoin (Retin A®, Avita®, Retin-A Micro®) is the most popular formulation. This drug is formulated as a gel, cream, and solution. It is usually applied at night, since contact with light inactivates the drug. Lower concentrations are used initially and the dose is gradually increased as tolerated. When first used, tretinoin may cause a worsening of the acne but this quickly subsides. Most patients experience some peeling and redness. If used consistently, this will stop. A new formulation, Retin-A Micro®, has recently become available and may be better tolerated by persons whose skin is sensitive to this medication. A pea-sized amount should be applied to the face and forehead. All the skin surface should be treated and not just the affected spots. The neck usually doesn't tolerate tretinoin very well, so applying it there is not suggested. The corners of the mouth, nose, and eyes may become inflamed with the use of this medication, but this is usually minor and can be remedied by simply avoiding these areas. The same is true for the eyelids. Some patients become more light sensitive by using tretinoin, but this is uncommon; use of a sunscreen will prevent any negative effects of sun exposure. Tretinoin works by causing the follicles to shed their cells normally and not become inflamed. It is one of the best preventative drugs known for acne, but is somewhat expensive. Most beneficial effects of this drug are found after it has been used for three to six months, so it is not for the impatient. The gel and cream are used mostly for the face; the solution is for large surface areas such as the back and chest. The gel has a drying effect and is better tolerated by persons with particularly oily skin. Tretinoin is safe both for short- and long-term use. Many patients use it for years or decades in an effort to prevent skin cancer and fight the effects of aging skin. It should be applied only by itself and washed off in the morning. Combining tretinoin with benzoyl peroxides or topical antibiotics may cause it to be inactivated or lose its strength.

The most potent retinoid for acne is isotretinoin (Accutane®). It is chemically almost identical to tretinoin but is taken in pill form. This medication is spectacularly effective, reasonably well tolerated, and the only successful medication for certain types of acne. The disadvantages are cost, the need for occasional blood work, an increase in sun sensitivity, and the drug's capacity to cause severe birth defects if taken during pregnancy. Side effects are the same as with large doses of vitamin A. These include chapped lips, mild muscle/bone/joint pain, headaches, dry eyes, mild hair thinning, and decreased night vision. Many of these symptoms improve after taking the drug for several months, but some do not. All side effects stop after the medication is discontinued. The most worrisome side effect is the consequences from exposure of unborn children to isotretinoin. Use of this medication during pregnancy may result in miscarriage, death of the fetus, or severe birth defects. Most women of childbearing age are required to sign release statements before beginning the medication that state that they are aware of this fact. Some dermatologists will not prescribe isotretinoin for women who have not either reached menopause or had a surgery that terminates their fertility (for example, tubal ligation). The blood levels of cholesterol and triglycerides increase in patients taking this drug, but this is rarely of significance. Effects on the liver and blood counts have been reported but are also rare. Routine laboratory evaluations in these patients help prevent significant problems. Isotretinoin is usually prescribed for patients with severe and disfiguring acne. In many cases, it is the only medication which is of any help. It is also very useful in persons with moderate acne of long standing who have had little success in treating their disease. Isotretinoin is usually given for five to six months at a dose of 1 mg per kg per day. Many patients tell dermatologists that they have been on this drug previously with good results but that their acne is coming back. On further questioning, they have almost always either been on too low a dose or treated for too little time. With a proper dose and length of therapy, acne relapses are very rare. This drug is the only known "cure" for acne; persons receiving it usually become permanently acne free.

The most recent addition to the retinoid-type class of drugs is adalapene (Differin®). This is actually a naphthoic acid derivative but is similar to the retinoids and vitamin A. This gel is also used for psoriasis, but it is most useful for acne. It is applied once daily, usually at night, just as with tretinoin. It is believed to work in a similar manner. It has some of the same side effects as tretinoin, such as mild irritation and burning, but overall seems to be better tolerated while working just as well. Adalapene is also useful when used in combination with other acne therapies.

Sulfa Drugs

The sulfones are a group of sulfa drugs used for certain infections and blistering diseases. The most commonly used member of this class of medications is dapsone. It is helpful in certain types of severe acne, particularly when isotretinoin cannot be taken. It is inexpensive, reasonably effective, and usually well tolerated. The major disadvantage of this drug is its effects on the blood. Almost all patients will develop a mild amount of anemia. In certain patients, particularly those that lack a blood enzyme called glucose-6-phosphate-dehydrogenase (G-6-PD), dapsone may cause the red blood cells to split apart, leading to a serious condition known as hemolytic anemia. More rarely, the drug may inhibit the bone marrow's capacity to make blood cells (aplastic anemia). Consequently, dermatologists follow these patients very carefully with appropriate blood work.

Hormonal Therapy

Since some acne is believed to be driven by the patient's hormonal imbalances, there is some practical benefit to treating the disease with oral hormones. In some women whose acne is worsened by oral contraceptives, it is helpful to change to a formulation with less progesterone. Estrogens are effective in men with severe acne but are rarely given since the side effects are usually unacceptable. Drugs known as antiandrogens block or incapacitate the effects of male hormones. These drugs are of some benefit for certain women with acne. They may have substantial side effects and patients are usually given very low doses and followed carefully. The antihypertension drug spironolactone exhibits some antiandrogen effects and may be useful in some older women with acne. Hormonal therapy is popular since better medications have become available.

Corticosteroids

These drugs are occasionally used in acne. Since they decrease inflammation, they are useful in severely inflammatory disease. Corticosteroids are given as pills or shots but are not meant for long-term control. If used for short periods, the side effects are minimal. Weak solutions of corticosteroids may also be injected into individual acne cysts to diminish their inflammation and pain.

Acne Conglobata

This acne variant is almost exclusively seen in males. Disease onset is later in life. Large cysts and comedones are found. Cysts may break down and drain. The lesions are very painful and heal with considerable scarring. The chest and back are extensively involved, and unusual areas for acne such as the legs and arms may show lesions as well. Treatment is almost exclusively with isotretinoin. Other medicines such as minocycline and dapsone may be useful. In acne conglobata, corticosteroids are used to calm the inflammatory aspects of the disease.

Acne Fulminans

Acne fulminans is probably the most worrisome of the acne variants. It occurs suddenly and explosively. Routine acne may have been present previously but often there is no warning. Teenage boys are almost exclusively affected. Patients run fevers and have increased white blood cell counts. Joint and muscle pain are present. X-rays may show erosions in certain bones. Draining acne cysts are seen as are large comedones. Scarring is usually widespread and severe. Corticosteroids are required to control the inflammation and antibiotics are usually started to control infection. Isotretinoin is begun after the disease has subsided.

Acne Excoriée

Patients, usually young women, who "pick" at their pimples have acne excoriée. While in some patients this indicates an underlying psychological illness, in the majority it does not. Most patients will admit to trying to pop their pimples to speed up their resolution. Acne excoriée is difficult to treat, since some patients are unaware that they are picking at their lesions.

Neonatal Acne

This disease affects infants and newborns. It is probably related to hormone levels in the baby which were produced by the mother. The pimples will go away on their own after a few weeks so therapy is not indicated. Treatment often makes the problem worse rather than better.

Steroid Acne

Patients who have been on high doses of corticosteroids or anabolic steroids will often break out with acne. This is also rarely seen in persons who have been applying very high potency corticosteroids to the face. These pimples often have small pustules and all appear to be in the same phase of development. Cysts and comedones are rare. Treatment involves stopping the corticosteroids if possible. Topical tretinoin and oral antibiotics are helpful. Steroid acne is one of the signs of anabolic steroid abuse among weight lifters and other athletes.

Acne Cosmetica

A number of products when applied to the skin result in the production of acne. This is most common with cosmetics and hair products, including hair spray. Discontinuing use of the offending agents and application of tretinoin are helpful.

Tropical Acne

Tropical acne is seen in patients who relocate to a tropical climate with high heat and humidity. Many of these patients have never had acne before. Covered areas such as the trunk and buttocks are affected. Cysts and comedones are seen. Discomfort may occur. Antibiotics are helpful, but ultimately the patient has to move to a cooler climate.

Acne Rosacea

Acne rosacea is called adult acne since it commonly begins in the forties and fifties. It starts as blushing and flushing of the face. Women are affected more often than are men. The sun plays some role in this disease. The actual cause is unknown. Various theories have been proposed, including infection with a skin mite called *Demodex folliculorum*, sun exposure, underlying infection, and genetic inheritance. As in acne vulgaris, there are several different types.

The clinical findings in rosacea are red skin, small dilated blood vessels called telangiectasias, pustules, and red bumps that look like acne. Initially, patients may only complain of excessive blushing or flushing of the skin. These may be provoked by spicy foods, alcohol, hot liquids, sun exposure, or emotion. The central face is most commonly involved. The blood vessels eventually become permanently dilated and the skin is continually red. Red bumps and pustules arise next, but blackheads are not present. The nose begins to appear slightly swollen. Some scalp involvement may be present with mild itching and scaling. The final stages of rosacea include swelling and deforming of the nose with large dilated pores (rhynophyma). This is occasionally called the "W.C. Fields" nose. Similar deformities may be seen on the forehead and ears. Acne rosacea also affects the eyes with mild inflammation and irritation.

Treatment and Care

Treatment is similar to that of acne vulgaris. Topical antibiotics are usually helpful. Topical metronidazole (MetroGel®, MetroCream®) is relatively new and effective. Tretinoin is of some benefit but not to the extent seen with acne vulgaris. Adalapene has not been tried in acne rosacea but might be useful in some patients. Antifungal agents such as ketoconazole (Nizoral®) are helpful, particularly with scalp scaling (shampoo form). Persons with acne rosacea should use sunscreen daily even if no outdoor activities are planned. Avoidance of even minute amounts of sunlight is important since it is cumulative. Dermatologists treat some patients with creams and shampoos designed to kill *Demodex* mites. This is very helpful in some cases, but not all. Topical steroids should not be used, since they may aggravate the formation of dilated blood vessels. These vessels may be obliterated with laser therapy or scarred down by insertion of a fine needle into the vein and application of a short burst of electricity. Although dietary restrictions are unlikely to help in acne vulgaris, they may be very useful with acne rosacea. Patients are urged to avoid foods which provoke flushing and blushing, as well as alcohol and tobacco, which may aggravate the disease.

Oral Antibiotics

These drugs are a mainstay of therapy. The tetracyclines are used as in acne vulgaris. Minocycline and doxycycline are particularly effective. If these medications fail, erythromycin and the sulfa drugs may be tried but these usually have little effect. Beta-lactams are ineffective. Unfortunately, patients have to be on these antibiotics for extended periods, and getting the patient to discontinue their use may be difficult. Oral metronidazole is used in recalcitrant cases. It takes up to two months to adequately control the disease and has some unpleasant side effects, but in certain patients it is a useful medicine.

Retinoids

Isotretinoin is helpful in almost all cases. There is some evidence that use of this drug in lower doses is effective. It is administered similar to that in acne. Topical preparations such as tretinoin (Retin-A®, Renova®), adalapene, and tazarotene (Tazorac®) may also be beneficial.

Surgery

Surgical treatment plays a role in this disease. Laser therapy may be helpful for the dilated blood vessels; however, this mode of treatment does nothing to prevent new telangiectases from developing. Rhynophyma may be removed with a cutting laser, scalpel, or electrical cutting loop. Again, preventing the early phases of acne rosacea is the best policy.

Other Forms of Acne Rosacea

Several variants of acne rosacea merit mentioning. Rosacea fulminans used to be called pyoderma faciale. It affects only teenage girls. The rosacea outbreak is severe and accentuated around the lower parts of the face. Nodules, cysts, drainage, and pustules are present. Stress seems to play some role in rosacea fulminans. Treatment is with isotretinoin and a short course of corticosteroids to diminish the inflammation. The prognosis is good if treatment is begun in time.

Steroid rosacea is essentially identical to steroid acne but evolves from topical use of corticosteroids. Stopping the steroid use is the first step in therapy, but often involves a dramatic worsening of the disease. Antibiotics and retinoids are used to control steroid rosacea.

Rosacea conglobata is a very severe form of acne rosacea with large nodules and scarring pustules. This is limited to the face and is controlled with isotretinoin.

AIDS-Related Skin Diseases

Acquired immunodeficiency syndrome (AIDS) is caused by infection with the human immunodeficiency virus 1 (HIV 1). This unusual virus, called a retrovirus, infects and disables a subset of white blood cells known as T-helper cells or CD4 cells. This, in turn, makes the patient susceptible to infection and malignancy from several types of cancer. This disease was first reported in the United States in the early 1980s. Initially, most infected persons were homosexuals, but it has since become clear that other groups of individuals are susceptible to this disease as well. Infection with the virus is transmitted in five major ways:

1. sexual contact of any form
2. perinatally (from infected mother to unborn child)
3. tissue transplantation (blood or blood product transfusion and solid organ transplantation)
4. drug use
5. infection in health care workers (puncture wound with contaminated needles)

There is also a subset of patients for whom none of these apply and who have acquired their disease by unclear means.

It is important to understand that not everyone infected with the HIV-1 virus has AIDS. AIDS occurs when HIV-1–infected patients meet certain criteria as defined by the Centers for Disease Control. It is conceivable that a person may be infected with the HIV-1 virus for years or even decades and manifest no symptoms. Consequently, he would not be designated as having AIDS and most likely would not know that he carried the infection. Worldwide, the number of persons with HIV-1 infection has grown from about 100,000 in 1980 to twelve million in 1992. Most of the infected patients are in Africa and Asia. By the turn of the century, it is estimated that up to 100 million persons will be HIV-1 positive and 20 million adults and three million children will have AIDS. Again, Africa and Asia will be hardest hit.

Like many illnesses, HIV-1 infection progresses through different stages. The initial stage is the original infection. Often the exact timing of infection is not clear, because the patient may exhibit no symptoms or the symptoms may be attributed to a cold or other viral illness. Classically, the initial HIV-1 infection produces symptoms similar to those of mononucleosis. The incubation period following exposure is approximately a month. Symptoms include fever, muscle aches, headache, sore throat, nausea, diarrhea, and loss of appetite. A fine red rash over the trunk and extremities may also occur. Testing the patient for HIV-1 antibodies will not normally be helpful before six weeks after the onset of the infection. Following this infection, the patient goes through what is termed *latency* in which the infection by the HIV-1 virus begins to take hold but the patient experiences few, if any, symptoms. This is probably the most dangerous stage, since persons may not only fail to receive therapy which could prolong their lives but may unknowingly infect other persons. Patients are occasionally diagnosed with their disease at this stage by a blood test for insurance physical, blood donation, military service, and so on. The next stage is termed asymptomatic disease. The CD4 count is continuing to fall and usually has reached the level of 500 to 750 cells per mm^3. Aside from some mild swelling of the lymph glands and fatigue, the patient feels well. Early symptomatic disease usually begins as the patient's CD4 count falls to between 200 and 500. This stage was previously called ARC (AIDS-Related Complex). Night sweats, fevers, headache, oral thrush (Candida infection) and persistent diarrhea are typical. Late symptomatic disease occurs when the CD4 count is between 50 and 200. Under some guidelines, these patients are considered to have AIDS. They develop Kaposi's sarcoma, Candidal infections of the esophagus, and chronic herpes infections and are at increased risk for lymphoma. Treatment in HIV disease is usually directed at the underlying infections and malignancies. There is some evidence that early therapy with zidovudin (Retrovir®) may slow the progression of the disease.

Infectious Complications

Viral Infections

The herpesvirus family includes:

1. Herpes simplex virus types 1 and 2 (HSV-1, HSV-2)
2. the varicella-zoster virus (chickenpox and zoster or shingles)
3. cytomegalovirus (CMV)
4. the Epstein-Barr virus (EBV; infectious mononucleosis)
5. human herpesvirus 6 (HHV-6).

Infection with HSV-1 and HSV-2 is commonly seen in HIV infection. As the body's immune system begins to fail, a person's capacity to fight these infections or at least keep them in check is compromised. Many healthy people have cold sores or genital herpes but experience only occasional outbreaks. Between outbreaks the virus is dormant in the nerves supplying the affected area of skin. Persons with diseases which affect the immune system commonly have herpes outbreaks that are difficult to control. HIV and AIDS patients may have large ulcers, nodules, or scabbed lesions which continue to grow and destroy the surrounding skin. These may also affect the mucous membranes of the mouth, esophagus, and genitalia. They are painful and may prevent the person from sufficiently eating or drinking. Additionally, these lesions shed a great number of virus particles, since the infection is going unchecked. Diagnosis may be made by culturing the lesions, biopsying them, or scraping them and checking for infected cells under the microscope. Treatment consists of oral administration of acyclovir (Zovirax®) in the doses usual for HIV-negative patients. If this is not effective, the drug may be given intravenously. Famciclovir (Famvir®) and ganciclovir (Cytovene®) are also useful. Occasionally, these medications are not effective because the virus has developed an immunity to the drug (drug resistance). In these cases, foscarnet (Foscovir®) is given intravenously. Unfortunately, resistance to foscarnet has been seen as well.

Varicella is another name for chickenpox. Herpes zoster is the official name for "shingles." In HIV-positive children, varicella is more symptomatic than in healthy children. In healthy adults, varicella is a serious disease and potentially life threatening in those who are HIV-positive. In HIV-positive patients, varicella may affect the internal organs, especially the liver, lungs, and brain. Normally, lifelong immunity to varicella infection takes place, but in the HIV-positive population, a second infection with a different strain may occur. The occurrence of zoster in healthy adults marks a drop in their ability to keep the virus in check, but usually does not indicate a serious problem with their immunity. In persons infected with the HIV virus, zoster is symptomatic and more widely breaks out. Normally, zoster affects a band of skin which corresponds to the area supplied by the particular nerve containing the virus. This is commonly on the trunk, but may be on the head and neck. In persons with damaged immune systems, widespread dissemination, as with chickenpox, may take place. The individual spots are red and blister. In HIV, these lesions may be large, may ulcerate, and may contain blood. They tend to last longer than in healthy persons and are more difficult to resolve. There is usually pain and/or itching which may remain after the eruption has cleared. Scarring may be seen. Most worrisome is involvement of the eye and other vital structures on the head and neck. The treatment is essentially the same as for HSV-1 and 2 but higher doses of acyclovir are used. Additionally, intravenous therapy is more common. The use of corticosteroids, common in healthy patients, is not usually appropriate for the HIV-positive population.

Infectious mononucleosis is caused by the *Epstein Barr virus*. It infects a type of white blood cells called B cells. Many persons have had EBV infections previously but were unaware of the illness, since it was mild and likely attributed to a cold or flu. In HIV disease, this virus plays a role in oral hairy leukoplakia (OHL) and some types of lymphomas. OHL manifests as a white fringe of tissue at the border of the tongue. It may also affect the cheeks and roof of the mouth. It is white to gray colored and slightly wispy. There are no symptoms. Diagnosis may be made by a biopsy but usually this is unnecessary. Treatment is difficult since OHL responds poorly to most therapies. Topical application of podophyllin or tretinoin (Retin-A®) may be helpful. Response following treatment with acyclovir, foscarnet, and zidovudine has been reported. Therapy with antifungal drugs has not been successful.

Cytomegalovirus is a common infection, particularly in those patients with advanced disease. This virus infects the eyes, gastrointestinal tract, and central nervous system. While it does involve the skin, the lesions are not specific. Diagnosis depends on a high index of suspicion and finding the typical features with a biopsy. Therapy with acyclovir has not been very helpful, but ganciclovir and foscarnet may be beneficial.

Human Papillomavirus

One of the most frustrating infections to treat in HIV-positive patients is that from the human papillomavirus (HPV) or warts. There are many different types of HPV, causing multiple kinds of warts. Some of these are associated with an increased risk of skin cancers. Condyloma acuminata or venereal warts are common in the HIV-positive population. These bumps range in size from that of a pinhead to a pencil eraser and tend to arise in and around the genitalia. Oral involvement is possible as well. Most are slightly red to purple or dark colored and scaling is uncommon. Sometimes they group to form very large lesions and interfere with urination and defecation.

Under the best of circumstances, these infections are difficult to treat (see section on warts) and they are even more so in HIV-positive patients. Liquid nitrogen, topical podophyllin, tretinoin, isotretinoin (Accutane®), electrofulguration (electric needle), interferon, and laser destruction are all effective in some patients but not in others. There appears to be no reliable means for predicting which patient will respond well to one therapy as opposed to another. Treatment is often a matter of trial and error. Surgical excision is used in persons with large warts but is obviously a last step. Common warts or verrucae are also frequently a problem in HIV disease. As with condyloma acuminata, they are difficult to eradicate; treatment is essentially the same. There is a theoretical possibility that these lesions will progress to skin cancer if they have arisen from the type of HPV associated with cancer (types 16, 18, and 31 to 35).

Molluscum contagiosum is a lesion that is common in children and sexually active young adults. It is transmitted by skin-to-skin contact and will resolve on its own over time. In persons with diminished immunity, these lesions may become very large, very numerous, and difficult to get rid of. They are caused by an infection with a poxvirus which is confined to the skin and mucous membranes. The individual lesions are flesh colored but may become inflamed and crusted. These bumps may grow to the width of a pencil eraser and usually have no symptoms. Molluscum contagiosum are not dangerous but are cosmetically disfiguring and a source of considerable concern in affected patients. In HIV disease they cluster over the head and neck, particularly in the shaving area of males and around the eyes. They are easy to diagnose by simple observation but a biopsy is occasionally done since skin infection with cryptococcosis, a serious fungal disease, may look identical to molluscum contagiosum.

Treatment is difficult because a single lesion may produce enough virus to reinfect the surrounding skin. Liquid nitrogen and laser destruction are popular. Freezing the lesions with ethyl chloride and quickly scraping them off the skin's surface is effective with a small to moderate number of lesions, but is uncomfortable and may produce significant bleeding in treated areas. Application of canthrone (Cantharadin®) to induce blistering is helpful and bloodless. After these small blisters resolve in a week the molluscum has been destroyed and is gone. Podophyllin is somewhat effective but not to the same degree as in condyloma accuminata, and it can't be used on sensitive skin areas such as the face. Topical anthralin (Drithocreme®) administration may also be helpful. Oral administration of griseofulvin (Gris-PEG®) has been effective. In some patients with recalcitrant disease, frequent office visits and application of liquid nitrogen keep the disease in check to an acceptable degree.

Fungal Infections

One of the most common infections in HIV disease and one of the defining criteria for AIDS is infection with the yeast *Candida* (candidiasis). This family of organisms is commonly found on the skin and mucous membranes of healthy individuals but rarely becomes a problem. As a person's immunity begins to fail, the balances that keep *Candida* in check are lost and infection occurs. In the latter stages of AIDS, almost all patients experience these infections.

The most common site of involvement is the mucous membranes, specifically the mouth. These infections present in several different patterns. One pattern, thrush, shows heaped-up aggregates of white to yellow colored material on the cheeks, palate, and back of the throat. There may be mild burning or pain and changes in the way food tastes or feels in the mouth. Involvement at the angles of the mouth is termed angular cheilitis. There is some redness, scaling, and cracking of the skin. It is mildly painful. Some infections in the mouth cause painful burning of the tongue and palate. Involvement of the esophagus is more common with later disease. This may produce difficulty in eating and discomfort such as heartburn. Candidal infection of the vulva and vagina is very common in HIV-positive women. Candidiasis of the nails and fingers (paronychia) is seen in children and adults. The nails show crumbling and thickening, with swelling of the surrounding skin.

Diagnosis of candidiasis is done by scraping some of the material off the skin and evaluating it under the microscope. A biopsy is also effective but usually unnecessary. Therapy includes antifungal medications such as ketoconazole (Nizoral®), itraconazole (Sporanox®), and fluconazole (Diflucan®). Once the infection is under control, prophylactic use of these drugs is begun. Topical medications such as ketoconazole may be used in angular cheilitis. Oral candidiasis is also treated with clotrimazole troches (Mycelex®) dissolved in the mouth and nystatin (Mycostatin®) suspension.

Dermatophyte infections are fungal infections of the nails, hair, and skin. There is probably no increased degree of infection with dermatophytes among HIV-positive patients; however, they are more difficult to clear. Infections of the skin (ringworm), hair (ringworm), groin (jock itch), and feet (athlete's foot) appear as they do in HIV-negative patients. Nail infection (onychomycosis) is more problematic and several different types are seen. Topical treatment of these infections is unlikely to be helpful and most patients require systemic therapy. Previously, most patients were treated with griseofulvin. There is some degree of resistance among these fungi to griseofulvin, however, and itraconazole and terbenefine (Lamisil®) are now more likely to effect a cure. Ketoconazole and fluconazole are also useful. Topical medications may be helpful for mild infections or prophylactically used. Ketoconazole and selenium sulfide shampoo (Selsun®) are useful.

Infection of hair follicles by *Pityosporum* organisms (Pityosporum folliculitis) is common in HIV-positive patients. These red bumps begin around hair follicles and may have pustules. They are usually on the upper trunk and arms. Symptoms include mild itching. Oral ketoconazole or itraconazole are used to treat this condition.

Another class of fungi, the deep fungi, also infect HIV-positive patients. These infections include histoplasmosis, cryptococcosis, blastomycosis, coccidiodomycosis, aspergillosis, and sporotrichosis. Ulcers, lumps, erosions, and patches of the skin are seen. These lesions may be various colors and most are symptomless. In short, these infections may present almost any appearance. If the patient is suffering from an acute or chronic infection, the diagnosis of the skin lesion is often suspected. However, many times the skin biopsy and/or culture are the first indication of the systemic spread of one of these infections. Therapy includes antifungal agents such as ketoconazole, itraconazole, fluconazole, and terbenifine. Intravenous administration of fluconazole is popular, since more medicine can be given.

Bacterial Infections

Bacterial skin infections are common in HIV-positive patients but are rarely different from those in healthy persons. Almost all bacterial organisms have produced disease in these patients at some time. The most common infecting bacteria is *Staphyloccocus aureus*. Folliculitis, cellulitis, and impetigo are all seen as are several other rarer diseases. Furuncles and carbuncles (boils) may also occur. Antibiotics such as cephalexin (Keflex®), amoxicillin/clavulanic acid (Augmentin®), and dicloxicillin (Dycil®) are effective treatments. Cultures may be performed to discover to what antibiotics the organism is resistant (if any). Prophylactic treatment with rifampin (Rifadin®) may help rid the patient of these bacteria on the mucous membranes and decrease the likelihood of infection. *Streptococcus pyogenes* is the second most common infecting bacteria in HIV disease and produces similar illnesses. A toxic shocklike condition with a red rash and mild scaling has been reported with this organism. Treatment is essentially identical for both bacteria.

Tuberculosis is common in HIV-positive patients. It is caused by infection with *Mycobacterium tuberculosis*, a member of the mycobacteria group of organisms. Disease is usually confined to the lungs, but skin involvement is seen in 20 to 40 percent of patients. These lesions appear as ulcers and swollen lymph glands with tissue breakdown, bumps, and small scaling patches. Diagnosis is made by skin biopsy. Skin lesions resolve as the underlying disease is treated. Other mycobacteria such as *Mycobacterium avium-intracellulare* (MAI), *Mycobacterium fortuitum*, and *Mycobacterium marinum* all produce cutaneous disease in the HIV-positive populace. These are rare and do not have a characteristic skin appearance. Antibiotic therapy depends on drug sensitivities and culture of the lesions is mandatory.

Bacillary angiomatosis is a newly described skin disease caused by *Rochalimaea henselae*; it is essentially restricted to HIV-positive patients. Skin lesions look like red bumps, which may grow to the size of a marble. The overlying skin may ulcerate and ooze. A few or many hundreds of lesions may be present. Involvement of internal organs and bone marrow is seen. A skin biopsy may be diagnostic. Erythromycin (PCE®) and doxycycline (Doryx®) are the preferred treatments and are usually very effective.

Coinfection with sexually transmitted diseases in HIV-positive patients is not uncommon. Syphilis is a particular problem, since the progression of the disease may not only be more aggressive but more difficult to detect. HIV-positive patients with syphilis have a greater number of symptoms and disability. Blood tests commonly positive in healthy patients may be negative in those with HIV, requiring more sophisticated testing. Therapy in these patients is protracted and difficult. Treatment failures are not uncommon. Patient follow-up is essential to ensure adequate therapy and prevent relapse.

Parasites

The most problematic parasitic condition in HIV disease is scabies. Scabies is caused by *Sarcoptes scabiei*, the itch mite. In healthy persons, only about thirty female mites attack a patient, but with HIV these organisms may number in the hundreds. They produce red bumps typically on the abdomen, between the fingers, and around the waist. Itching is the most common symptom and usually lesions are excoriated. Diagnosis is made by scraping a lesion and looking for the mite under the microscope or doing a skin biopsy. Topical application of lindane has been the therapy of choice but treatment failures are common and most dermatologists prefer to use topical 5% permethrin cream (Elimite®). In healthy adults, a single application is usually effective, but with HIV-positive patients, multiple treatments may be needed. Crotamiton (Eurax®) may be used but is less likely to succeed. Ivermectin (Stromectol®) has recently been shown to be an effective oral therapy for scabies.

About 50 percent of the population in the United States has been infected with *Toxoplasma gondii*. In healthy patients, the infection is dormant and causes no problems. However, in persons with HIV disease, the infection may be reactivated and spread. This worm traditionally affects the central nervous system; however, skin lesions and a rash have also been reported. Treatment is with sulfadiazine and pyrimethamine (Daraprim®).

For obvious reasons, infectious diseases, more than most other aspects of skin disease, are more prevalent in HIV-positive patients. Almost every infection with cutaneous involvement has been described as occurring in HIV disease. Additionally, many infectious disorders of the skin look considerably different than in healthy persons. For this reason, dermatologists who take care of HIV-positive patients have adopted an "anything can be anything" attitude toward skin conditions that they see. Liberal use of biopsies, cultures, and antibiotics are often the rule in such patients.

Noninfectious Skin Eruptions

Most of the cutaneous diseases in HIV-positive patients are not much different from those in healthy patients. However, they tend to be exaggerated and more difficult to clear. Often chronic therapy is needed to prevent acute relapse and serious symptoms.

Psoriasis

There is no more psoriasis in HIV-positive patients than in the general populace, but it is usually much more difficult to control. Persons with mild disease before they are infected often have explosive psoriasis following infection. The skin changes are essentially identical to routine psoriasis and include red, scaling areas over the elbows, knees, and trunk. Itching is usually minimal. Psoriatic arthritis is also seen and may be severe. Treatment of these patients must take into account their immune status. Topical therapy is stressed, since many oral medications for psoriasis interact with the immune system. Topical corticosteroids and calcipotriol (Dovonex®) are useful as are tars, anthralin, and ketoconazole shampoo. Ultraviolet light therapy is very useful. Psoralens and ultraviolet light (PUVA) has also been used successfully. Retinoids are not believed to affect the immune system and consequently have been popular in treating widespread disease.

Reiter's disease is a condition very much like psoriasis. The skin findings are almost identical except that involvement of the palms and soles is generally more severe, a condition called keratoderma blenorrhagicum. Scaling and redness on the head of the penis (circinate balanitis) is also found. Additionally, arthritis and inflammation of the urethra (urethritis) and iris of the eye (iritis) are seen. These patients are often infected with other bacteria such as *Chlamydia*, *Shigella*, or *Salmonella*.

Treatment is similar to psoriasis with an emphasis on retinoids. Topical therapy with corticosteroids is helpful but usually the disease is too severe. Moisturizers containing urea or lactic acid may decrease the thick scaling of the palms and soles. Most dermatologists consult with a rheumatologist and ophthalmologist for management of joint and eye disease.

Seborrheic Dermatitis

This eruption affects primarily the face, scalp, groin, and upper chest areas. There is mild to moderate scaling which often has a thick or "greasy" quality. The rash is a light red or pink color but symptoms are uncommon. Some patients have disease restricted to the scalp which may appear as bad dandruff. This eruption is very common in HIV disease. In healthy patients, mild topical corticosteroid preparations and ketoconazole-containing shampoo usually suffice to control the disease. However, in HIV-positive patients, oral ketoconazole, itraconazole, or fluconazole may be required.

Eosinophilic Folliculitis

This disease was originally seen primarily in healthy children and is known as Ofugi's disease. It is very common in HIV-positive patients, particularly with advanced disease. The eruption involves the hair follicles on the trunk, extremities, and face. There is mild redness and itching. The diagnosis is usually made with a biopsy. Treatment consists of antibiotics such as erythromycin and tetracycline (Sumycin®). Topical corticosteroids and oral antihistamines are useful for preventing itching. The most effective therapy is ultraviolet light B (UVB) treatments given several times a week. This disease is difficult to control and practically impossible to cure.

Oral (Aphthous) Ulcers (Canker Sores)

Most persons experience an oral ulcer or canker sore at some point in their lives. In patients with severe immune system disease, such as HIV, these ulcerations may be persistent, large, and very painful. They occur on the mucous membranes of the mouth and throat. They are more common in later stages of the disease. Lesions may be the size of a quarter or even larger. Aside from discomfort, the real concern with aphthous ulcers is that they will impede eating and drinking. Treatment is difficult. Topical corticosteroid preparations such as gels may be applied to the ulcer. A suspension can be used which bathes the ulcer while being held in the mouth. Injecting a corticosteroid suspension is effective, but painful. Thalidomide is often helpful but is not available in the United States. Colchicine (ColBENEMID®) and zinc sulfate are alternative therapies that usually don't interfere with the patient's damaged immune status.

Drug Eruptions

Drug eruptions are frequent in a healthy population. In the HIV-positive population, they are even more common and frequently more severe. Almost any medication may be responsible, but some are more likely than others to cause problems. Sulfonamides, particularly trimethoprim-sulfamethoxazole (Bactrim®), are used in HIV disease to treat pulmonary pneumocystis infection and toxoplasmosis. Adverse reactions to these drugs occurs in about half the patients treated. The eruption is similar to most drug allergies and includes red spots on the trunk and extremities. Fever and other symptoms may occur.

Therapy includes avoiding these drugs if possible or gradually desensitizing the patient if necessary. A short course of oral corticosteroids or a corticosteroid injection may also be helpful. Pentamidine is an alternative medication in the treatment of pneumocystis pneumonia, but unfortunately about a fifth of these patients also react to this medication. Severe skin eruptions such as toxic epidermal necrolysis, erythema multiforme, or blistering drug eruptions are also common in HIV-positive patients. These arise not only from the usual medications but also with drugs less suspect in healthy patients. Most patients with HIV are taking zidovudine; this drug is capable of causing skin changes as well. The most common change is increased pigmentation of the nails. Affected fingernails and toenails become dark and streaked with pigment in up to 40 percent of treated patients. Generalized skin discoloration, vasculitis, itching, hives, and acnelike eruptions have also been described.

Xerosis (Dry Skin)

Xerosis, or dry skin, is common in HIV-positive patients. Mild scaling and itching is seen. This is a particular problem in the late stages of the disease. Malnutrition and chronic illness likely underlie the condition. Treatment centers around use of skin lubricants and emollients.

Many different skin diseases such as granuloma annulare, pityriasis rubra pilaris, atopic dermatitis, porphyria cutanea tarda, vitiligo, and alopecia have been reported in HIV-infected persons. Whether these and other diseases are more common with HIV infection is unclear, however, most any disease process will be more difficult to manage in these patients and the available therapies will be limited.

Malignancy

Kaposi's Sarcoma

This is the most common malignancy in HIV disease and one that has become a hallmark of this illness. This tumor is believed to result from malignant proliferation of cells which form the lining of blood vessels called endothelial cells. Karposi's sarcoma (KS) is divided into four groups—classic KS (men of Mediterranean and eastern European descent), AIDS-associated KS, endemic KS (children and adults from central Africa), and immunosuppression-associated KS (persons with organ transplants or underlying cancer). In HIV disease, KS is most commonly seen as the disease progresses. Almost all patients are homosexuals or bisexuals. It is unclear what causes this disease, but an infectious agent besides the HIV is suspected. There also seems to be some inherited susceptibility.

Kaposi's sarcoma begins as a small red to purple patch which gradually enlarges and develops a thickened or nodular appearance. The patches commonly arise on the trunk, extremities, and mouth. Lesions may also occur on the face and may be disfiguring. Symptoms are rare. As the lesions age they may become scaly, and some skin swelling may be seen. The internal organs may be involved, particularly the gastrointestinal tract and lungs. Internal bleeding is seen occasionally in these patients. In relatively healthy populations, KS is not considered dangerous; however, in HIV-positive patients it is a marker for severe disease. Patients may die of the KS itself or other HIV-related processes.

Therapy is difficult. Some patients benefit by beginning zidovudine if they are not already on it. Radiation therapy is a preferred method; it is bloodless, painless, and relatively easy to administer. For cosmetically unacceptable lesions, this is the treatment of choice. Unfortunately, it does not work on all lesions and may be expensive if used over a large area. Liquid nitrogen is effective if the areas to be treated are not numerous or large. Injecting interferon alpha (Intron-A®) into the lesion is also effective but is limited by cost and degree of skin involvement. Chemotherapy agents may be injected into the KS lesions. This therapy has met with some success but is expensive and uncomfortable, particularly if the lesion is in a sensitive site. An interesting therapeutic option involves iontophoresis along with the chemotherapy agent vinblastine (Velban®). Iontophoresis is a process whereby a small electrical current is used to drive medications across the skin barrier. This treatment method is time consuming but is safe, essentially painless, and reasonably effective. It is most useful in persons with a few easily visualized lesions. Systemic therapy is indicated if the patient has numerous tumors, is symptomatic from internal lesions, or if topical therapy has failed. New drugs are becoming available which "jump start" the body's capacity to make white and red blood cells. Use of these medications in conjunction with chemotherapy may make KS easier to treat.

Skin Cancer

Nonmelanoma skin cancer, basal cell carcinoma (BCC), and squamous cell carcinoma (SCC) may occasionally be more prevalent in persons with damaged immune systems. Not surprisingly, HIV-positive patients tend to have more of these cancers. In healthy persons, these rarely metastasize or threaten the patients' health but with HIV disease metastasis is not uncommon. Squamous cell carcinoma also occurs in areas not routine for healthy patients.

Melanoma, the deadliest form of skin cancer, is believed to be more common in HIV-positive patients. Additionally, these tumors tend to have invaded more deeply than in healthy patients.

Lymphoma

Cancer of the lymph glands and white blood cells is more common in HIV disease. These tumors may involve the brain and central nervous system as well as other internal organs. Treatment in healthy patients involves radiotherapy and chemotherapy. While radiation therapy is mostly inconsequential in HIV-positive patients, chemotherapy is not. Lymphomas result in the death of about 5 percent of HIV patients.

Bacterial Skin Infections

Almost everyone will experience a bacterial skin infection at some point in their lives. These can be anything from a minor inconvenience to a life-threatening condition and occur when bacteria overcome the body's capabilities to prevent infection. Bacteria are normally found on the skin; they vary in type and amount depending on the person's age, gender, physical condition, and environment. Normally, the skin is protected from infection by these organisms; antibacterial substances and the acidic pH of the skin impede bacterial growth. Additionally, the presence of certain "good" bacteria stifles the growth of other bacteria (bacterial interference).

Two conditions must be present for a bacterial infection to begin—a break in the skin surface or the presence of a foreign body. Normally, the skin's own construction protects it from irritation, such as from clothing. When the skin is breached by a cut, insect bite, or abrasion, however, it is easy for resident and opportunistic bacteria to gain a foothold. Similarly, when a foreign body such as a splinter or suture invades the skin, it breaches this protective barrier and brings with it bacteria, fungi, and viruses, which may then cause infection. Persons with underlying illnesses such as cancer, diabetes, AIDS, and so on are often troubled by skin infections.

There are many different kinds of bacterial skin infections. Some involve only the skin and have few, if any, systemic symptoms. Others arise from internal infections in which skin involvement is secondary. Bacteria are divided into several categories, the oldest being gram negative and gram positive. Most of the bacteria that infect the skin are gram positive; they are relatively easy to eradicate. Gram-negative infections are more common in patients with underlying diseases and tend to be more difficult to treat.

Impetigo

Impetigo contagiosa is a bacterial infection of the superficial layers of the skin. It is caused by the gram-positive bacteria *Streptococcus viridans* (Group A Streptococcus) and *Staphylococcus aureus*. *S.* aureus causes most impetigo worldwide. Other groups of *Streptococcus* occasionally cause disease, but this is uncommon. This infection predominantly affects children, usually in the late summer and fall. It is extremely contagious and spreads rapidly through classrooms, day-care facilities, and homes. Poor hygiene has traditionally been blamed for inducing these infections, but it arises in healthy, well cared for children as well. Crowding and malnutrition also play a role. The infection begins on the skin and then spreads to the nasal passages (streptococci) or originates in the nose and subsequently spreads to the skin (*S. aureus*). Minor trauma to susceptible skin surfaces may initiate the infection, but other skin diseases such as chickenpox and scabies may also be a trigger. The lesions begin as small blisters which become cloudy and quickly break down to form shiny golden-yellow crusts. The central face is typically involved but the scalp and other areas are susceptible as well. The infection may be spread by contaminating the fingers with the bacteria and then touching another area of the body. There may be itching and pain, but it is usually minor. Systemic symptoms are very rare. A variant of impetigo called bullous impetigo shows larger lesions with blisters; these may look like burn blisters. As the lesions of impetigo clear, the central area returns toward normal. This gives the appearance of a "ring," and ringworm may be incorrectly diagnosed.

Therapy involves penicillin and penicillinlike medications. These may be injected, but oral therapy is less expensive and just as effective. Erythromycin (EryPed®) may also be used but some strains of bacteria are resistant to this drug. Culturing the crusts or exudates will determine what medications will be effective. Most physicians, however, prefer to use whatever antibiotic has been most recently successful in treating similar patients. Cephalosporins and dicloxacillin (Dycil®) are also effective. Amoxicillin-clavulanic acid (Augmentin®) is an oral antibiotic to which few bacteria of this type have become resistant; it is widely used. Topical therapy with mupirocin (Bactroban®) has been advocated as being as effective as oral therapy; however, it is messy and somewhat expensive. Other topical treatments containing bacitracin (Polysporin®) or silver sulfadiazine (Silvadene®) may be helpful but are unlikely to clear the infection. Topical washes containing hexachlorophene (pHiso-Hex®) and chlorhexidine (Hibiclens®) similary are beneficial but won't usually clear the infection. Removing the crusts is important to many parents. Left alone, the lesions will drop off after several days of antibiotic therapy but this may be hastened by *gentle* use of warm water and a soft washcloth. The only long-term concern with impetigo is the rare case of infection with a strain which also induces inflammation of the kidneys (nephritic strain). These patients may develop diminished kidney function and total failure is a possibility. Fortunately, better medications are available today and this complication is rare. Prompt treatment of impetigo, however, is encouraged. Persons who develop impetigo on a regular or recurrent basis may benefit from regular application of mupirocin ointment in the nose. Using a cotton-tipped swab to apply the ointment to the nasal cavity twice daily five days a week may, over several months, lead to a reduction in impetigo outbreaks.

Cellulitis

This infection involves the deeper structures of the skin. The same organisms which cause impetigo are responsible for most cases of cellulitis. The typical case involves an area of skin which is red and feels thick. The extremities are most commonly affected, but any skin area is susceptible. The leading edge of the infection advances slowly. Clearing of the infection in the center of the lesion is occasionally seen. The overlying skin is normally uninvolved except for the color and texture. Some cases, however, show a mild exudate which may be yellow to pink. Blisters and skin breakdown are also rarely present. Red streaks may extend from the involved area and represent involvement of the lymphatic vessels. These streaks are commonly called "blood poisoning" because of their resemblance to infected blood vessels. The skin itself is mildly to moderately tender and hot to the touch. Symptoms such as fever, chills, nausea, vomiting, and loss of appetite are common with cellulitis as the bacteria begin to invade the body. Swollen lymph nodes often arise in areas adjacent to the infection. Cellulitis usually begins after some trauma, such as a cut or abrasion, but often, no inciting event can be recalled. There are several subtypes of cellulitis, including perianal cellulitis, which is seen most often in children and saphenous vein cellulitis, which begins in the area of vein donation for heart bypass surgery. Cellulitis may also begin in areas where there is chronic swelling from radiation therapy for a malignancy.

Unlike impetigo, this infection may be serious and life threatening. It may cause elevated white blood cell counts and decreased blood pressure. Culturing the exudate on the skin's surface will occasionally identify the causative organism, but culturing the patient's blood may be more effective. Antibiotic therapy may be done on an outpatient basis using oral medications, but often hospitalization with intravenous medication is needed. The antibiotics used are essentially the same as for impetigo but patients usually need to remain on them for ten days to two weeks depending on the severity of the infection. It is important that a *full* course of medication be taken to prevent relapse, possibly with a resistant strain of bacteria. Local care of the skin is another therapy. This may relieve some discomfort but will not effect a cure. Keeping the skin clear of crusting can be done with warm compresses using a washcloth.

A variant of cellulitis affects children's faces and is called facial cellulitis. This disease does occur in adults, but usually only in those over the age of fifty. The skin findings are essentially the same as in routine cellulitis but patients are usually much more ill. Children with facial cellulitis are infected with the gram-negative bacteria *Haemophilus influenzae*. Most patients are under three years of age and have had a recent upper respiratory infection. They develop swelling and redness of the face, particularly around the eyes and upper cheeks. They have fevers and may be lethargic. This is an emergency, and prompt antibiotic therapy must be instituted. Antibiotics are almost always given intravenously. *H. influenzae* is resistant to most standard antibiotics. Consequently, cephalosporins such as ceftriaxone (Rocephin®) and cefotaxime (Claforan®) are recommended. Chloramphenicol (Chloromycetin®) is useful in persons with penicillin allergy. Other family members are often treated with rifampin (Rifadin®) to prevent the illness. Immunization is now available for this bacteria, but it cannot be given until the patient is eighteen to twenty-four months of age.

Erysipelas

This disease is technically a form of cellulitis in that the invading organisms infect the deeper tissues of the skin. The infecting organism is almost always *S. viridans*. Rarely, *S. aureus* may be responsible. Erysipelas begins as an area of redness and warmth over the upper cheeks. The patient may have had a recent upper respiratory illness such as sinusitis or bronchitis. A breach in the skin's surface is the most common way for the organism to infect the skin. In infants, involvement of the abdomen occurs around the umbilical stump. Fevers and chills may be profound and patients are often quite ill. The patient's white blood cell count is elevated, indicating an infection. The skin is very thick and hard. It is hot to the touch and the redness advances forward as the bacteria invade adjacent areas of the face. The skin may be painful. There is occasionally mild blistering of the skin and scaling as the infection subsides.

Surprisingly, in the days prior to antibiotics, most of these patients did well and the illness resolved on its own in a week or so. Occasionally, however, it would soon recur or produce more deep-seated disease with greater symptoms and risk. Antibiotics are given as for cellulitis and impetigo. Therapy is normally by mouth if the patient is otherwise healthy and not particularly symptomatic. If the infection is worrisome, however, antibiotics are given intravenously and the patient is hospitalized. The symptoms begin to subside in about forty-eight hours.

A similar-sounding infection called erysipeloid also is caused by a gram-positive bacteria (*Erysipelothrix rhusiopathiae*) but is more commonly seen on the hands of housewives, fishermen, and butchers. This organism lives in the slime of aquatic animals such as fish and crabs as well as in pigs. Infection comes from handling infected material such as meat. The skin becomes a brilliant reddish purple with mild swelling. It is hot and tender. The infection is usually limited to the skin of the hands but variants of erysipeloid involve other skin surfaces as well as the heart valves. Penicillin given in high doses intravenously is curative. Erythromycin and vancomycin (Vancocin®) may be substituted in penicillin-allergic persons.

Ecthyma

In ecthyma, patients develop open sores with crusting and weeping. Some blistering may also occur. These arise after mild trauma such as insect bites or scratches and usually occur on the extremities. They enlarge to the size of a silver dollar or bigger within several days. Mild pain and itch may be present. Ecthyma usually arises in children or patients with poor hygiene, such as the homeless. Group A streptococci are almost always responsible. Treatment includes improvement of hygiene and antibiotics such as cephalosporins, erythromycin, penicillins, or topical application of mupirocin ointment. Medications must usually be continued for several weeks, since the lesions are slow to heal.

Erythrasma

Erythrasma is a bacterial infection of the superficial skin. It is not dangerous but may cause some mild itching and burning. Most patients are young adults. The armpits, groins, and spaces between the toes may be affected. The skin is pink to brown with some mild scaling. It is often misdiagnosed as jock itch or another fungal infection. Erythrasma is caused by infection with a bacteria called *Corynebacterium minutissimum*. If a black-light lamp is held up to the skin it will glow or fluoresce a bright red color. Treatment consists of oral erythromycin for a week. Applying topical erythromycin (ATS® Solution) or clindamycin (Cleocin®) is also helpful.

Furuncle/Carbuncle

These are often called "boils." Furuncles are deep-seated infections of single hair follicles, whereas carbuncles are similar infections involving several adjacent hair follicles and are larger. The infecting bacteria is almost always *S. aureus*. These lesions typically appear on the buttocks, the armpits, the neck, and the trunk. They only occur where hair follicles are found. Patients with diabetes, alcoholism, cancer, malnutrition, AIDS, and those taking chemotherapy drugs are particularly susceptible to these lesions; however, practically anyone can develop a furuncle. The lesions are large red nodules and may show a pustule at the apex. Rupture expresses masses of pus and a "core" of harder material. Mild to moderate discomfort is typical. Carbuncles, on the other hand, are more dangerous, since patients may run fevers. After resolution of the lesions, there may be significant scarring. If the infection has not been adequately treated and scarring is considerable, the infection may "smolder" in the tissues of the skin. It almost always will recur and may require prolonged courses of antibiotics to fully eradicate it.

Treatment used to consist of warm compresses to soften the nodule, allowing it to rise to the surface where it would either rupture spontaneously or be surgically drained. Antibiotics are used almost universally now and if given early in the disease, may cause the furuncle to subside without developing a pustule. The antibiotics mentioned for other staphylococcal diseases are helpful here as well. Given the seriousness of this infection, many physicians use drugs to which the bacteria are unlikely to be resistant, such as amoxicillin-clavulanic acid or dicloxacillin. Therapy is usually done on an outpatient basis, but if the patient is particularly ill or has an underlying disease, hospitalization with intravenous antibiotic therapy is appropriate. Surgically opening the furuncle/carbuncle is helpful in certain cases, but only under sterile conditions and only if the patient is receiving antibiotics.

Furuncles/carbuncles arising around the mouth and on the lips are a concern since if bacteria spread from these lesions into the bloodstream, they may cause an infection in the brain. Consequently, these lesions are treated very carefully and surgical drainage is used only as a last resort. Persons who develop chronic disease are believed to carry the bacteria in their nasal passages or groins and continually reinfect themselves. These sites are usually cultured and if *S. aureus* is confirmed in the laboratory, a course of rifampin is given for several weeks to eradicate the bacteria. Use of antibacterial ointments such as mupirocin or bacitracin in the nasal passages is also begun. These patients are encouraged to use an antibacterial soap such as chlorhexidine, change bedding and clothing often, and frequently wash their hands. Care of any underlying illnesses is also necessary. Some patients have had a similar but harmless strain of bacteria called *S. aureus* 502A inoculated into their nasal passages in an effort to crowd out the disease-causing bacteria, but this treatment is not used much anymore.

Scarlet Fever

This disease is well known to older persons who remember epidemics in the preantibiotic era. Scarlet fever is seen in persons infected with *S. viridans* capable of producing a toxin called erythrogenic toxin. Not all strains of this bacteria can make this protein, so not everyone with strep throat or some other type of strep infection develops scarlet fever. Persons usually only get scarlet fever once, so some type of immunity probably develops. This disease is seen most often in children but adults may also develop it. The most common infection is pharyngitis or a sore throat. The sore throat is similar to most strep throat but after two to four days, a fine red rash arises on the neck and spreads to the extremities. The palms and soles are not involved. The rash spreads for about a day and a half and then stops. The face is involved but classically the area around the mouth is spared (circumoral pallor). The rash usually lasts for four or five days. The tonsils are enlarged, red, and coated with pus. The tongue initially is white with red speckles on the top and sides ("white strawberry tongue") but after several days the white color fades and it becomes bright red ("red strawberry tongue").

Administration of appropriate medications for the strep infection such as penicillin, erythromycin, or cephalosporins will dramatically alter the skin rash. As the fever, chills, and sore throat of the strep infection subside, so does the rash. Mild scaling after several days will usually be seen.

Staphylococcal Scalded Skin Syndrome

Staphylococcal scalded skin syndrome (SSSS), or Ritter's disease, affects two groups of persons—infants and persons with kidney disease. The skin in these patients begins to peel off in large sheets following infection with certain subtypes of *Staphylococcus aureus*. The infection is usually not in the skin but rather in the sinuses, ears, or elsewhere. The infecting bacteria produce a toxin known as exfoliatin, which causes the most superficial layers of the skin to peel in thin sheets. Since kidney function in these patients is not sufficient to excrete this protein, it builds up in the body and exerts its influence. The skin is red and tender but heals quickly. The neck, groin, and armpits are involved. There may be fever but patients are not usually seriously ill. Since the lost tissue is so superficial, there is little danger. Treatment consists of therapy for the underlying staphylococcal infection, such as cephalosporins or dicloxacillin. Routine care is all that's required since the skin will repair itself in a few days.

Toxic Shock Syndrome

Toxic shock syndrome was well publicized several years ago following numerous infections in menstruating women using tampons. This disease has continued to be a problem and principally involves women during the first six days of their periods, but it also affects persons with infections of the bone and lungs, women using contraceptive sponges, and patients who have had their nasal passages packed after surgery. Toxic shock syndrome arises after infection with *Staphylococcus aureus* and some strains of *S. viridans*. A toxin is apparently produced by the offending bacteria to which the patient reacts violently. There is an acute onset with evidence of liver and kidney involvement, diminished blood pressure, vomiting or diarrhea, fever, and decreased blood cell counts. The skin is usually fiery red and begins to scale and slough after a week or two. This is particularly prominent over the palms and soles. This disease is considered an emergency and hospitalization is required. Therapy consists of aggressive antibiotic administration and management of any underlying kidney and liver disease.

BIRTHMARKS

The word *birthmark* means different things to different people. Some envision a large red patch over a person's face, whereas others think of almost any discolored area present since childhood. By definition, these lesions are present at birth or develop within a few months. Almost all are benign, but only a few will subside with time. Most are composed of blood vessels, pigment-producing cells (melanocytes), or fibrotic tissue. The following "birthmarks" are listed in order of their approximate frequency of occurrence.

Capillary ("Strawberry") Hemangioma

These lesions arise at birth or shortly thereafter. They are raised and may even be nodular. The head and neck are the usual sites but they also arise elsewhere. Usually only a single hemangioma is present. The lesions may initially grow very quickly but then begin to subside. If the hemangioma is around an eye or other vital structure, the growth may occlude it. In developing children, occlusion of the eye can cause blindness, so this situation is considered an emergency. Lesions are pink to red and may be purple. They are symptomless but may ulcerate if they become too large.

Therapy for hemangiomas is somewhat controversial. About 75 percent of these lesions will slowly resolve over five to ten years. They do so with some mild scarring and/or discoloration, but the cosmetic result is considerably better than the original lesion or the scar of a surgical excision. Therefore, if the hemangioma is not blocking an eye or impairing the patient's ability to eat, breathe, defecate, or urinate, most dermatologists advise allowing the lesion to resolve on its own. If the hemangioma has ulcerated and poses an infection risk or if it is rapidly enlarging, oral corticosteroids may be used. These drugs impede the growth of hemangiomas and are useful for short-term therapy. Topical corticosteroids are not effective and oral administration cannot be given without risk or for prolonged periods. Injection of corticosteroids can also help. Laser therapy is useful for some lesions. The pulsed-dye laser is effective but may not penetrate deep enough into the lesion to treat the affected blood vessels. The argon laser penetrates deeper but may cause some scarring.

Two syndromes involving capillary hemangiomas merit mentioning. Diffuse hemangiomatosis is a disorder in which patients develop multiple hemangiomas. They may involve the internal organs and bleeding is a problem. Many of these patients die. Kasabach-Merritt syndrome is a condition in which the blood platelets become entrapped in a large hemangioma and compromise the blood's capacity to clot. This is considered an emergency, but fortunately is very rare.

Nevus Flammeus/Port Wine Stain

A nevus flammeus, or port wine stain is among the most common birthmarks. These appear as flat patches of red-colored skin, mostly over the face and neck. They may also be pink and purple and usually fade when pressure is applied. Lesions on the extremities and trunk are occasionally seen. On the eyelids, they may be called "angel kisses" and on the nape of the neck they are often known as "stork bites."

The lesions tend to fade with time but in a certain percentage of patients they remain and may become thickened. Unless the lesions are very large and unsightly, the best treatment option is to leave them alone and allow them to resolve on their own. Having a large visible lesion can be psychologically traumatic and therapy may be indicated in some patients. Previous therapies included camouflage (makeup [Covermark®, Dermablend®], pigment tattooing), excision when feasible, cryosurgery, and x-ray therapy. Now, the best results are achieved using lasers such as the copper vapor, pulsed-dye, and krypton laser. These lasers destroy the enlarged blood vessels in the skin which impart the red color. Discomfort is minimal, scarring is uncommon, and each treatment does not involve much time. Precautions to safeguard a patient's vision must be taken if the nevus flammeus is around the eyes. Multiple treatments may be needed and are expensive, but laser therapy is a giant step forward in the management of port wine stains.

Cavernous Hemangioma

These lesions are very similar to strawberry hemangiomas but are larger and arise deeper in the skin. They are rare and occur more often in childhood than in infancy. The head and neck are most commonly involved. The lesions are usually dark red to purple and nodular. They may badly distort sites such as the ear or eye. The lesions are compressible when pressure is applied but slowly fill back up and return to their original shape. They are rarely symptomatic and infrequently ulcerate. These lesions are also seen in blue rubber bleb nevus syndrome, Mafucci's syndrome, Riley-Smith syndrome, and Bannayan syndrome. All are very rare.

Unlike capillary hemangiomas, cavernous hemangiomas grow very slowly and do not resolve on their own. Consequently, corticosteroids are not as likely to be effective. If a solitary lesion is fed by a single blood vessel, surgeons may be able to destroy the vessel. Laser therapy is also occasionally effective, but much less so than with capillary hemangiomas because the blood vessels are much deeper in the skin. Excision of the lesion is an option, but results in a scar and may not be possible depending upon where the hemangioma has arisen. Use of tight-fitting garments and dressings help to some degree; however, this requires a significant investment of time and energy.

Congenital Nevi

Congenital nevi (or moles) are very common. They are formed as are most nevi by the aggregation of melanocytes, the pigment-producing cells in the skin. These moles have several different names such as garment nevus, giant nevus, and "bathing suit" nevus. They may be present at birth or develop in the first few years of life and are larger than routine moles. These nevi are usually divided into small congenital nevi (less than 20 cm in diameter) and large congenital nevi (greater than 20 cm in diameter). They increase in size with the patient and may show considerable growth during infancy and early childhood. Congenital nevi occur in about 1 percent of the populace. There seems to be an inherited tendency in some cases. Most are small and single and are round or oval. Some display a significant amount of hair, but many are hairless. Usually the surface is rough or cobblestoned; it is rarely flat. They tend to be the same color throughout and are well demarcated from surrounding normal skin. Some are dark brown to black, and freckling may be noted. Congenital moles may be found on almost any area of the body. The pigmentation lightens with time in some lesions. There is an association in some cases with other congenital deformities, but this may be coincidental. Lesions on the head and neck may have an increase in melanocytes along the coverings of the brain and spinal cord (leptomeninges). While this usually causes no problems, occasionally the accumulation of melanocytes is so great that it blocks the flow of cerebrospinal fluid and causes hydrocephalus. These patients may develop brain damage, seizures, and mental retardation.

The management of these lesions is a problem. The most worrisome aspect of these nevi is the potential they have to become malignant (melanoma). If the nevus is small and single, the most expedient thing to do is measure it and observe it for any unusual symptoms or rapid growth. The real question regarding these lesions is whether to surgically excise them. Surgery is usually performed after the child is six months of age and before the age of twelve. If the nevus appears abnormal, dermatologists often recommend immediate removal, since fatal melanoma has developed in infants. Measuring the lesion and taking photographs are good means of following these nevi. Large congenital nevi have a greater tendency to become cancerous than small congenital nevi. The estimated lifetime risk for large lesions to develop a melanoma is between 5 and 10 percent. It is less for small congenital nevi. Worrisome signs include itching, ulceration, bleeding, and the development of a nodule or lump in the nevus. If these occur, a biopsy is necessary to evaluate for malignant changes. If a melanoma has developed, treatment will usually be the same as for older patients. Larger congenital nevi are sometimes removed in a series of surgeries to avoid a melanoma, but for the largest lesions and those in cosmetically sensitive areas (the face, groin, hands, and so on), this may not be possible. Some techniques expand the tissues with the placement of a gradually enlarging balloon and stretching the skin. This allows for more normal skin to be available at the time of surgical removal of the mole so that repair of the defect is easier. Removing the lesion and grafting skin into the area is popular, but obviously results in significant scarring. There is hope that in the future lasers may be used to destroy the melanocytes in these lesions and render them incapable of becoming cancerous.

Cafe au Lait Spots

These lesions are most typical of what is termed a "birthmark." They are light brown in color and appear at or shortly after birth. They rarely are much larger than a quarter. Cafe au lait spots tend to develop on the extremities. They have smooth to jagged borders and may darken with sun exposure. They usually are single but some patients have several. In patients with more than five or six, there is the possibility that they have neurofibromatosis (Von Recklinghausen's disease). These patients may also have freckling under the arms. Treatment of the isolated cafe au lait macule is rare since they do not become cancerous. They may be surgically excised if desired, and some types of laser treatment also may be useful. In addition to neurofibromatosis, these lesions may also be seen in Albright's syndrome, Bloom's syndrome, Fanconi's syndrome, tuberous sclerosis, and ataxia telangiectasia.

Nevus Sebaceus

This is technically an epidermal nevus but it has some features which set it apart from other lesions. These are normally present at birth or develop during childhood. They are almost always on the scalp but the forehead, neck, and face are also sites of involvement. They are pink to slightly yellow in color, are raised, and are slightly cobblestoned to the touch. As the patient passes through puberty they may become more prominent and wartlike. Scaling is occasionally seen. They cause no symptoms. These lesions are composed of aggregates of sebaceous or oil glands which normally appear in the skin. They occasionally develop benign and malignant skin tumors, so excision is usually recommended. The malignant tumors are not different from routine skin cancers and excision is curative.

Mongolian Spots

Mongolian spots are large (palm-sized) areas of darkening usually found on the trunk. They may not be visible at birth but appear in the weeks following. They fade in most cases over months or years. They are more common in Orientals, blacks, and Hispanics. A major concern is that they may be mistaken for bruises from child abuse. They have no potential to become malignant.

Epidermal Nevi

These lesions are called nevi, but they do not have the proliferation of melanocytes seen in congenital nevi or nevi acquired during life. Epidermal nevi occur sporadically in about 1 per 1,000 births. Most are present at birth or develop shortly thereafter, but they may also occur during childhood. They rarely arise after puberty. Epidermal nevi are tan to brown and raised, and they have a wartlike surface. As they develop, they may become very scaly. They are usually set close together in a linear pattern. Some itching may occur, but they are not usually symptomatic. Rarely, a skin cancer may arise in epidermal nevi.

A rare condition known as epidermal nevus syndrome is seen in some patients with this disease. This is a constellation of findings which include other birthmarks such as cafe au lait spots, hemangiomas, and routine melanocytic nevi. Most worrisome, however, is the association with neurological defects such as seizures, mental retardation, visual deficits, and paralysis. The patient's bone structure may also be defective with finding such as scoliosis, spina bifida, and enlarged bones. Patients with large epidermal nevi are usually evaluated for this syndrome.

Treatment is almost solely surgical. If the lesions are itching, topical corticosteroids may help and exfoliating creams containing lactic acid (Lac-Hydrin®) or alpha hydroxy acids may be useful for scaling. Excision of the lesion is most effective but is only done if the epidermal nevus is particularly objectionable, since the surgeon will have to cut deep into the tissues to completely remove it. Liquid nitrogen, dermabrasion, and laser therapy may also be useful if the lesion is small. Destroying epidermal nevi by applying trichloroacetic acid or phenol may also work. If the lesion develops a skin cancer, it must be surgically excised. Symptoms of this complication are a rapid increase in size, bleeding, and breakdown of the tissues.

Lymphangiomas

A lymphangioma is the lymphatic vessel counterpart to a hemangioma. Lymphatic vessels carry tissue fluid which has leaked out of blood vessels. Lymphangiomas are present at birth or may appear in early childhood. Girls are affected more frequently than boys. There are several different types; the most common is called lymphangioma circumscriptum. These lesions are composed of a mass of clear to reddish purple nodules which may appear blisterlike. They commonly arise on the buttock or extremity but may occur essentially anywhere. Lymphangioma circumscriptum are superficial in the skin but are still not easily surgically removed. Cystic hygromas are very large cystic structures that arise on the neck or under the arms of infants. These are painless and flesh colored, but may become so large that they impair breathing and eating. Lymphangioma cavernosum, as the name suggests, is a deep-seated lesion that does not affect the overlying skin. The deeper tissues are enlarged and spongy to the touch. All of these lesions are difficult to remove because the structures involve the deep tissues; if they are not completely removed they recur in a matter of months or years. Laser therapy is not usually helpful.

Connective Tissue Nevus

The connective tissue nevus, like the nevus sebaceus or epidermal nevus, is not composed of melanocytes. Rather, it is derived from proliferation of the connective tissue (collagen) normally found in the skin. Since the superficial aspects of the skin are not involved, these lesions look like nodules or large tumors under the skin. They arise on almost any surface but the trunk is a common site. They are usually flesh colored but may be slightly brown or yellow. There are no associated symptoms. Lesions are present at birth or develop during childhood. A distinct type of connective tissue nevus known as a shagreen patch is seen in patients with tuberous sclerosis. This lesion is about the size of a half or silver dollar and commonly is on the back. It has a slightly knobby appearance. Connective tissue nevi do not become cancerous, but patients who have them often have underlying diseases such as Buschke-Ollendorf syndrome. These lesions may be excised, but this is not necessary since they remain benign.

Aplasia Cutis Congenita

While this is not usually considered a birthmark, it is present in children at birth and leaves a lifetime scar. Aplasia cutis congenita is seen almost exclusively on the scalp. The area is hairless, skin colored to slightly red, and mildly depressed. When the child is born the area may be ulcerated; later it may heal with scarring. Aplasia cutis congenita arises when layers of the skin fail to properly form. If the superficial aspects of the skin are missing, the lesion will heal with scarring but no other problems. If the deeper parts of the skin are involved, plastic surgery may be required to cover the defect and allow it to heal. These areas are occasionally mistaken for trauma from the obstetrical delivery.

Nevus Comedonicus (Comedone Nevus)

These unusual tumors are found at birth or in childhood. They arise on the face, neck, and trunk and are linear, slightly raised, and pink to brown. An unusual feature is that as the nevus ages, comedones ("blackheads") are seen. These comedones do not appear greatly different from those seen in acne or old age. While nevus comedonicus is a benign tumor, the comedones may rupture into the skin just as in acne and cause inflammation and infection. Treatment is surgical excision. Tretinoin, although very effective in comedonal acne, is not helpful with these lesions, but they do not become malignant.

Ash Leaf Macules

These spots occur in tuberous sclerosis, a disease with mental retardation and seizures. They arise on the trunk and are the size of a thumbprint or the leaf of an ash tree. They are lighter colored than surrounding skin (hypopigmented) and flat. They are usually single but multiple lesions may occur. Ash leaf macules do not fade with time and do not become cancerous; treatment is not necessary.

Cutis Marmorata Telangiectatica Congenita

This is an unusual birthmark in that it involves the blood vessels of the skin. These vascular structures are dilated and therefore appear more prominent. The affected skin looks "mottled" with a net or spiderweblike appearance. It is reddish pink to blue colored and typically affects an extremity or the trunk. A similar eruption occurs in newborns and adults when they become cold (cutis marmorata) but resolves upon warming. In cutis marmorata telangiectatica congenita, the lesions are permanent and gradually expand during the first few years of life. They do not fade with time or warming. Treatment is difficult; surgical excision is usually out of the question since the lesions are too large. Laser therapy might be of some help but has not yet been attempted.

BLISTERING DISEASES

Diseases that result in blistering (bullous disorders) are some of the most difficult and dangerous illnesses in dermatology. Previously, patients with these diseases would easily develop infections and many, if not most, died. The development of corticosteroids in the 1940s dramatically reduced the mortality rate of some blistering diseases. Today corticosteroids are the mainstay in treatment of bullous disorders and numerous other drugs have been found effective as well. Blisters may involve the skin, the mucous membranes, or both.

The skin is divided into several layers and different diseases affect different layers. Consequently, some bullous diseases have large tense blisters which spread to become palm sized or greater, whereas in others the blisters are so fragile that they easily rupture and result in sores or erosions. Most of these conditions are diagnosed with specialized types of skin biopsies called immunofluorescent biopsies. Sometimes the patient's blood is analyzed for the antibodies causing the blistering. The bullous diseases represent true emergencies; in few other aspects of dermatology is it as important to reach a definite diagnosis, since therapies for these disorders may be quite different. Appropriate management may require multiple biopsies and the use of several different, and occasionally dangerous, medications. In many patients it is possible to effect a cure and see the skin return to normal. The healed skin may be temporarily discolored, but with a few rare exceptions, scarring is unusual.

Pemphigus

This disorder is actually a grouping of diseases with similar features in the disease process and on skin biopsy. Pemphigus is considered an autoimmune disease; the patient's immune processes have turned on themselves and are now attacking certain parts of the body. In the case of pemphigus, the immune system is making antibodies that attack the skin and cause it to blister.

Pemphigus Vulgaris
Pemphigus vulgaris is the most common of the pemphigus diseases but is still relatively infrequent. It usually affects young to middle-aged adults, especially Jews and those of Mediterranean descent. It typically begins as erosions in the mouth; most

patients will eventually have oral involvement. These areas are actually blisters, but since the mouth is constantly traumatized by everyday activities, they are never actually able to form an intact blister. Other mucosal surfaces such as the genitalia, nasal passages, bronchi, esophagus, eyes, and anus may be involved as well. Erosions are painful, red, and can be as large as a quarter. They interfere greatly with eating and drinking. Skin lesions are more likely to look like a blister, but they are fragile, and erosions and ulcerations are usually seen. Crusting and scabbing are common. The trunk and extremities are most often involved, but virtually any skin surface is at risk.

Pemphigus Vegetans

This condition is essentially the same as pemphigus vulgaris but the skin lesions are thick, heaped-up crusts which may have a foul odor.

Neonatal Pemphigus

Neonatal pemphigus occurs when mothers with this disease give birth to children with similar lesions. Children improve as the level of antibodies in their bloodstream subsides.

In all variants of pemphigus, lesions heal without scarring. Patients are sensitive to heat and many are intolerant of sunlight. Diagnosis is made by skin biopsy and, in some cases, analysis of the patient's blood for evidence of the antibodies attacking the skin.

Treatment of these patients is difficult but considerably easier than in the past. Previously, a diagnosis of pemphigus vulgaris was tantamount to a death sentence; recovery was infrequent. Survival today is almost universal. Treatment of infecting bacteria with an antibiotic effective against *Staphylococcus aureus* and *Streptococcus viridans* is usually required. Patients may be malnourished and dehydrated, depending on the degree of involvement of the mouth and esophagus. Hospitalization for a few days is frequently helpful to control the disease and educate the patient regarding follow-up care. The treatment of choice for control of pemphigus vulgaris is corticosteroids. Intramuscular triamcinolone (Kenalog®), intravenous hydrocortisone or methylprednisolone (Solu-Medrol®), or oral prednisone/prednisolone (Deltasone®/Prelone®) are all effective but must be given in high doses (prednisone 60 to 120 mg per day or higher). Doses of corticosteroids are tapered slowly over weeks to months after the disease has been brought under control, but some patients may have to remain on corticosteroids indefinitely. These medications are not without significant side effects at these doses, and intolerance may occur.

If corticosteroids are not effective or cannot be used, another medication must be employed. Azathioprine (Immuran®) is a popular second choice. In addition to helping control the disease, this drug may allow the prednisone dose to be lowered. Azathioprine is well tolerated in many patients but may have dangerous side effects. Close monitoring of bone marrow, liver, and kidney function is required. Other immune-suppressing drugs such as methotrexate (Rheumatrex®), cyclophosphamide (Cytoxan®), chlorambucil (Leukeran®), and gold (Myochrisine®) are useful in selected patients but have significant side effects of their own. Again, they may allow the corticosteroid dose to be lowered.

An unusual form of therapy involves removing the offending antibodies in a process known as plasmapheresis. In this procedure the patient has blood removed from a vein, the antibodies responsible for causing pemphigus are removed, and the blood cells and serum are returned to the bloodstream. This treatment is often combined with drugs and is generally only indicated for patients in whom other therapies have failed. It is considered reasonably safe; however, it is time consuming, expensive, and offered only in a few medical centers.

Children with neonatal pemphigus may require no treatment other than application of a potent topical steroid preparation to their lesions.

Skin lesions begin to heal relatively quickly after beginning corticosteroids and/or immunosuppressants but topical skin care is still important, particularly in pemphigus vegetans. Moisturizing bath oils may help debride the skin of dead tissue and foul-smelling crusts. Topical antibiotics such as bacitracin (Polysporin®) or silver sulfadiazine (Silvadene®) help diminish local bacteria counts and decrease odor. Corticosteroid medications for oral ulcerations with topical anesthetics (lidocaine) allow patients to eat and drink. With increased skin metabolism and the loss of fluids, good nutrition and adequate fluid intake are important.

Pemphigus Erythematosus, Pemphigus Foliaceus, and Fogo Selvagem

These two conditions are often linked together since the findings on skin biopsy for both illnesses are essentially identical. Pemphigus erythematosus demonstrates almost solely erosions and ulcerations, since the blister formation is so superficial that rupture of each lesion is just about guaranteed. This disease is also known as Senear-Usher syndrome; there is an association with the symptoms and findings of lupus erythematosus. Pemphigus erythematosus is generally localized to one area, typically the face and upper chest. It is not usually considered dangerous and management is relatively easy. Pemphigus foliaceus also rarely demonstrates intact blisters. These patients usually have disease localized to the face and upper trunk but they may experience widespread almost total body involvement. Pain, itching, and burning are common, and there is scaling and crusting. Heat and sun exposure make this disease worse. Neither disease has the mucosal involvement that occurs with pemphigus vulgaris.

Fogo selvagem is also known as endemic pemphigus foliaceus. It is seen almost exclusively in the rain forests of Brazil. Younger patients, including children, are susceptible. It is thought to be caused by the bite of certain insects found in this region. The disease tends to run its course but may take many years to resolve.

The treatment of these diseases is essentially the same as for pemphigus vulgaris/vegetans. However, pemphigus erythematosus/foliaceus are usually less serious illnesses and aggressive measures may not be necessary. Prednisone is the drug of choice, but the high doses needed for pemphigus vulgaris/vegetans may not be required. Topical corticosteroids, antimalarial medications, and dapsone all play a role in treatment.

Drug-Induced Pemphigus

Occasionally pemphigus results as a side effect of a medication. The disease is most like pemphigus foliaceus and shows similar features on biopsy. Penicillamine (Cuprimine®) and captopril (Capoten®) are the most common drugs associated with this disorder, but rifampin (Rifadin®) and penicillin have also reportedly caused it. The treatment is the same as for other forms of pemphigus, but discontinuing the medications is most important. The skin changes subside as the medication leaves the body.

Paraneoplastic Pemphigus

Paraneoplastic pemphigus is a blistering disease most like pemphigus vulgaris which arises in patients with cancer. The skin lesions may also resemble those seen in lupus erythematosus and erythema multiforme. Most cancers associated with this skin eruption arise in the bone marrow and lymph glands (lymphomas and leukemias) but other types of cancer have been involved as well. Treatment of the underlying malignancy is the best means of controlling the skin eruption; therapy otherwise is similar to that for other forms of pemphigus. There is a high mortality rate with this disease.

Pemphigoid

This group of blistering diseases consists of bullous pemphigoid, cicatricial pemphigoid, herpes gestationis, and epidermolysis bullosa acquisita. With the exception of herpes gestationis, most of these diseases are more common in elderly patients. These blisters result from a split in the skin which is deeper than in pemphigus and as a result they are tense and more difficult to break. Erosions are less likely but healing takes longer. As in pemphigus, these diseases arise when the body's immune system begins to make antibodies against itself. The site of attack is different than that in pemphigus, but skin biopsies usually distinguish between the diseases.

Bullous Pemphigoid

Bullous pemphigoid is unusual in persons under sixty years of age. Tense blisters appear in the folds of the body such as the groin, neck, and under the arms. Involvement of the mouth and other mucous membranes is much less common than with pemphigus, occurring in less than a quarter of patients. Lesions may itch or burn. Commonly, the bullae first appear as hives and over the ensuing days begin to develop large blisters. There is usually mild surrounding redness to the skin. These lesions may burst, but less so than in pemphigus, and they range in size from that of a pencil eraser to several inches. Some suggest that bullous pemphigoid occurs more frequently in patients with underlying diseases such as cancer, rheumatoid arthritis, diabetes, and ulcerative colitis; however, these ailments may simply be more common in the elderly population. The diagnosis is evident in most patients, but in some cases skin biopsies and blood are subjected to immunofluorescent testing for confirmation. Some patients develop bullous pemphigoid after they have been treated with furosemide (Lasix®) and other medications.

Treatment is similar to that for pemphigus vulgaris. Prednisone or other corticosteroids are usually begun but generally not in the high doses needed for pemphigus. Topical corticosteroids are useful for mild mucosal and skin disease. Generally, however, another immunosuppressive drug such as azathioprine or methotrexate must be used. This allows for lower corticosteroid doses. Dapsone and sulfapyridine are effective in certain patients as is tetracycline (Sumycin®) and minocycline (Minocin®). Tetracycline and niacin 500 mg four times daily have been very helpful in some cases. Niacin occasionally causes mild flushing of the skin but is otherwise well tolerated. This regimen is both safe and inexpensive. Plasmapheresis may also be useful. The prognosis for bullous pemphigoid is good, particularly compared to that of pemphigus vulgaris; many patients will go into remission even without therapy and most today can be cured with proper therapy. Treatment may be required for several years, however, before the disease subsides.

Cicatricial Pemphigoid

This disease is also called benign mucosal pemphigoid and involves the mucosa of the mouth, esophagus, eyes, genitalia, and anus. Its name is inappropriate since this disease is anything but benign. "Cicatricial" means scarring, and these patients have blisters which heal with scars. Mucous membranes, especially the mouth, are affected. About two-thirds of patients have eye lesions. Blisters do not last long and painful erosions and ulcerations are seen. There are the usual blisters seen with bullous pemphigoid. This disease shows little tendency to resolve on its own. Unfortunately, the scarring may be very damaging to the eye and loss of vision occurs in some patients, and strictures in the esophagus and the vaginal canal may occur. Cicatricial pemphigoid is difficult to control. If there are few lesions, injection of corticosteroids into the surrounding tissues may be helpful as may use of potent topical creams and ointments. Consultation with an ophthalmologist is recommended. Usually, high doses of corticosteroids and immunosuppressants are required for disease control; unfortunately, these medications are not always successful and the eye disease progresses.

Herpes Gestationis

Herpes gestationis is also inappropriately named. This disease has nothing to do with herpesvirus infection but acquired its name from the appearance of the skin blisters. Herpes gestationis occurs almost exclusively in pregnant women, although it may occur when patients take birth control pills. It is relatively rare, occurring only about once in 25,000 to 50,000 pregnancies. It most commonly arises during a patient's first pregnancy and may develop in subsequent pregnancies as well. The skin blisters are essentially identical to those of bullous pemphigoid but do not become so large. The initial skin findings are redness and itching hives or burning. The mucosa of the mouth and genitalia are spared. The disease subsides within a few days of delivery but may recur with menstrual periods or use of oral contraceptives. Children born to mothers with this disease may have some hives or blisters but their disease is usually not severe; it requires little therapy aside from topical corticosteroids and will slowly subside on its own. Herpes gestationis does not affect the mother's health but there is some debate about whether there are adverse effects on the unborn child.

Treatment is limited because of the ongoing pregnancy. Topical corticosteroids are sometimes enough to control the blistering and make the patient more comfortable, but if systemic therapy is required, prednisone is the preferred medication. The high doses required for pemphigus vulgaris or bullous pemphigoid are not necessary; most patients can be controlled with 40 mg per day or so. Almost all other medications usually used for blistering diseases are toxic to the unborn child and cannot be used.

Epidermolysis Bullosa Acquisita

Epidermolysis bullosa acquisita (EBA; dermolytic pemphigoid) is a rare cause of skin blistering. In some patients, it is difficult to distinguish from bullous pemphigoid or cicatricial pemphigoid and can only be diagnosed using sophisticated procedures. The most common type of EBA, however, shows skin blistering and erosions over areas subjected to mild trauma. The hands, toes, knuckles, elbows, and knees are most commonly involved. The skin is thinned, scarred, and slow to heal in the ulcerated areas. Healing takes place with the formation of minute cysts (milia, "whiteheads") in the skin. Nail loss and scalp scarring with hair loss are also seen, and these areas are uncomfortable. EBA is seen with various diseases of the immune system, but especially with lupus erythematosus and inflammatory bowel disease. In some patients, it becomes impossible to distinguish between bullous pemphigoid or cicatricial pemphigoid and EBA. Treatment is very difficult because epidermolysis bullosa acquisita responds poorly to most drugs. High doses of prednisone are effective in some patients but most other immunosuppressants have not proven helpful. Cyclosporine shows the most promise but cannot be used for extended periods and is dangerous for persons with high blood pressure or kidney disease. Good skin care, avoidance of excessively hot water and harsh soaps, and use of appropriate clothing are probably the most important aspect of treatment.

Familial Benign Pemphigus (Hailey-Hailey Disease)

As with cicatricial pemphigoid, this disease is misnamed; it is not benign and is inherited in less than half the cases. Hailey-Hailey disease affects patients in their teens and twenties. It consists of small blisters or erosions that aggregate and become crusted and scabbed. Most affected are the folds of the skin in the groin and under the arms, but the neck and trunk may also show lesions. There is mild itching and pain, but the most significant complaint is odor. The disease is more common in warm weather. Hailey-Hailey disease is not an autoimmune disease but its cause is unclear.

The disease plaques are commonly infected and antibiotic treatment may be required before significant healing can take place. Tetracycline may be useful as in bullous pemphigoid to treat the infection and for long-term suppression of the disease. Other antibiotics such as doxycycline (Doryx®) and minocycline (Minocin®) may be similarly used. Topical corticosteroids and topical mupirocin (Bactroban®) are effective but oral corticosteroids are occasionally required. Dapsone and methotrexate may also be helpful.

Epidermolysis Bullosa

Epidermolysis bullosa (EB) is a group of diseases which have as a central feature skin fragility, ulceration, and blistering. There are over twenty subtypes of this disease and most are extremely rare. They are usually inherited and are classified based on where the split occurs in the skin. The nails, hair, and teeth may also be affected.

Scarring is often widespread, and in patients with long-standing disease, skin cancers may develop. In certain cases the skin is so fragile and the skin sloughing so profound that open areas are subject to continual infection and death may occur. The most common variant of the disease is called epidermolysis bullosa simplex. Only the skin is affected and only to a limited degree. Blistering and skin separation mostly occurs over the elbows, fingers, and toes, and lesions are more common in warm weather. Healing is uneventful and without scarring.

Treatment is similar to that for any blister and includes keeping the area clean, covered, and coated with a layer of antibiotic ointment such as mupirocin or bacitracin. Keeping the patient in a cool, dry environment is also helpful. Careful surveillance for evidence of infection is important. Topical corticosteroids may relieve some discomfort but will not speed healing. Medications to prevent blistering are not available, although for some of the more severe variants of EB, phenytoin (Dilantin®) may be given to stimulate skin healing. Good nutrition and dental care are vital in persons with widespread disease. Patients with different subtypes of EB need to know the inheritance patterns for the disease since the possibility exists that they may pass it on to their children.

Dermatitis Herpetiformis (Duhring's Disease)

Dermatitis herpetiformis (DH) is an autoimmune disease found in young people, including children, which is inherited and associated with diet. Persons with DH have a high incidence of certain proteins on the surfaces of their bodies' cells. The profile of these proteins is inherited; most patients have a protein called HLA-B8. Additionally, a protein found in wheat, rye, and barley known as gluten may induce or aggravate DH in some patients. Dermatitis herpetiformis usually arises in young adults as very itchy, small red bumps on the elbows, buttocks, lower back, and knees. If left alone, many of these lesions will blister but finding one intact is rare, since they are so uncomfortable that patients usually excoriate them. There may be a burning sensation. The disease may be worsened by eating wheat-containing foods and beverages such as breads and beers. Iodide-containing substances and nonsteroidal pain relievers may also exacerbate DH. Some patients relate complaints of gastrointestinal symptoms such as diarrhea, gas, bloating, and pain but many have no symptoms at all. The disease is simply an aggravation in most persons but there is a small risk that in certain patients a lymphoma of the intestines may develop.

Avoidance of dietary gluten is important in therapy. Gluten-free diets, however, are unpopular due to the number of foods excluded from them. Several companies make gluten-free bread and cracker products. The most effective medication for DH is dapsone. This drug is occasionally used for diagnostic purposes in patients suspected of having this disease since one or two doses may effect a dramatic decrease in symptoms. Sulfapyridine is sometimes substituted for dapsone. This medication is inexpensive, easy to take, and safe for extended periods, however, there is some risk of certain types of anemia. Dapsone is given at 100 to 150 mg per day. Topical corticosteroids may help with itching and redness but oral preparations are not effective. Other immunosuppressants are not usually helpful. Colchicine and cholestyramine (Questran®) have also been used successfully.

Bullous Disease of Childhood

This is a blistering disease seen in children prior to puberty. Affected children average about five years of age. Large tense blisters similar to those of bullous pemphigoid develop in the groin and around the lower trunk. They are usually red and tissue breakdown with erosion and ulceration are seen. Scabbing, scaling, and itching are present. The mucous membranes may be involved, particularly in patients with lesions around the mouth. The disease is self-limited and will resolve within twenty-four months but may be very debilitating. It is not dangerous, but some lesions become infected, requiring antibiotic therapy. Dapsone and sulfapyridine are the most popular therapies, but the same risks and precautions must be addressed as when using them for adults. Oral corticosteroids are useful in some patients, and topical preparations may also play a role in treatment.

Subcorneal Pustular Dermatosis (Sneddon-Wilkinson Disease)

Subcorneal pustular dermatosis (SPD) is believed by some dermatologists to represent a variant of pustular psoriasis; others consider it one of the blistering diseases. SPD is more common in adult women before the age of forty. Lesions begin as small blisters which become cloudy as the pustules form. These blisters enlarge to form rings, some of which have clearing in their centers. Rings may be several inches in diameter. The surrounding skin is mildly red to normal in color. As the lesions resolve, they become crusted and thickened. The disease may subside for weeks or months only to become active again for unknown reasons. The groins, upper thighs, arm folds, neck, and under the breasts are most often affected. There is a characteristic burning pain along with modest itching. The disease may begin following an infection such as bronchitis or influenza. Dapsone and sulfapyridine are the drugs of choice and are given in the same manner as with dermatitis herpetiformis. Topical corticosteroids (particularly very potent preparations) may help with discomfort, but there is little role for oral corticosteroids in treatment. Acitretin (Soriatane®) may be helpful in certain patients.

Burns

Thermal burns or those from a source of intense heat such as a fire, scalding liquids, or a stove element are common. Most simply cause discomfort, but each year about 12,000 people die from their injuries. Burns have traditionally been divided into three categories:

1. A first degree burn, the most common, means that the most superficial parts of the skin have been damaged. The skin turns red and hairs have usually been singed but blisters do not form. Pain lasts for several days and healing takes place within a week or so; scarring does not occur.

2. Second degree burns are more serious. The damage extends into the underlying part of the skin called the dermis and blisters form. The skin is usually red but may blanche white. Healing takes between three to four weeks but scarring, if present, is usually minor. Pain is the biggest problem. If the wound is deep enough, a large scab called an eschar will form and healing may take months. In this case, the scarring may be significant.

3. Third degree burns have penetrated into the fat underlying the skin and may have gone through muscle all the way to the bone. The skin is usually blanched to pink and the wound itself may be black and charred. Healing is very slow and always involves significant scarring.

Most burns are of the first degree type and can be taken care of at home. It is important to remember that if the area which has been burned involves a sensitive organ such as the eyes, mouth, or genitalia, evaluation by a physician is in order. Otherwise, treatment is usually fairly easy since the problem will take care of itself in a few days. Putting the burned area under cold running water or applying ice packs helps relieve the swelling and discomfort. Acetaminophen (Tylenol®) or ibuprofen (Advil®, Motrin®) are good at blunting some of the pain, but in some instances patients may need more powerful analgesics such as codeine (Tylenol #3®) or hydrocodone (Vicodin®). Quick application of a very potent steroid cream or ointment within minutes of the burn may help slow down the inflammation and reduce the pain. Pramasone® cream or ointment has a mild numbing medicine and is also useful.

Second degree burns are the type most often seen in emergency rooms, since they cause blistering. Applying cold water compresses or ice bags is helpful but it is important to *not burst the blisters*. When the blisters are opened, the skin underneath has lost its protective covering. Burned patients are at risk of skin infections so keeping this covering intact is very crucial. If the blisters become too large and uncomfortable they may be drained with a sterile needle and then a thick coating of antibiotic ointment applied. The preferred antibiotic for covering burn wounds is silver sulfadiazine (Silvadene®) cream. Other antibiotic ointments such as bacitracin and mupirocin are also useful; these burns should be kept covered until they heal. Pain medications are usually appropriate. If the wound is severe enough, a skin graft may be necessary. This may be a substantial operation and require hospitalization. The use of a compound called Silastic® has greatly aided in the care of burns and burn patients. This is poured into the wound and allowed to "cure." It forms a hard covering under which the tissues can heal. At the time of grafting it is removed and the skin graft placed in the wound to heal it. Obviously, substantial scarring will take place both at the site of the burn and the area where the normal tissue was taken (the donor site). Research is developing techniques to allow pieces of laboratory-grown sterile skin to be applied to the burn with no donor site necessary.

Third degree burns are the most worrisome; they are considered medical emergencies. Patients are almost always hospitalized and many do not survive their wounds. Adults and the elderly have a higher mortality rate than do young people. A rule of thumb is that the risk of burn mortality is the sum of the patient's age and the percent of the body surface area involved. The major problem is either shock, in which the blood pressure gets extremely low, or infection after the patient has been hospitalized for several days. There are specialized burn units in most major medical centers designed to care for these patients. Providing an intact skin surface depends almost entirely on skin grafting.

Chemical burns need special treatment. Most chemical burns happen on the job and are usually treated by physicians familiar with the industry. The therapy for chemical burns usually involves application of a dilute acid if the burn is alkali in nature or dilute alkali if the offending substance is an acid. Since it may be difficult to immediately know whether the chemical is an acid or alkali, a good rule of thumb is to irrigate the area with large amounts of water while arrangements are being made to have the burn evaluated either in an emergency room or the plant infirmary. Burns caused by quicklime (calcium oxide) are an exception to this rule. Irrigating the area with water will cause the material to liquefy and worsen the burn.

Dermatitis

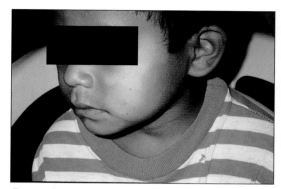

Figure 1 Pityriasis alba

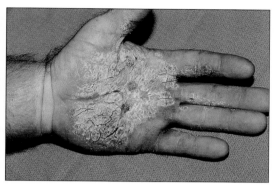

Figure 2 Hand dermatitis due to chromate allergy

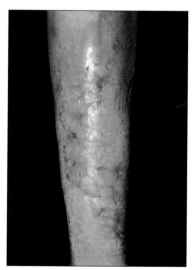

Figure 3 Winter itch ("eczema craquele")

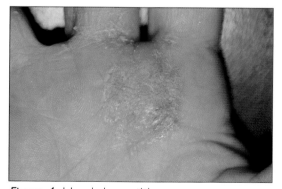

Figure 4 Hand dermatitis

Dermatitis

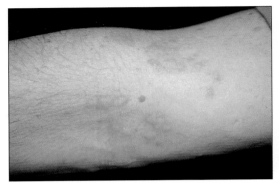

Figure 5 Contact dermatits from poison ivy

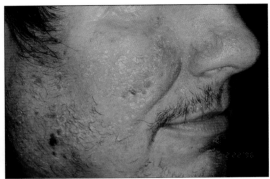

Figure 6 Seborrheic dermatitis

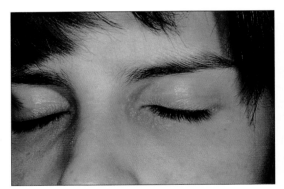

Figure 7 Eyelid dermatitis

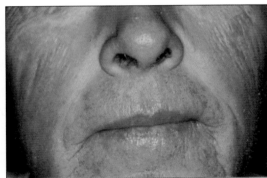

Figure 8 Photodermatitis

Skin Cancer

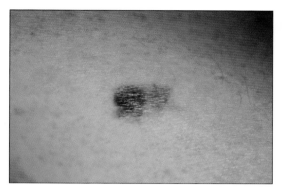

Figure 9 Melanoma

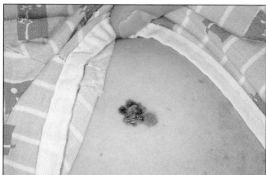

Figure 10 Melanoma

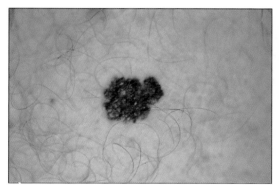

Figure 11 Lentigo maligna melanoma

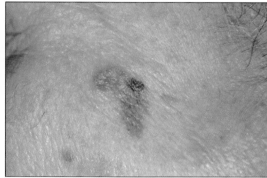

Figure 12 Lentigo maligna melanoma

Skin Cancer

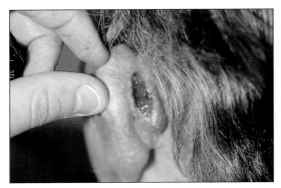

Figure 13 Basal cell carcinoma

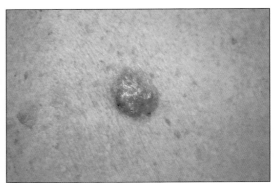

Figure 14 Basal cell carcinoma

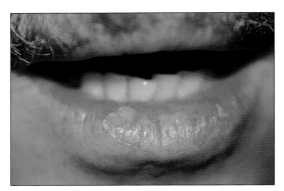

Figure 15 Squamous cell carcinoma

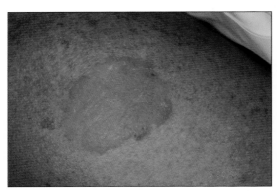

Figure 16 Bowen's disease (squamous cell carcinoma in situ)

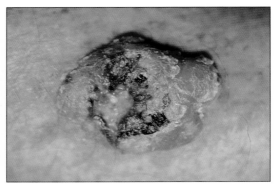

Figure 17 Squamous cell carcinoma

Skin Cancer

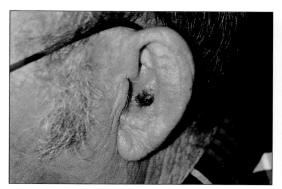
Figure 18 Squamous cell carcinoma

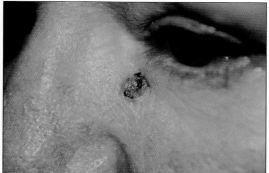
Figure 19 Basal cell carcinoma

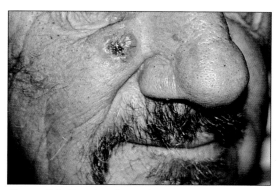
Figure 20 Basal cell carcinoma

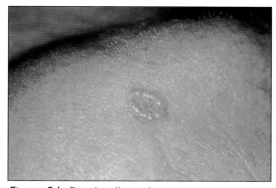
Figure 21 Basal cell carcinoma

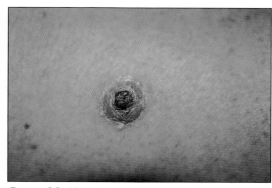
Figure 22 Keratoacanthoma

Skin Diseases and Conditions

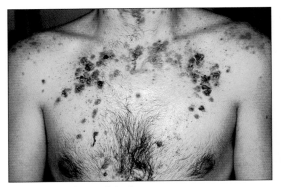

Figure 23 Acne fulminans

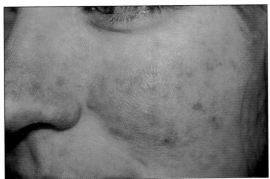

Figure 24 Acne rosacea

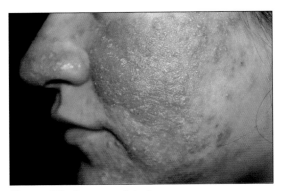

Figure 25 Rosacea fulminans

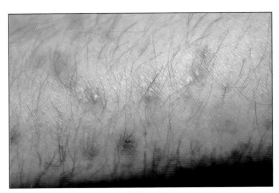

Figure 26 Bacterial folliculitis

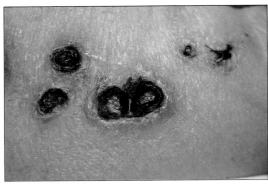

Figure 27 Echthyma (bacterial infection)

Skin Diseases and Conditions

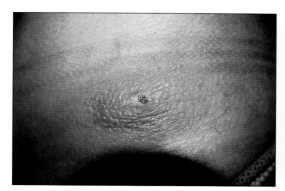

Figure 28 Furuncule (boil)

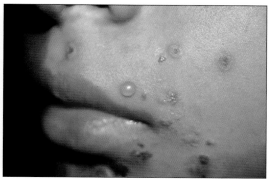

Figure 29 Impetigo (bacterial infection)

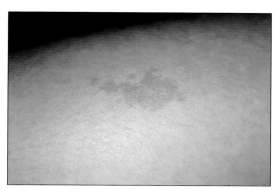

Figure 30 Café au lait macule (birthmark)

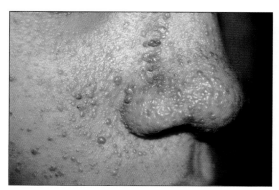

Figure 31 Adenoma sebaceum of tuberous sclerosis (blrthmark)

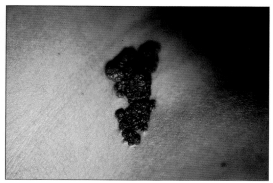

Figure 32 Epidermal nevus (blrthmark)

Skin Diseases and Conditions

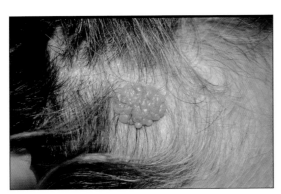

Figure 33 Nevus sebaceus (blrthmark)

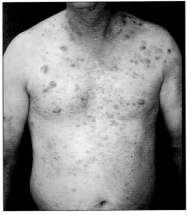

Figure 34 Pemphigus vulgaris (blistering disease)

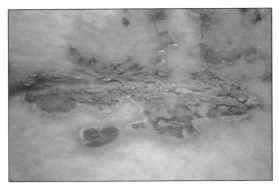

Figure 35 Benign familial pemphigus (Hailey-Hailey disease)

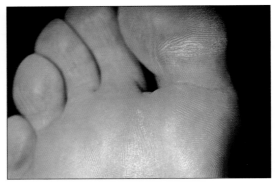

Figure 36 Callus

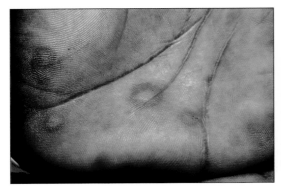

Figure 37 Erythema multiforme

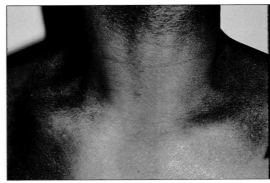

Figure 38 Erythema dyschromicum perstans ("ashy dermatosis")

Skin Diseases and Conditions

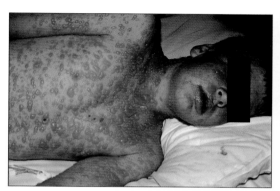

Figure 39 Stevens-Johnson syndrome

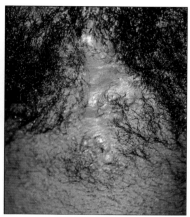

Figure 40 Folliculitis keloidalis

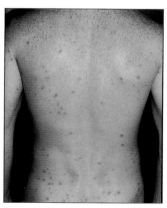

Figure 41 Hot tub folliculitis

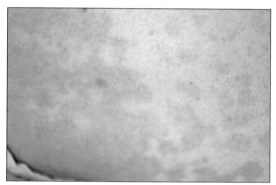

Figure 42 Tinea versicolor (skin fungus)

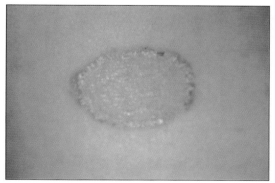

Figure 43 Ringworm (tinea corporis)

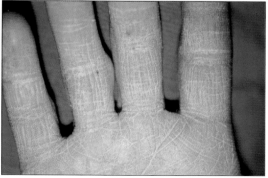

Figure 44 Fungal infection of the palms (tinea manum)

Skin Diseases and Conditions

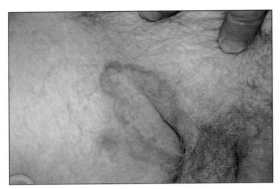

Figure 45 Jock itch (tinea cruris)

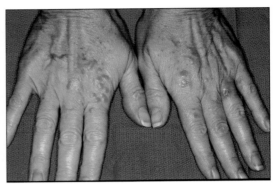

Figure 46 Granuloma annulare

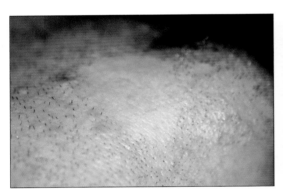

Figure 47 Alopecia areata

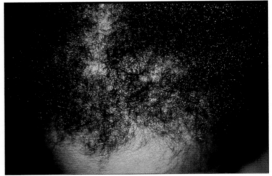

Figure 48 Traction alopecia

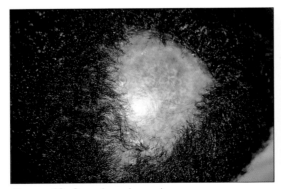

Figure 49 Scarring alopecia

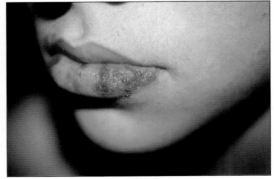

Figure 50 Herpes labialis (cold sore)

Skin Diseases and Conditions

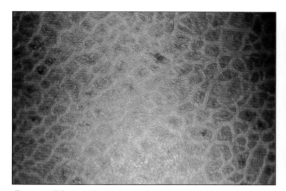

Figure 51 Ichthyosis vulgaris

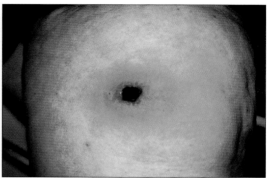

Figure 52 Brown recluse spider bite

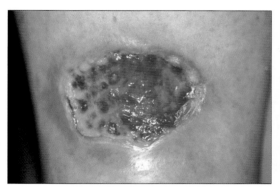

Figure 53 Leg ulcer

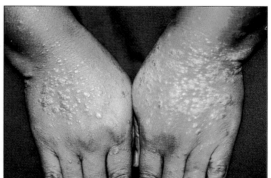

Figure 54 Lichen planus

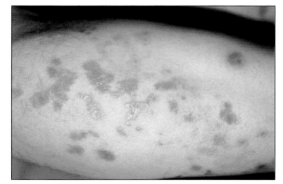

Figure 55 Lichen planus

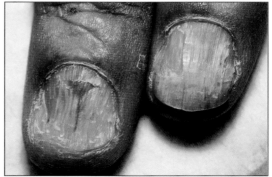

Figure 56 Lichen planus of the nails

Skin Diseases and Conditions

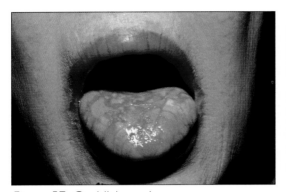

Figure 57 Oral lichen planus

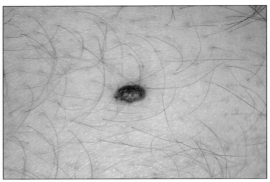

Figure 58 Senile angioma

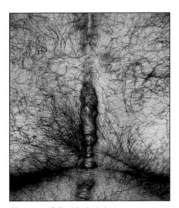

Figure 59 Keloid

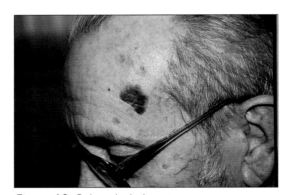

Figure 60 Seborrheic keratoses

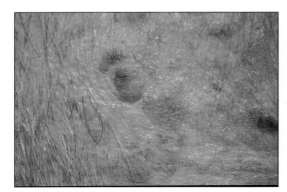

Figure 61 Seborrheic keratoses

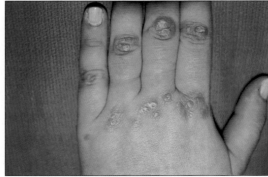

Figure 62 Gottren's papules of dermatomyositis (lupus)

Skin Diseases and Conditions

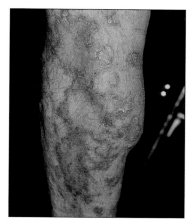

Figure 63 Subacute cutaneous lupus erythematosus

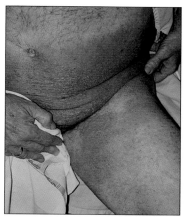

Figure 64 Mycosis fungoides (cutaneous T-cell lymphoma)

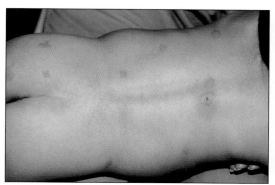

Figure 65 Mastocytomas

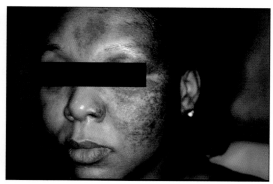

Figure 66 Nevus of Ota

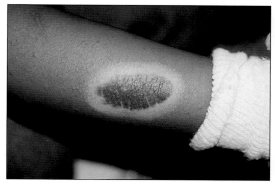

Figure 67 Halo around a congential nevus

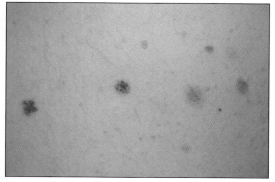

Figure 68 Dysplastic moles

Skin Diseases and Conditions

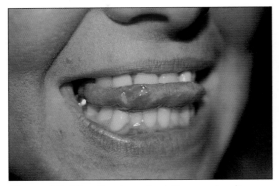

Figure 69 Mouth ulcer (aphthous ulcer)

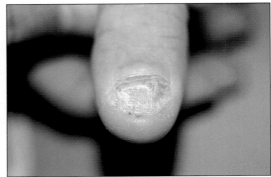

Figure 70 Fungal infection of the nails (onychomycosis)

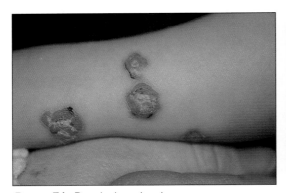

Figure 71 Psoriasis vulgaris

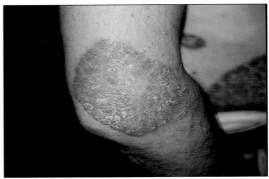

Figure 72 Psoriasis vulgaris

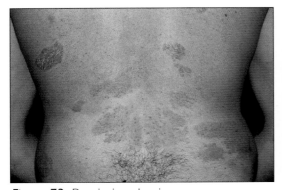

Figure 73 Psoriasis vulgaris

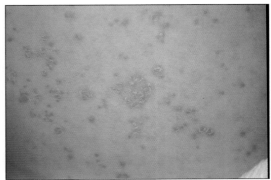

Figure 74 Guttate psoriasis

Skin Diseases and Conditions

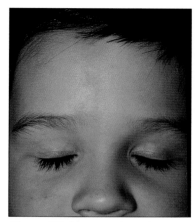

Figure 75 Linear scleroderma (coup de sabre)

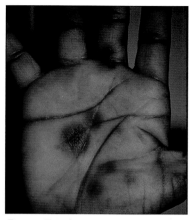

Figure 76 Secondary syphilis

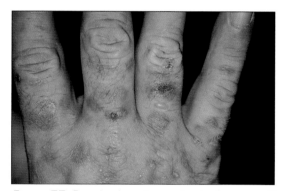

Figure 77 Porphyria cutanea tarda (sun sensitivity)

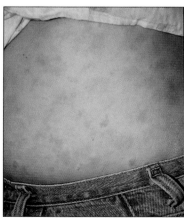

Figure 78 Urticaria (hives)

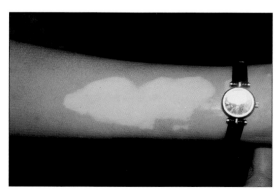

Figure 79 Vitiligo

Skin Diseases and Conditions

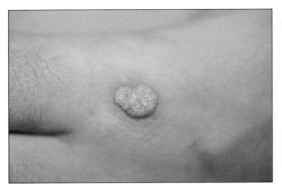

Figure 80 Verruca vulgaris (wart)

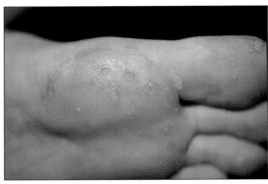

Figure 81 Verruca plantaris (plantar wart)

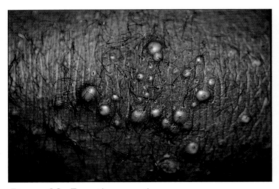

Figure 82 Eruptive xanthoma

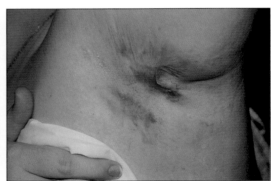

Figure 83 Hidradenitis suppurativa

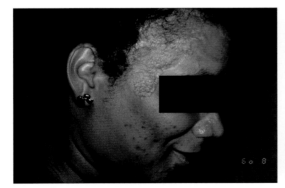

Figure 84 Sarcoidosis

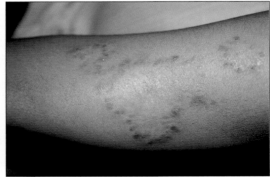

Figure 85 Sarcoidosis

Callus and Clavus

A callus occurs on the skin when it is subjected to friction. Calluses most typically are on the hands but may be on the feet. They protect the skin in that they prevent outside friction from making the skin peel and blister. A clavus (corn) occurs when pressure is applied to the skin, either from the outside or the inside. They are most common on the feet and between the toes. Hard corns are thick and tough; they are usually on top of the toes or on the balls of the feet. Soft corns usually occur between the toes, generally between the fourth and fifth digits. They are mushy with wet, soggy skin overlying them. Corns arise under areas where the bones or bone spurs are pushing from underneath the skin, and shoes, particularly those that do not fit well, are pushing from the outside. Corns can be painful and may limit one's choice of footwear. Women are affected more than men because of the types of shoes they wear. It's important to distinguish corns and calluses from plantar warts. Plantar warts usually have small black dots in them ("seeds") but corns and calluses do not.

Plasters are available to treat calluses. These are 40% salicylic acid (Sal-Acid Plaster®) and may be applied to the callus. They are cut to fit the skin being treated and are applied for twenty-four to forty-eight hours. When the tissue is soft after a bath or shower, a pumice stone or emery board may be used to gently scrape away the dead skin cells. Applying a pad around the callus protects the skin from friction and allows it to gradually subside. The easiest method for treating a callus is to pare it down using a very sharp blade such as a razor. Obviously, this must be done very carefully and if the treated skin is subjected to friction again, the callus will not be present to protect it.

There are a few more treatment options for corns. The lesions will subside on their own if the underlying bone problem is solved or if better-fitting footwear is used. One of the most popular methods of therapy is using circular "doughnuts." These may be purchased over the counter (Dr. Scholl's®) to protect the corn. Salicylic acid plasters also work very well and are used the same way as for calluses. Salicylic acid in solution (Occlusol HP®, Salactic® Film, Sal-Plant®) may also be used. Paring down corns is another option and may be done safely by a podiatrist or dermatologist.

An important point to remember for anyone with foot problems is that if diabetes is present, it is crucial to be careful when treating corns and calluses. Diabetic foot ulcers are occasionally an unintended complication of trying to remove these lesions at home. If a person with diabetes needs treatment for corns and calluses, the safest method is a consultation with a podiatrist or dermatologist.

CANDIDA INFECTIONS

Candida infections are caused by fungal organisms from the *Candida* family. The most common pathogen is *Candida albicans*, but there are numerous other members of this family that can cause infection in humans. These are often seen in persons who have a damaged immune system from cancer, chemotherapy, diabetes, genetic diseases, or HIV infection. Conditions that make persons susceptible to infection are listed in Table 21.

C. albicans is found in and on the mucous membranes of most people. Because it requires a somewhat moist environment, it is not commonly present on dry skin. Multiple factors hold this organism in check and prevent its excessive growth and involve the white blood cells and various proteins produced by the body. In the conditions listed in Table 21, something happens to alter this balance and the organisms begin to proliferate unchecked. In most healthy patients this is not a major problem; antifungal antibiotics are effective in clearing the infection. In persons who have very low white blood cell counts such as following chemotherapy, however, *Candida* infections may be fatal.

Symptoms

There are a number of different ways *Candida* may infect the skin and mucous membranes. One of the most common manifestations is intertrigo. Intertrigo may be due to organisms other than *Candida*. It occurs when an area of skin is subjected to moisture, such as perspiration, and then is occluded, usually by a fold of skin. Common areas include the skin under the breasts, in the folds of the groin, under the arm, and under overlapping folds of abdominal skin. These sites, particularly in warm weather and among diabetics or persons who sweat a lot, are prime areas for *Candida* infection. The affected skin becomes red with small spots at the edge of the rash. Mild scaling and buildup of dead skin are common. There may be itching or burning, but in many patients there are no symptoms. Odor may be mild to severe. Scraping exfoliated skin cells and examining them under the microscope will often show fungus.

Treatment usually involves oral antifungal medications such as ketoconazole (Nizoral®) and fluconazole (Diflucan®) taken for ten days or so. Terbenifine (Lamisil®) and itraconazole (Sporanox®) are also effective. Topical antifungal medications such as ketoconazole, econazole (Spectazole®), and clotrimazole (Lotrimin®) are helpful if applied sufficiently but this may prove difficult. Over-the-counter antifungal medications are unlikely to be effective. Prevention is the most important aspect of therapy. Weight loss, a cool environment, and use of loose-fitting clothing will help, as will control of any underlying diseases such as diabetes. Areas which are occluded by folds of skin should be dried completely after bathing. This may be accomplished using a handheld hair dryer placed on the cool setting. Dry the affected area as much as possible with a towel and then use the hair dryer to finish evaporating any residual moisture. Zeasorb® is an absorbent powder which may help keep the skin dry; Zeasorb AF® contains miconazole, a weak antifungal agent. These won't usually cure an active infection but are useful for prevention and may be used on almost any skin surface.

Other Forms of Infection

An unusual type of infection called a paronychia involves the nails and the tissues surrounding them. The cuticle and skin becomes red, swollen, and painful and may exude pus when pressure is applied. This disease is most common in persons whose hands are frequently or continually wet such as homemakers, bartenders, or fishermen. *Candida* organisms invade the skin and alter the formation of the nail so that it appears deformed. This condition may be acute, or can be chronic when the fingers are continually in wet environments. The ultimate therapy is avoidance. Treatment with topical antifungals is unlikely to be effective and oral medications are required.

Another common *Candida* infection is a type of diaper rash; this is covered in the section on diaper rash.

Candida most commonly presents itself in the mouth and mucous membranes. This is known as thrush or acute pseudomembranous candidiasis. It is usually seen in infants and newborns and in persons with deficient immune systems. Most people have white to gray material which builds up on the tongue, cheeks, and palate. It looks like stuck-on bits of food but when removed there is underlying redness and mild bleeding may occur. Other types of oral candidiasis are very red without buildup of material (atrophic candidiasis), or they demonstrate profound thickening of the tongue, which has a black discoloration (black hairy tongue). Atrophic candidiasis is commonly seen on the palate and gums of persons who wear dentures. Perleche is an irritation at the corners of the mouth that is due to *Candida* infection. This occurs most often in persons with poorly fitting dentures or redundant skin which overlaps and occludes the area; this keeps the area continually moist

Table 21 **CONDITIONS IN WHICH**
CANDIDA INFECTIONS ARE COMMON

Age extremes

Burns

Cancer

Diabetes

Down syndrome

HIV infection

Inherited immune deficiency diseases

Kidney failure

Malnutrition

Medications
    Antibiotics
    Birth control pills
    Chemotherapy
    Corticosteroids

Menstruation

Occlusion (clothing, dentures, excess skin, and so on)

Pregnancy

Radiation therapy

Thyroid failure

and creates an ideal breeding ground for yeast. The area is mildly red and scaly. None of these conditions are particularly uncomfortable but patients may experience some burning and irritation. Alteration in taste sensation is possible as well. Treatment centers around correcting ill-fitting dentures and redundant skin folds if possible and, more important, treatment of any underlying illnesses predisposing the patient to these conditions. Oral nystatin (Mycostatin®) suspension held in the mouth and swallowed four times daily is helpful. Drops may be used for infants and children. Nystatin is also made as a pastille. One or two of these may be placed in the mouth four to five times per day and allowed to slowly dissolve. A similar product made of clotrimazole (Mycelex® Troches) may be used. Oral ketoconazole and fluconazole may be required in more resistant cases. Itraconazole and terbenifine may also be effective but have not as yet been tested for this disease.

Candida infection is a common cause of vaginitis. Women experience itching and burning and sometimes painful urination. A discharge is common and may be very thick. This infection can spread to skin surrounding the labia and anus. Women with diabetes, who are pregnant, or who take birth control pills are particularly susceptible. Some patients have these infections repeatedly and are seemingly chronically infected. The sex partners of these women must be evaluated for evidence of *Candida* infection, since sexual transmission is possible. Treatment is with clotrimazole vaginal suppositories or a course of oral antifungal medications as for oral candidiasis. A similar disorder of the male genitalia may be present. This is seen as red spots with some scaling on the penis. Heaped-up debris as in thrush may also be present. In persons with underlying disease and occlusive clothing, the scrotum and groin may become infected, resulting in red, painful skin. Oral anti-Candidal preparations are usually effective but intermittent therapy may occasionally be needed to prevent recurrence.

An unusual and rare group of patients are those with chronic mucocutaneous candidiasis. This disease is actually a complex of diseases; their common theme is chronic and recurrent involvement of the skin, nails, and mucous membranes with *Candida.* The disease may begin in childhood. Patients have crusted, deformed nails and red, thickened skin lesions. *Candida* infections involving the mouth and mucous membranes are also seen. These patients are often otherwise well. Sometimes onset is in adulthood and is associated with underlying malignancies such as a thymoma, or disease of the endocrine system such as hypothyroidism or diabetes. Some patients have immune system deficiencies. Therapy almost always involves oral anti-Candidal medications, since topical therapy is unlikely to be effective. Most important is control of any underlying diseases.

Diaper Rash

Diaper rash is also called diaper dermatitis or napkin dermatitis. It is one of the most common skin eruptions in infants but may also be present in some adults, usually those wearing incontinence protection garments. In almost all cases it is merely an annoyance and associated with no worrisome diseases. There may be some instances, however, in which the child is uncomfortable to the point of being unable to urinate.

The most common type of diaper rash is due to the irritant effects on the skin of being in contact with a wet surface. There is a component of irritation caused by the urine but most of the problem results simply from wetness and friction of the skin as the child moves about. The areas subjected to friction are most affected. A subset of irritant diaper dermatitis is called Jacquet's dermatitis. In this disorder cutaneous nodules develop, some of which have begun to ulcerate. Diaper dermatitis due to irritation may very quickly improve or worsen.

Contact dermatitis also causes diaper rash. Irritant contact dermatitis is much more common than the allergic type. These may come from the use of harsh soaps, topical moisturizers, detergents, and medicinal creams or ointments. The folds of the skin tend to be spared since they are protected to some extent. Patients may be uncomfortable, especially if the skin begins to ulcerate.

One of the most common types of diaper dermatitis is due to *Candida* infection (see section on candida infections). Other fungi such as those that cause athlete's foot or jock itch may also involve the diaper area but are much less usual than *Candida*. This disease occasionally occurs after a course of antibiotics for an upper respiratory infection. The bacteria which hold these fungi in check are destroyed and the *Candida* finds a home in the moist, covered areas under the diaper. The skin may show deep red, raised areas with scale and small pustules. The presence of these pustules several inches away from the main body of the rash is a key finding. Thrush in the mouth may also be present. The diagnosis may be made from a scraping of the skin.

Other varieties of diaper dermatitis are more rare. Seborrheic dermatitis is generally considered a type of atopic dermatitis (eczema) and in children may involve the diaper area. There is usually evidence of involvement elsewhere, such as the scalp and face. This rash is less red and the child less uncomfortable. The scale in seborrheic dermatitis is thick and possesses a "greasy" character. Psoriasis in infants may occur in the diaper area and is often seen elsewhere including the nails.

Intertrigo is an infection by bacteria of sodden and irritated skin. The skin is weepy and may ulcerate. Intertrigo commonly occurs in hot weather and when children wear too many clothes.

Several nutritional deficiencies can cause diaper dermatitis, including zinc deficiency (acrodermatitis enteropathica) and biotin deficiency.

Treatment of diaper dermatitis may be simple and effective or difficult and frustrating depending on the child and the cause of the skin irritation. Frequent diaper changes prevent continuous contact with wet diapers and are the mainstay of therapy. Allowing the child to remain without a diaper is very helpful but not always feasible. Dusting powders such as Zeasorb® are useful; they allow for absorption of moisture and diminish the friction between the skin and the diaper. It does not seem to make much difference whether cloth or disposable diapers are used. Creams containing zinc oxide may help protect the skin and allow healing. *Candida* infections are best treated with topical antifungal agents such as nystatin (Mycostatin®). If there is a bacterial infection such as in intertrigo, antibiotics will be required but these may worsen a *Candida* infection. If the dermatitis is particularly severe, as with Jacquet's dermatitis, application of wet compresses may help (see the section on wet dressings). Topical corticosteroids are generally not useful. Hydrocortisone will diminish the irritation but potent preparations may make the dermatitis worse and can be absorbed into the bloodstream. Preparations containing an antifungal medication and topical corticosteroid (Lotrisone®, Mycolog®) should not be used.

Erythema Multiforme, Stevens-Johnson Syndrome, and Toxic Epidermal Necrolysis

These three diseases are closely related. With these conditions, the skin becomes red and is reacting to some outside force or influence. Usually, this outside influence is a medication or infection that has nothing to do with the skin. These diseases have been present since antiquity but only recently have their effects on the skin become better understood. Recovery is complete for most patients, but the disease may recur in some persons and can be fatal in others. Diagnosis of these conditions is sometimes difficult and skin biopsies are usually performed.

Erythema Multiforme

Erythema multiforme (EM) is responsible for about 1 percent of visits to dermatologists. Most patients are under age fifty, but disease in children is unusual. Men are more commonly affected than are women. Incidence of the disease increases in spring and fall.

Symptoms

Lesions are classically found on the palms and soles as red spots with the appearance of a "target" or an "iris." The extremities are involved more than the trunk. Other lesions appear as red nodules or blisters. The mucous membranes of the mouth and genitalia may show some lesions but extensive involvement usually denotes Stevens-Johnson syndrome (SJS). The spots will resolve in a few days if the inciting cause is corrected. Some crusting and scaling may be present. Patients may also experience fever, fatigue, swollen lymph nodes, and/or symptoms of an upper respiratory infection such as cough, runny nose, or sneezing. The skin eruption arises quickly and spreads in crops. The lesions may itch or burn, but some patients have no symptoms at all. If the inciting cause is not corrected or discovered, this cycle of skin eruption may occur with regularity; some persons experience as many as a dozen or more episodes per year.

Causes

As mentioned, the cause of EM is usually a medication or infection. The list of medications that can provoke this disease is essentially endless. The most common culprits include allopurinol (Zyloprim®), barbiturates, penicillin and penicillinlike drugs (cephalosporins), antiseizure drugs, sulfa drugs, and oral antidiabetes medications. The most common infection is herpes simplex. This may occur after a fever blister or outbreak of genital herpes. Typically the eruption of EM follows the fever blister by ten to fourteen days. The second most common infectious cause is pneumonia due to *Mycoplasma* organisms ("walking pneumonia"). Infections with different bacteria, fungi, parasites, and viruses have also been implicated in EM. Other precipitants of this disease include autoimmune diseases such as lupus erythematosus, leukemias, and lymphomas, and endocrine factors such as pregnancy or menstrual periods. In a number of patients, no precipitating cause can be determined. Some dermatologists believe that these patients actually have an active herpes simplex infection somewhere in the body for which there is no evidence. When the infection flares, the erythema multiforme recurs.

Therapy

Treatment of this disease is somewhat controversial. Many dermatologists find that a short course of oral steroids such as prednisone (Deltasone®) or an injection of triamcinolone (Kenalog®) is helpful for acute symptoms. In some instances, however, the EM remains the same when the medications are stopped. In this case, a long-term course of steroids must be considered. There is no evidence that these medications help eradicate the disease more quickly and many dermatologists do not use them. Topical steroids, on the other hand, may be very helpful in alleviating the symptoms and making the lesions appear less red and angry. They are also useful in controlling the blisters that sometimes occur with EM. Medications causing the disease should be discontinued, if possible, and all infections must be addressed with appropriate measures. For persons with recurrent disease, some dermatologists prescribe acyclovir (Zovirax®) to be taken prophylactically. This is continued for six to twelve months. If the patient remains free of disease the medication is discontinued.

Stevens-Johnson Syndrome

This syndrome is often called "erythema multiforme major" to distinguish it from routine erythema multiforme. As the name suggests, this condition has some of the same signs and symptoms as EM but is usually much worse. The disease is most common in younger patients. Most severe cases seem to be in children and young adults.

Symptoms

About half of affected patients experience a viral-like illness before onset of the skin eruption. Symptoms include fever, loss of appetite, headache, nausea and vomiting, cough, and sore throat. This may last up to two weeks. The skin findings are similar to that for EM but tend to be more widespread. Blistering and oozing is possible, and pain, itching, and burning are present. The most important aspect of SJS is the involvement of the mucous membranes. This is usually widespread, severe, and explosive. Painful erosions and blisters may be seen on virtually all mucous membranes, making eating and drinking difficult or impossible. Some internal organs may also be affected.

Causes
The causes of SJS are similar to those for EM. Medications, particularly sulfa drugs, are the most common culprits. Antiseizure drugs, antibiotics, and anti-inflammatory medications are also known to cause SJS.

Therapy
Therapy commonly involves hospitalization, frequently in the burn unit since these physicians and nurses are experienced in dealing with patients afflicted by the loss of large amounts of skin. Persons with SJS usually have difficulty eating and drinking so dehydration quickly becomes a problem. Intravenous fluids are usually given in large amounts. There is controversy as to whether administering steroids is helpful or harmful in SJS. While these drugs decrease the associated inflammation and discomfort, they may also make the person more susceptible to infection. Avoidance of precipitating medications and treatment of inciting infections is important.

Stevens-Johnson syndrome takes longer to recover from than EM. Patients usually require three to six weeks to clear the skin and for many it is months before they completely return to normal. There is about a 10 percent mortality rate from the disease, usually from infections that arise when so much of the skin's protective properties are lost. Scarring may take place, particularly on and around mucosal surfaces. Rehabilitation services may be required.

Toxic Epidermal Necrolysis

Toxic epidermal necrolysis (TEN) is a severe form of skin loss that usually results from a drug allergy. Sulfa drugs, allopurinol (Zyloprim®), antiseizure medications, and anti-inflammatory drugs are the most common culprits. Infections are much less likely to induce TEN, but in some cases no cause can be found. Affected patients often have kidney disease; this may prevent them from excreting medications that bother their skin.

Symptoms

The skin initially become red and tender. Over the following hours and days there is a "shedding" of the skin in large sheets. Some small blisters may be seen. Patients experience burning and significant discomfort. Secondary bacterial infection is common and contributes to a 20 percent mortality rate. TEN may be explosive, with the skin going from normal to almost total blistering in twenty-four to thirty-six hours. Other body systems are involved including the heart, lungs, kidneys, and gastrointestinal tract.

Therapy

Patients are usually treated in burn units and hospitalization may be extensive and complicated. Treatment is essentially the same as for SJS, with careful attention paid to the prevention and early treatment of any signs of infection. If the patient is kept in good health, the skin will recover in a few weeks. Scarring may be extensive and rehabilitation is required by some patients.

FOLLICULITIS

Inflammation of a hair follicle or follicles is called folliculitis. Some types of folliculitis such as eosinophilic, pityosporum, and furuncles/carbuncles have been discussed elsewhere in this text.

Bacterial Folliculitis

This disease is somewhat like furuncles in that it involves *Staphylococcus aureus* infection of a hair follicle. In folliculitis, however, the disease is not so deep or uncomfortable. Folliculitis begins with redness and mild swelling of the skin around a hair follicle. Over time, a small pustule may occur but "blackheads" are not seen. The trunk and proximal extremities are most often involved. Folliculitis is a particular problem in persons with a lot of hair. There are two forms of folliculitis, superficial (Bockhart's folliculitis) and deep (sycosis barbae). The latter principally involves the face and neck. This infection is relatively benign and may be effectively treated with cephalosporins, erythromycin (PCE®), clarithromycin (Biaxin®), and penicillins such as dicloxacillin (Dycill®) or cloxacillin. Long-term use of tetracyclines (Sumycin®) and antibacterial soaps are effective in persons prone to develop folliculitis. Topical erythromycin (ATS®), clindamycin (Cleocin®), and mupirocin (Bactroban®) may also be useful. Hot packs are helpful for symptomatic relief in the deep variant of folliculitis but antibiotics are faster and more effective. Scarring is seen with sycosis barbae but not in superficial folliculitis.

Hot Tub Folliculitis

An unusual variant of folliculitis is known as "hot tub" folliculitis. This is caused by a gram-negative bacteria (*Pseudomonas aeruginosa*) found in contaminated hot tubs. Red, swollen lesions arise around the follicles on the trunk and extremities. They itch and may be painful. They arise several days after the use of a hot tub or jacuzzi; however, public swimming pools or dirty whirlpools may also provoke this disease. The folliculitis will resolve on its own in one to two weeks but ciprofloxacin (Cipro®), lomefloxacin (Maxaquin®), floxacin (Floxin®), and enoxacin (Penetrex®) are all effective against the bacteria and will cure the disease faster.

Gram-Negative Folliculitis

Gram-negative folliculitis occurs in patients with acne who have been on antibiotics, particularly tetracycline, for prolonged periods. Follicles around the nose and mouth and on the neck and trunk are affected. The involved follicles are red and demonstrate pustules. Culture of the material in the follicles may be helpful. Treatment with isotretinoin (Accutane®) is usually very effective. The problem antibiotics must be discontinued and are usually replaced with medications effective against gram-negative bacteria such as amoxicillin-clavulanic acid (Augmentin®) or trimethoprim-sulfamethoxazole (Bactrim®). Theoretically, the same drugs used for hot tub folliculitis should be effective in this disease.

Demodex Folliculitis

The demodex mites, *Demodex folliculorum* and *Demodex brevis*, are common inhabitants of the skin in adults. They live in the follicles and oil glands and, for the most part, have no effect on a person's health. Some patients, however, develop an inflammation of affected follicles, usually on the face. Most are older women who have been applying thick, occlusive creams. Redness develops around the hair follicles and some pustules may be seen. The rash feels like the surface of a nutmeg grater. Mild itching may be present. Inflammation of the eyelids with scaling and redness may also be present. The diagnosis is made by gently scraping some of the inflamed follicles and looking for mites under the microscope. Discontinuing the offending creams will help, but some dermatologists use antiscabies medications such as permethrin cream (Elimite®) for a few days.

Acne Varioliformis and Acne Necrotica Miliaris

These variants of folliculitis are seen on the scalp. In acne varioliformis (AV), small pustules develop on the scalp, usually at the back. Men are more commonly affected than women and patients are usually middle aged. Some mild itching may be present. The diagnosis may be confirmed by a biopsy but this usually is not necessary. Treatment consists of tetracycline or tetracycline-type antibiotics. Isotretinoin has also been helpful. Topical antibiotics may be useful but are not usually the first treatment of choice.

Acne necrotica miliaris (ANM) is probably a variant of AV. It is seen most often in older men. The number of lesions are less than with AV and the symptoms are problematic. There is itching and burning. Crusting is common, and if the lesions are constantly scratched, there may be mild ulceration. Biopsies can aid in making the diagnosis. Treatment is difficult; tetracyclines and other oral antibiotics are occasionally helpful but fail in many patients. Isotretinoin is considered the drug of choice; the medication is given at the same doses as for acne and for the same length of time.

Perforating Folliculitis of the Nose

The involved follicles in this disorder are at the tip of the nose. Painful lesions are initially found in the cavity of the nose and some pus may be present. In some cases, the infection tracks along the root of the hair and is seen on the *external* skin of the nose. This appears as a red bump which eventually shows some pus and inflammation. Removal of the involved hairs and application of topical antibiotic cream (bacitracin and mupirocin) are the best means of therapy.

Stye

This is also called a hordeolum and is technically an inflammation of the hair follicles along the margin of the eyelid. A red, tender swelling arises in this area and a pustule may be present. Crusting of the eye may also occur. Some patients have chronic problems with mild redness and scaling of the eyelids (blepharitis); this is thought to play a role in these lesions. Treatment consists of applying warm (not hot) compresses to the area. Application for a few minutes per hour is the preferred method. This should cause the stye to "point," or drain. Application of antibiotic ointments to the area is also helpful, but must be selected carefully since some of the ointment will invariably get into the eye. Trying to "burst" or "pop" the stye is discouraged; this may cause the surrounding skin to become more inflamed.

Fungal Infections of the Skin

There are many different types of fungal infections involving the skin but only the most common will be discussed here. The most prevalent type of infection is from a group of fungi known as dermatophytes. These fungi have received this name because of their preference for infecting the skin, hair, and nails. There are some reports of these fungi infecting internal organs, but this is rare and usually occurs in people who have a poorly functioning immune system (patients with cancer, AIDS, taking chemotherapy, and so on). There are more than twenty-five different dermatophyte organisms but all are members of three families known as *Epidermophyton*, *Microsporum*, and *Trichophyton*. Some of these fungi prefer to live on animals, some in the ground and on vegetation, and some on humans. Infection with dermatophytes is encouraged by hot weather, high humidity, occlusion of the skin, and probably most important, a suitable host. The fungi that cause these infections can be found just about everywhere, so coming into contact with them is probably a daily occurrence. These infections commonly go by the name "tinea." A word of caution: If these infections are treated with topical corticosteroid preparations, they will likely become less red and scaly but the corticosteroid will not get rid of the infection. In fact, it will cause it to worsen. While this is not dangerous, it does delay treatment and cure.

Athlete's Foot (Tinea Pedis)

This infection involves the soles and webs between the toes. Infection of the palms (tinea mannum) is also caused by the same organisms. One in ten people have these infections at any given time. Symptoms include mildly red and scaly skin. Some people have a "moccasin" type of rash that extends up the sides of their feet. Heaped-up dead skin with ulcers may be seen between the toes. Sometimes this is such a problem that infection by a bacteria is found as well. Some patients have mild blistering; itching is occasionally a problem, but often patients have no symptoms at all and may not know they are infected. Despite its name, this disease is not more common in athletes. It is rare in children before puberty. A diagnosis may be made by scraping some of the loose skin onto a glass slide and looking at it under the microscope. Sometimes cultures of the skin scraping are done but these often take weeks or months to grow and are expensive.

Treatment

Topical antifungal creams and lotions (see Table 22) are useful in helping to clear the skin but are usually too weak to do so by themselves. Most patients have to be given oral medications. Previously, the only suitable drug was griseofulvin (Gris-PEG®) and patients had to take multiple daily doses for months. Even so, treatment failures were a common occurrence. Recently, however, there have been better medications developed and cures are more likely. Ketoconazole (Nizoral®), itraconazole (Sporanox®), fluconazole (Diflucan®), and terbenifine (Lamisil®) are oral medications that can be used to treat these infections. Washing the skin with antifungal shampoos such as selenium sulfide (Selsun®) and ketoconazole (Nizoral Shampoo®) will probably not cure an infection but may prevent its recurrence once the fungus has been eliminated. If a bacterial infection is present between the toes it must also be treated.

Because the fungi that cause these diseases are so prevalent, it is difficult to prevent infection or reinfection. Routine washing with antifungal soaps/shampoos and application of antifungal dusting powders (Zeasorb AF®) can be useful. Some dermatologists give patients a short prophylactic course of oral medications every few months. Some patients with athlete's foot have significant sweating of the feet; because they are always wet they are more susceptible to tinea pedis. Frequent sock changes can help and some topical medications such as aluminum chloride (Drysol®) may decrease sweating.

Ringworm (Tinea Corporis)

Ringworm is a common name for a dermatophyte infection of the skin (tinea corporis). This disease has nothing to do with an infection from a worm—the infecting organisms are fungi. It derives its name from the fact that the skin lesions are round or ring shaped. These occur on the skin of the arms, legs, and trunk. Lesions are usually circular and red with some scaling. Itching is usually mild. In the center of these circles there may be a return of the skin to normal color and consistency. Sometimes infection of hair follicles occurs and appears as red bumps. The surrounding skin may or may not be red and flaky. Scraping the scale off and examining it under the microscope will usually show organisms. Tinea barbae is a subset of tinea corporis. It involves the beard area and affects only males.

Treatment is essentially the same as for tinea pedis with one exception. If the infection is not too extensive and doesn't involve the hair follicles, a cure may be effected using only topical medicines. Oral medications are more effective, however, and are more likely to completely rid the skin of the infection. Again, the fungi that cause this disease are so widespread that prevention is difficult. The patient may

Table 22 TOPICAL ANTIFUNGAL AGENTS

Generic	Brand
Ciclopirox	Loprox®
Clotrimazole	Lotrimin®
Econazole	Spectazole®
Ketoconazole	Nizoral®
Naftifine	Naftin®
Oxiconazole	Oxistat®
Sulconazole	Exelderm®
Terbenifine	Lamisil®

have picked up the infection from a cat or dog in the home. Having animals checked by a veterinarian may be helpful. Avoiding contact with known infected items or persons can help, as can prophylactic use of antifungal shampoos such as selenium sulfide or ketoconazole.

Nail Fungus (Tinea Unguim/Onychomycosis)

Fungus infection of the nails is very common. Between 5 and 10 percent of the population has an infected nail at some time in their lives. One-third of persons with fungal disease affecting other body sites also have nail involvement. Almost all cases occur in adults. While this is not a life-threatening illness, it may be painful and does cause a substantial degree of psychological trauma since fingernails are exposed in public. Dermatophyte organisms cause most of these infections, but yeasts such as *Candida* and others may also be responsible. Occlusive footwear and trauma are believed to predispose a person to infection, but there likely is an inherited susceptibility as well. There are different types of nail fungal infections but the most common show crumbling and distortion of the nail. Discoloration may also be prominent and is classically yellow-brown. Nails are thickened and may be difficult to clip. The nail may separate from the underlying skin back toward the cuticle and in some cases falls off altogether. Diagnosis is usually made by scraping the nail debris and either looking at it under a microscope, culturing it, or both.

Treatment is essentially restricted to oral antifungal agents. Topical creams and lotions are easy to use and safe but almost never potent enough to get into the crevices of the diseased nail and destroy the fungus. There is one exception to this rule: Topical terbenifine cream in some instances may clear a nail infection by itself. Over-the-counter medicines are essentially useless. The standard treatment until recently has been oral griseofulvin for six to eighteen months. While this may be effective, there is a high failure rate and many patients are unwilling to undertake such a regimen. Ketoconazole, itraconazole, fluconazole, and terbenifine are all very effective when given orally and there are several different schedules for administering these drugs. Some dermatologists surgically remove the nail and begin the patient on oral antifungal antibiotics. This allows the nail to regrow in a fungus-free environment. Whatever the treatment, there is a good chance that the fungus will return, so prophylactic use of creams or courses of antifungal antibiotics is recommended.

Hair Infections (Tinea Capitis)

Infections of the hair and scalp are not as common as they once were. Previously, infection of the scalp by one of the more aggressive dermatophytes could result in such a degree of inflammation that as the infection cleared significant scarring occurred and the patient would be left with permanent hair loss. The introduction of griseofulvin to treat these infections has significantly reduced the incidence of this disease. Tinea capitis was and remains largely an infection of children, and boys are more often affected than girls. Uninfected persons may carry the dermatophytes and infect other susceptible persons.

Tinea capitis presents in several different ways on the scalp. The classic infection is a large raised area with ulcerated skin and scabbing. This area of inflammation is called a kerion. Some patients have a patch of scalp with hair loss and "black dots" on the skin. These "dots" harbor the fungus. Other patients show simple hair loss with some mild scaling. There may be pain and itching depending on the degree of inflammation. Swollen and tender lymph nodes in the neck are common. Diagnosis involves obtaining some of the infected hairs and either examining them under the microscope or culturing them, since the inflamed skin, scabs, and pus do not normally have large numbers of fungal organisms. Holding a fluorescent lamp called a Wood's lamp over the affected area may show fluorescence of certain fungal species.

Treatment involves dealing with both the fungus and the bacterial infection that usually involves the surrounding skin. Since most cases of tinea capitis occur in children, the mainstay of therapy has been liquid griseofulvin (Grifulvin V®). This works reasonably well but has to be given for six to eight weeks, so some treatment failures occur when the drug is not given for the full course. There has been some success using a large single dose of the drug. Some strains of fungus are resistant to griseofulvin and oral ketoconazole must be used. There is no children's suspension of this drug but it may be compounded by a pharmacist. Oral fluconazole (which does come in a suspension), itraconazole, and terbinafine are also very effective. Since the infection is so deep seated, there is usually little help from topical antifungal lotions or creams. Oral antibiotics such as cephalexin (Keflex®) or amoxicillin/clavulanic acid (Augmentin®) are usually sufficient to eliminate contaminating bacteria. The inflammatory reaction may be so severe that the dermatologist will give the patient several days of prednisone therapy to calm the reaction. Scarring usually occurs at the infection site and hair loss may be permanent.

Antifungal shampoos (ketoconazole, selenium sulfide) may be used by family members who might be infected or are carriers of the disease. Objects which come into contact with patients such as clothing, hats, toys, telephones, and so on can spread disease and these objects should be disinfected.

Jock Itch (Tinea Cruris)

Tinea cruris is a dermatophyte fungal infection involving the groins and genitalia. It is almost exclusively a disease of men. The affected area is red and scales are seen on the leading edge of the rash. It typically involves the inner aspects of the thighs but can extend around to the buttocks. The shaft of the penis and the scrotum are almost never affected. Tinea cruris occurs in warmer months when sweating increases, in persons who wear occlusive clothing, and in individuals with fungal infections elsewhere, such as the feet and nails. Itching is the most common symptom but if the infection is severe, there may be pain as well.

Treatment is the same as for tinea corporis, although topical medications may play a greater role in jock itch. Dusting the skin with absorptive powder containing antifungal medicines (Zeasorb-AF®) may help prevent a recurrence.

Tinea Versicolor (Pityriasis Versicolor)

This is a fungal infection that involves the trunk, upper arms, and neck. It usually occurs in the warmer months and especially in areas with high humidity. This is not caused by a dermatophyte but by a yeast called *Pityosporon*. This fungus is normally found on the skin. For unknown reasons, in certain patients it begins to infect the skin's uppermost layer. It is commonly discovered when affected skin fails to tan with sun exposure. The skin is darkened with mild scaling, and there are no other symptoms except for occasional mild itching. Diagnosis is accomplished by examining skin scrapings under the microscope.

There are numerous treatments for tinea versicolor. Ketoconazole given in a single dose or for a few days is usually effective. Selenium sulfide shampoo may be curative when applied to the affected areas for about five minutes twice a week. Ketoconazole shampoo can be used the same way. Ketoconazole cream will work but there may be such a large area to cover that application of sufficient medicine may be too expensive. Itraconazole and fluconazole when given by mouth are also successful.

Sporotrichosis

This disease is different from the others previously discussed in that the fungus is not a dermatophyte or yeast, and it infects deeper parts of the skin. Sporotrichosis is caused by *Sporothrix schenckii*, an organism that lives on plants and in the soil. Persons infected with it have usually been active outdoors (gardening, hiking, and so on). This disease is very common in Africa and South America but infections are reported in the United States as well. While there are several different forms of sporotrichosis, the most common involves an initial area of infection that spreads up an extremity. The initial site of infection becomes red and develops into a hard nodule. It turns somewhat dark and may break down. In the following weeks, new lesions appear up the arm or leg and go through the same cycle as the initial spot. Variations include a type with only a single lesion and one in which multiple nodules with crusts break out over wide surface areas of the body. A diagnosis may be made if the patient can relate some risk factors for infection (for example, working in the garden, getting stuck with a plant thorn, and so on). Skin biopsies may help with the diagnosis but the organisms are usually few in the tissue and easy to miss on examination. Culturing some of the infected tissue can also help but is time consuming and requires special culture media.

Treatment has for many years centered around using oral potassium iodide in gradually increasing doses. This has to be continued for about a month. Amphotericin B (Fungizone®) is effective but an unpleasant medication. Interestingly, application of heat to the infected skin has been shown to help eradicate the fungus. Itraconazole is probably the drug of choice since it is easy to take, has few side effects, and is very effective. Ketoconazole may also be helpful.

Granuloma Annulare

Granuloma annulare (GA) is an eruption with several different symptoms or manifestations and for which a definite cause has not been found. Fortunately, there are few symptoms and the eruption tends to subside on its own. The rash, however, may be cosmetically disfiguring.

Symptoms

Granuloma annulare occurs in younger patients, particularly children. Women are affected twice as often as men. There are several different variants of the disease. Localized GA consists of a single lesion or perhaps a few. These typically arise on the hands, feet, arms, and legs, but symptoms are rare. The lesions are red to pink and slightly thickened. They are raised and circular or ringed. They vary in size from that of a pencil eraser to a silver dollar. If they are large enough, some clearing of the skin in the center of the lesion will occur. This gives the lesions a targetlike appearance. Persons with multiple (usually more than ten) lesions may have generalized GA. This form of the disease usually occurs in children and older adults. Hundreds to thousands of lesions may be seen over the entire body, including the head and neck. Generalized GA may be associated with diabetes or underlying cancer. Most lesions are small and may not be as red or pink as with localized disease. Subcutaneous granuloma annulare occurs as deep lumps in the skin. It is usually present on the extremities and scalp. The lesions are without symptoms and are usually about the size of a pea. Some redness may be present, but most sites are skin colored. Most types of GA may be diagnosed with a simple skin biopsy.

Causes

The cause of granuloma annulare is not clear. There are some relationships to diabetes and rheumatoid arthritis but these diseases are certainly not seen in all persons with GA. It has been reported to follow insect bites, sun exposure, and viral infections but a clear-cut cause of GA has not been found. It is likely that the skin is reacting to some provocation and does so by forming the typical skin lesions. There is evidence that the body's immune system is involved in producing the rash.

Treatment

The treatment options are numerous. Many persons do not want or require therapy since the skin lesions will eventually disappear with time. Persons with numerous or disfiguring lesions usually require treatment. Oral corticosteroids are useful but have too many side effects for prolonged use. If there are few lesions, corticosteroid injections are helpful as is the topical application of very potent corticosteroid creams. PUVA therapy (the combination of *P*soralens and *U*ltraviolet Light A—see section on psoriasis) has been used successfully but is expensive and time consuming. Numerous systemic medications have been shown to be successful in some patients including pentoxifylline (Trental®), nicotinamide, isotretinoin (Accutane®), hydroxychloroquine (Plaquenil®), potassium iodide, dipyridamole (Persantine®), dapsone, and chlorambucil (Leukeran®). These medications have a variety of side effects and the benefits of treatment must outweigh the side effects of their use.

HAIR LOSS AND HAIR DISEASES

Hair disorders and diseases are common reasons to visit the dermatologist, making up about 5 percent of patient visits. There has been significant research in the area of hair diseases in the past decade and the medications and surgical procedures available to help these patients have considerably improved. The body is capable of producing several different types of hair but the most common is called a terminal hair. These hairs are found over most body surface areas except for mucous membranes and the palms and soles. They are thick, pigmented, and large. They grow at varied rates depending on their anatomic locations and many are very sensitive to hormonal changes. It is important to note that a hair *follicle* is the anatomic organ which gives rise to hair *shafts*. Most persons simply use the word *hair* to refer to the visible product of hair follicles and unless otherwise specified, this section will follow the same pattern.

There are three stages of follicles that produce hair. The anagen follicle is actively growing. At any given time, about 85 to 90 percent of follicles on the scalp are in the anagen phase of growth. This phase lasts about 1,000 days, or three years. The next phase is called catagen and lasts only a few weeks. Few follicles (less than 5 percent) are in catagen at any given time. The telogen phase lasts about three months and about 10 to 15 percent of follicles are in this stage. Follicles in telogen are resting until they are replaced by new, growing anagen follicles. These phases usually progress appropriately but if one or more is delayed or prolonged, the result can be a significant change in the appearance of the scalp hair.

Hair loss may take place for numerous reasons including illness, drug intake, underlying diseases, hormonal abnormalities, and more. These categories are usually divided into those which result in scarring of the scalp (in which case regrowth is unlikely) and those without scarring (in which case regrowth is potentially possible). Theoretically, in nonscarring alopecias (causes of hair loss), if the underlying problem or problems can be reversed the hair may regrow naturally and assume its former state. Unfortunately, in some of these instances the process has gone on too long and the capacity for regrowth of new hair follicles has diminished.

Male Pattern Baldness (Androgenetic Alopecia)

This is the most common type of hair loss and one for which millions of dollars are spent annually to reverse its effects. Male pattern baldness usually begins in the twenties or thirties with some thinning of the hair at the back of the scalp and along the front and sides. There may be a slight recession of the frontal hairline. For some patients this is all the hair loss they experience. For others, however, the disease progresses and results in greater amounts of hair loss. Men may experience balding in their teens but it rarely begins after age forty. Almost all men will experience some thinning of the hair by age fifty. The affected hairs are transformed from the normal thick terminal hairs to smaller, lighter versions called vellus hairs. The follicles which produce these hairs are sensitive to hormonal changes; these are believed to cause androgenetic alopecia. This susceptibility is genetically controlled. Men inherit male pattern baldness more from the mother's side than the father's. The other key ingredient is male hormones. Testosterone and other male hormones must be present for the hair loss to continue. Apparently the follicles of some men are more sensitive to these hormones. This sensitivity is controlled by the person's genes. There is no evidence that dandruff, the type of shampoo used, hair treatments, or styling play any role in the beginning or progress of androgenetic alopecia. Making the diagnosis of male pattern baldness may not necessarily be easy, particularly in patients with no family history of hair loss. A skin biopsy may be useful but needs to be evaluated by a dermatopathologist familiar with biopsies done for hair loss.

Treatment for androgenetic alopecia has traditionally been frustrating. Many highly touted solutions and potions have been produced with the claim of being able to regrow hair. The most recent medication to become available is finasteride (Propecia®). This drug inhibits the action of testosterone on the hair follicle and prevents it from being lost. Finasteride is well tolerated and causes some mild impotence or loss of sex drive in less than 2 percent of patients.

The only other medication proven to help male pattern baldness is minoxidil (Rogaine®). This drug is now available without a prescription and can be used indefinitely on the scalp. It must be applied twice daily and aside from an occasional rash it is well tolerated. About a third of patients will receive no improvement, about a third will notice that hair loss either stops or slows considerably, and about a third will have some new hair growth. The major disadvantage to topical minoxidil use is expense. A month's worth of medicine costs between $40 and $50. Since the drug must be used indefinitely, the cost is continual.

A hair transplant or scalp reduction flap, while costing several thousand dollars, is usually a one-time expense and may be a more cost-effective means of addressing this problem (see section on cosmetic dermatology). Other options include hairpieces and hairweaves.

Remember, there have been no proven pills, lotions, devices, or treatments aside from what has just been discussed ever proven to be of use in treating male pattern baldness. While numerous companies claim to have a product to treat this problem, none have ever been able to demonstrate a significant degree of benefit when subjected to traditional scientific testing.

Androgenetic alopecia also occurs in women. In female patients, the cause is an inherited susceptibility to the disease and, in some cases, an increased amount of male hormones in the blood. In some patients this may be caused by underlying tumors secreting male hormones, but this is rare. Most women with male pattern hair loss are overweight; and it is thought that some female hormones are converted to male hormones more rapidly in obesity. Weight loss is usually helpful to some extent. Androgenetic alopecia in females appears slightly different than it does in males. The hair loss is on top of the scalp and toward the frontal hairline. Frank balding does not often occur but thinning of the hair is common. Treatments are similar but some antihormonal therapies such as cyproterone acetate (not available in the United States) and spironolactone (Aldactone®) are useful. Finasteride can deform unborn children and may not be used by pregnant or nursing women.

Alopecia Areata

This is the second most common form of hair loss. The capacity for a patient's hair to regrow is much better in alopecia areata than in androgenetic alopecia; however, the potential for rapid and complete hair loss is greater as well. Alopecia areata refers to persons with scattered areas of hair loss on the scalp or beard area. Alopecia totalis describes the condition of total or near total hair loss of the scalp. Alopecia universalis occurs in persons who have lost most or all of their body hair including eyebrows, eyelashes, and pubic hair. Some persons develop small pits in the nails but other skin disease is not seen.

The cause of this hair loss in not known but seems to center around an abnormality in the immune system whereby the body's immune cells begin attacking the hair follicles. Some types of autoimmune diseases include a higher incidence of this type of hair loss as well. There is a genetic factor, since alopecia areata runs in some families. Persons with an atopic background (a history of eczema, asthma, and seasonal allergies) have more alopecia areata. Stress, which has often been cited as a factor in alopecia areata, probably does not cause the disease but may worsen it. There are some conditions associated with alopecia areata such as some thyroid diseases and types of anemia. These may be evaluated with appropriate blood tests.

Alopecia areata has a good prognosis for most patients, particularly if hair loss has begun after puberty. In children, the loss of hair may be permanent and difficult to treat. Even without therapy, however, most hair loss will resolve at some point. Regrowth is often very fine or downy and usually white colored. The emotional impact of considerable hair loss, particularly in women or girls, is underestimated. Therapy is therefore indicated in virtually all cases of alopecia areata. Early treatment is best, since it increases the odds for complete regrowth of hair. There is a variety of patterns of hair loss and each has a different chance for treatment success or failure.

Corticosteroids are the most commonly used medication. Initial therapy, particularly in persons losing large quantities of hair, may be with oral prednisone (Deltasone®). This drug is not intended for long-term use but may blunt or terminate the inflammation around the hair follicles. Topical corticosteroids are not usually of much benefit as they are not strong enough. Only the most potent preparations are likely to be of any help. Since their application for prolonged periods may result in thinning of the skin and other unwanted side effects, they should not be used for longer than three weeks. Application under plastic wrap may be more effective but this is difficult to accomplish on the face or scalp. Injection of corticosteroids has become one of the mainstays of treatment. Different concentrations are used on different body sites with a limitation on the total amount of corticosteroid injected. This is the most efficient means of therapy, particularly for an isolated spot or two. There are few side effects aside from some occasional sinking in of the skin about a month after the injection, and this usually resolves with time. This treatment may be repeated at monthly intervals. Photochemotherapy (PUVA) is popular and has a reasonably good success rate. There must be twenty to forty treatments to obtain adequate results (longer than for psoriasis), and it has the same disadvantages as in treating other disorders. This therapy is better suited for persons with extensive hair loss. Cyclosporin (Sandimmune®) is usually helpful when orally taken. The hair loss tends to relapse, however, when the medication is discontinued. The drug is also very expensive and has a number of unwanted side effects. Topical cyclosporin is much safer and less expensive but does not work as well. Minoxidil has been used extensively for alopecia areata with mixed results. It works well in some patients, particularly when a 5% solution is used. It must be applied for three to twelve months, however, for an adequate response and many patients won't or can't wait that long for relief. The medication is expensive, although it is available without a prescription. Topical anthralin (Drithoscalp®) is useful for small patches of alopecia areata. Since it tends to stain the skin, its use in persons with white or blond hair or on facial lesions is not well accepted. It supposedly stimulates hair regrowth by inducing a mild degree of irritation and inflammation in the skin.

Telogen Effluvium

Telogen effluvium is a state of hair loss caused by large numbers of hairs entering the telogen or shedding stage of growth. As mentioned, only about 10 to 15 percent of hairs at any one time are in the telogen phase. They account for the hair loss we experience from day to day (about 100 hairs per twenty-four hours). If a larger percentage of the scalp's hair follicles enter this stage, say 25 percent, then the loss of hair may be enough to be noticed by the patient and result in visible thinning (150 to 400 hairs per twenty-four hours). Telogen effluvium is most often noticed by persons with darker hair since their hair has likely been very thick and any thinning is very noticeable. Pushing more follicles into the telogen phase may have a number of causes including pregnancy and childbirth, a serious illness (particularly if accompanied by a high fever), severe mental or emotional stress, stopping or starting certain medications such as corticosteroids or birth control pills, and severe dieting or starvation. This hair loss results in an even thinning throughout the scalp but baldness does not result. Hair regrowth is usually complete but may take six to twelve months. In some patients, the hair may never be as thick as it once was. There is no treatment per se, however, but for patients who have a prolonged course, topical minoxidil may be helpful.

Anagen Effluvium

This form of hair loss occurs when the follicles are damaged over a short period of time and are forced to stop growing. The result is the follicles' death and loss of the hair shaft. The classic example is the hair loss resulting from chemotherapy. Certain chemotherapeutic drugs such as cyclophosphamide (Cytoxan), actinomycin, doxorubicin (Adriamycin®), and nitrosourea are more likely to cause this than others but almost any drug may induce alopecia in certain patients. The hair loss begins about two weeks after taking the medications and peaks at about two months. The hairs become weak and fragile and fall out with routine care such as washing and styling. There is no therapy for this condition; the hair will regrow normally after the damage has stopped.

Traction Alopecia

This hair loss occurs when the hairs are pulled from the scalp. It does not result in scarring and if the behavior is stopped the hair will regrow. The most common type of traction alopecia occurs in girls and women who have their scalp hair too tightly braided, as with "corn rows." Ponytails may also cause stress on hair shafts along the frontal hairline and result in their breakage and loss.

A more unusual form of traction alopecia is called trichotillomania and results from an emotional or mental illness in which the patient consciously or unconsciously pulls at the scalp and facial hair with resultant hair loss. The diagnosis may be made by biopsying a portion of the scalp at the border of the balding areas. Some patients respond well to counseling or medications aimed at relieving them of their underlying stress.

Alopecia from Underlying Disease

Many diseases demonstrate a loss of hair as a component of their effects on the body. These include thyroid disease, infections such as syphilis and AIDS, certain medications, and nutritional deficiencies such as of proteins, fats, or vitamins. The hair loss is generally diffuse throughout the scalp, does not commonly result in complete hair loss, and stops when the underlying disease state is resolved.

Scarring Alopecia

Hair loss that occurs with significant scarring in the skin will result in the destruction of hair follicles and the loss of the ability to regrow hair. This has numerous causes including some unusual skin diseases involving the scalp, infections, tumors, and physical agents. There are a few conditions, however, which primarily affect the scalp and result in permanent hair loss.

Dissecting cellulitis of the scalp also goes by the name perifolliculitis capitis abscedens et suffodiens and almost exclusively affects young black males. The scalp becomes very boggy with numerous deep collections of pus. This pus may leak through to the surface and can be expressed by pressing on the scalp. The hair loss is permanent and usually occurs over a period of a few weeks to a few months. Some discomfort is present. Several different bacteria have been implicated but treatment with antibiotics is usually disappointing. Oral corticosteroids are helpful as is griseofulvin (Gris-PEG®). The treatment of choice, however, is isotretinoin (Accutane®). This drug is given in the same doses used for cystic acne. This will stop the hair loss within a few weeks of beginning the medication.

Folliculitis decalvans is an inflammatory response in hair follicles on the scalp. This eruption begins over the back of the scalp and spreads with a gradually increasing area of scarring. At the leading edge of this scarring are red, inflamed follicles which may have some pus in them. This is believed to be some type of infection since antibiotics are useful in some cases. Folliculitis decalvans is difficult to treat and isotretinoin seems to be the most helpful medication.

The follicular degeneration syndrome is also known as hot comb alopecia and primarily affects black females. It was previously believed that heat and oils from hot combs used in this population made their way down the hair shaft and damaged the follicle. The crown of the scalp is primarily involved.

Lichen planopilaris (Graham-Little-Feldman syndrome) is thought to be a form of lichen planus which affects the scalp. Some follicles are plugged as with blackheads or open comedones. The hair of other body parts may also be affected and the typical skin changes of lichen planus are occasionally seen. Treatment is difficult and centers around the same therapies used for lichen planus including oral corticosteroids, isotretinoin, and PUVA therapy.

Lupus erythematosus, particularly the discoid variant, commonly involves the head, neck, and scalp. These patches possess the same features as those elsewhere. The scarred skin shows increased and decreased pigmentation with mild scaling. Treatment is with antimalarial medications and corticosteroids.

Hair Structure Defects

Patients with these conditions have defects of the hair shaft structure. These are relatively rare and some are inherited. Patients develop fragile hair that is difficult to style and easily breaks. As a result, most patients have short hair with an unusual texture and appearance. Common diagnoses include monilethrix, pili torti, pili annulati, trichorrhexis nodosa, and trichorrhexis invaginata. Diagnosis is usually made by looking at a few hairs under the microscope. Treatment is difficult, especially for genetic diseases in which most if not all follicles are involved. Biotin for strengthening hair and nails may be of some use.

HERPES INFECTIONS AND SHINGLES

The herpesvirus group is composed of several different viruses. The best known are the herpes simplex virus type 1 and 2 (HSV-1, HSV-2) and the varicella-zoster virus (VZV) which is responsible for chickenpox (varicella) and shingles (zoster). They have different manifestations but somewhat similar treatment. Cytomegalovirus is another herpesvirus which has become important in recent years. Other herpesvirus diseases are discussed in the section on viral infections.

Herpes Simplex

These infections are caused by two different viruses, termed Herpes simplex-1 (HSV-1) and Herpes simplex-2 (HSV-2). In general, HSV-1 is responsible for producing cold sores or fever blisters, whereas HSV-2 is responsible for causing genital herpes. This is not absolute, since some overlap does occur.

Herpes Labialis (Cold Sores)

Cold sores occur when a person has a recurrence of the viral outbreak. These are routinely found on the lips and central face. This disorder affects one-fourth to one-third of the populace. The outbreak takes place after the initial infection, known as primary gingivostomatitis. This takes place when the virus initially comes into contact with a previously uninfected person through mouth-to-mouth or other physical contact. Typically, it is seen in children and young adults. They may run high fevers and have sore throats with small blisters, or there may be almost no symptoms at all. The fever blisters that then occur on the lips in years to come are a *recurrence* of that infection. Not everyone who has been infected experiences a recurrence, but most do. The viruses reside in the nerves. When they come to the surface of the skin in the form of a fever blister they do so in the same spot each time. Most affected persons have a few eruptions over the course of their lifetimes but some people have three or four per year. The symptoms of a recurrence become well known to affected patients. Typically, the involved area begins to tingle, itch, or burn about a day or so before the skin becomes affected. The skin begins to turn red and then forms blisters. Eventually a scab forms, and in a week to ten days the skin has quieted down and returned to normal. During the first three to four days of the cold sore it is possible to transmit the virus to uninfected persons. When patients have open cold sores, they therefore are encouraged to avoid personal contact with others, particularly young children or those with damaged immune systems in whom an infection could be very serious. Cold sores are provoked by a variety of different causes such as trauma, illness, sun exposure, stress, menstruation, and fatigue.

TREATMENT The traditional method of treatment has been acyclovir (Zovirax®) tablets, liquid, or cream. The only cream available until recently was acyclovir, which while very convenient, does not work as well as the liquid or tablets. A new product, however, penciclovir cream (Denavir®) has recently come on the market and is reportedly more effective. It must be applied every two hours while awake and is expensive; however, it essentially has no side effects. The dose for acyclovir liquid and tablets is usually 200 mg five times daily. This will cut down on the duration of the outbreak and its discomfort. It will also diminish the amount of virus shed from the cold sores so that infection of other people is less likely. Sunscreen-containing lip balms aid prevention if sunlight is likely to provoke an outbreak, as are antianxiety medications for stress. For those extremely susceptible to outbreaks, oral acyclovir daily has been useful. Acyclovir is helpful for the initial infection, but this is often a difficult diagnosis to make and so treatment is rarely begun. Similar medications such as famciclovir (Famvir®) and valacyclovir (Valtrex®) are used for genital herpes and shingles (herpes zoster) but may help some patients with fever blisters. Over-the-counter medications are available for fever blisters (Herpecin-L®, Tanac Gel®, Zilactin Gel/Liquid®). These contain a sun-protective agent or mild numbing medication. They are generally harmless but will not provide the relief or resolution that acyclovir will provide.

Genital Herpes

Genital herpes is usually due to HSV-2. This is the most common cause of genital ulcers in the United States and is a risk factor for HIV infection, since the virus of HIV may infect persons through the open skin of an ulcer. The small blisters and ulcers occur three to fourteen days after contact with an infected sexual partner. The first sign of infection is a gathering of small blisters which soon break and become painful or itchy. Infected women typically complain of pain when urinating. The lymph nodes in the upper thigh and groin may become swollen and painful. With the initial infection other symptoms, such as stiff neck and headache, may also occur. The symptoms peak at eight to ten days and the lesions heal by three weeks in most cases. Persons are usually the most infectious (capable of transmitting the infection) during the first ten days. After the lesions have crusted, the ability to infect another person is considerably reduced.

Recurrent herpes simplex is the most common form of this disease and affects about 25 million Americans. It is more common in men but is more uncomfortable in women. If a person has recurrences of these lesions (not all infected patients do), he will have, on average, about three to four outbreaks per year. Some persons will have as many as eight to ten per year. The eruption occurs in the same spot each time since, like the HSV-1 virus causing cold sores, this virus lives in nerves and travels to a specific area of the skin. The symptoms are the same as for the initial infection but may be less severe; the fever, stiff neck, and headaches of the primary infection almost never recur. An initial pain, tingling, numbness, or itch in the area commonly arises several hours or days before the small blisters appear. They rupture and heal in about a week to ten days. During the first three to four days of the eruption there is the greatest likelihood of infecting another person. All areas of the genitalia may be involved including the cervix. Cervical infections are not necessarily uncomfortable and women may have this infection without knowing it. Consequently, an examination of the cervix is crucial to detecting the presence of this virus. Persons with an active outbreak of genital herpes should refrain from sexual activity at least until the blisters have crusted and are in the process of falling off. It is also a good idea to wash hands thoroughly after using the toilet since it is possible to pass this virus to others by the hands.

TREATMENT The treatment of genital herpes simplex uses similar medications to that for cold sores. Acyclovir is the oldest and best-known medication. The cream is useful but not as much as the pills or suspension. The oral dose is 200 mg five times per day for ten days. The drug works best if taken when a person feels an outbreak beginning. Acyclovir shortens the outbreak period, decreases the numbers of "shed" viruses and thereby lessens the likelihood of infecting someone else, and reduces the associated discomfort. Valacyclovir and famciclovir are also used to treat genital herpes. As with acyclovir, there are few side effects, but they are expensive. They are taken orally but fewer times per day.

Two other forms of herpes simplex bear mentioning. Cutaneous herpes simplex is similar to cold sores but the affected skin is on the arm or trunk. This is not of any significance except in persons who have a great deal of body contact with others. Herpes gladiatorum is a form of cutaneous herpes simplex seen in wrestlers and rugby players. These persons spread the virus by skin-to-skin contact, particularly if the skin has been cut or scraped. Lumbosacral herpes simplex is a variant of genital herpes simplex but involves the lower back and buttocks. This usually occurs in persons over forty years of age; outbreaks are triggered by the same causes as genital herpes and fever blisters. The blisters are similar to genital blisters. A key feature of lumbosacral herpes simplex is the pelvic pain that accompanies an outbreak. One to three days before the outbreak patients will experience very disabling deep pain in the pelvis and occasionally radiating down the back of the leg (sciatica). The treatment for these two disorders is similar to that for fever blisters and genital herpes.

Chickenpox (Varicella)

Chickenpox, or varicella, is one of the most common childhood diseases and is considered highly contagious. It is seen worldwide and occurs almost exclusively in children under the age of ten. For most persons, an infection is uncomfortable and distracting but not dangerous. In adults and those persons with damaged or defective immune systems, however, it may be life threatening. The skin rash occurs ten to twenty-one days after exposure to an infected person (usually about two weeks). The first finding is a rash consisting of small red bumps, which shortly become blistered. Fever is prominent along with headache and muscle aches. The skin in the area of the rash is slightly reddened ("dewdrops on a rose petal") and is usually very itchy. The blisters come out in waves or "crops." The rash tends to occur on the face and protected parts of the body. Areas subjected to mild trauma such as the diaper area are also common sites. Mucous membranes in the mouth, genitalia, and eyes may be affected. The blisters eventually become cloudy as they form pustules. They then become crusted and fall off in one to three weeks. Patients are considered no longer infectious when the rash has become crusted. The typical runny nose, cough, and congestion seen with colds and flu are usually not present. Infection produces lifelong immunity and second infections rarely occur.

There are few complications of this disease in children. Scarring is the most worrisome outcome, particularly if there is a lot of facial involvement. If the blisters are not traumatized, the chances of scarring are greatly reduced. This rash is usually very itchy, however, and preventing children from scratching is difficult. Occasionally some of the blisters may become infected with bacteria, particularly if they have been scratched. While this is rarely dangerous, it greatly increases the chances of scarring and may require an antibiotic.

Varicella in adults is much more dangerous. The rash tends to be more involved and more complicated. Although the death rate is only 1 in 50,000 for children, it is about 1 in 1,500 for adults. Involvement of the lungs (varicella pneumonitis) is the most worrisome complication in otherwise healthy adults. Another important complication is Reye's syndrome, which causes liver damage in persons with chickenpox who have taken aspirin. As mentioned, persons with diseased immune systems such as AIDS or cancer have increased problems when they develop this disorder. A vaccine for varicella has recently become available and is indicated for persons in whom this disease would be either dangerous or very inconvenient (children with two working parents who can't take time off). It is not clear if a booster shot will have to be given after a certain number of years or if this will have any effect on herpes zoster (shingles), which is the recurrence of this virus in the skin.

Treatment

The treatment of varicella is usually directed at making the patient comfortable while the disease runs its course (see Table 23). Fevers and muscle aches should be treated with acetaminophen (Tylenol®, Panadol®). Aspirin should never be given. Lots of fluids and rest are also helpful. Itching is usually the most unpleasant symptom and the one which requires the most treatment. Clipping the patient's nails short helps prevent scratching. Antihistamines such as hydroxyzine (Atarax®) and diphenhydramine (Benadryl®) are beneficial as are the others recommended for atopic dermatitis. Topical antihistamines such as diphenhydramine are not particularly useful and are better avoided. Topical corticosteroids are also not a good idea, although Pramasone®, which contains an anti-itching medication and hydrocortisone is useful for controlling the itching. Sarna® lotion and Aveeno Anti-Itch® cream are available over the counter and may be applied as often as needed. Calamine lotion may also help. Frequent baths with one-quarter cup cornstarch or Aveeno® bath lotion or powder will relieve itching and are safe.

Acyclovir by mouth is very helpful for treating the infection. This medication comes as a suspension and may be given to children. Many pediatricians and dermatologists prefer to let the disease run its natural course, believing that it may help solidify permanent immunity. Acyclovir and presumably valacyclovir or famciclovir are more commonly given in cases of adult chickenpox, since these patients are usually sicker and more likely to experience serious complications. The doses are the same as for herpes simplex infections. These medications are also sometimes given intravenously in persons with damaged immune systems. Immunizations should be considered for persons who are known to not have been previously infected and who have AIDS or cancer. There are a few other antiviral medications which may be used including foscarnet (Foscavir®) and vidarabine (Vira-A®), but these are only given if the infection fails to respond to the more usual medications.

Varicella Zoster (Shingles)

Varicella zoster is also known as shingles. An outbreak represents a recurrence of the virus. This disorder is more common in the elderly but with the increased number of patients with poorly functioning immune systems it is being seen more frequently in younger persons. For the most part, it manifests as an uncomfortable skin rash but in some persons can cause long-lasting discomfort.

Table 23 TREATMENT OPTIONS FOR CHICKENPOX (VARICELLA)

Antihistamines	Diphenhydramine
	Hydroxyzine
Baths	Cornstarch
	Baking Soda
	Aveeno Bath Powder and Bath Oil
Anti-Itch Creams	Pramasone® Cream/Ointment (Rx)
	PramaGel® (Rx)
	Sarna® Lotion
	Aveeno Anti-Itch® Concentrated Lotion
	Calamine Lotion

Most affected patients are over fifty years of age. The eruption occurs in the skin supplied by the nerve that contains the virus. As a result, the blisters are usually restricted to a band across the trunk which does not cross the midline. The trunk is the most common site of involvement, but the arms and legs may also be affected. The most worrisome pattern of shingles involves the head and face. In this case the eyes may be affected, with scarring and loss of vision. In those who are old or sick, the eruption may occur all over the body and appears somewhat like chickenpox. Before the outbreak, the skin may become very tender and sore; this may last a week or more before the red bumps and blisters appear. As in chickenpox, the eruption only occurs once but may later arise at a different site. Persons with an outbreak of shingles may transmit chickenpox to susceptible patients.

In most cases, an outbreak of shingles lasts several weeks and amounts to little more than an unpleasant experience. In some people, however, the pain of the rash lasts long after the blisters have subsided. This is called postherpetic neuralgia and it may be quite debilitating. It is seen in 10 to 15 percent of patients, particularly those over sixty years of age or with head and face involvement. Some skin scarring may occur as well if the outbreak has been particularly bad or the eye is involved. Sometimes nerves on the face are affected and the muscles are weakened or palsied. Most patients eventually recover their ability to move the muscles.

Treatment

Therapy for shingles is similar to that of chickenpox. Acyclovir is given but usually at a higher dose. If the person is old or particularly sick, it may be intravenously administered. Famciclovir and valacyclovir are also useful for shingles and have the advantage of having to be given less frequently. Other medications such as interferon (Intron-A®) and vidarabine (Vira-A®) have also been used. A controversial point in the treatment of shingles is whether giving corticosteroids is helpful. There is some evidence that patients given prednisone (Deltasone®) by mouth or triamcinolone (Kenalog®) by injection tend to have less postherpetic neuralgia. If there are no contraindications to prednisone, many dermatologists give the drug hoping that it will prevent this side effect.

Postherpetic neuralgia is difficult to treat. The use of antidepressants such as amitryptyline (Elavil®) and fluphenazine (Prolixin®) have been helpful in alleviating the pain in some patients. The antiseizure drug carbamazapine (Tegretol®) has also demonstrated some usefulness but must be given with great care and the patient carefully monitored. Some dermatologists have obtained good results by injecting corticosteroids into the areas of discomfort. The over-the-counter cream capsaicin (Zostrix®) applied several times daily for several weeks may decrease sensitivity in the area. Finally, remember that if the eye or the structures around it are involved with shingles, an evaluation by an ophthalmologist must be done right away.

Cytomegalovirus

This is probably the least known of the herpesvirus family, yet it is a very common virus and almost everyone has been infected by it at some time. Infection usually occurs in children or sexually active young adults. The symptoms of infection are not very specific and are typical of a cold or flu. For healthy patients, infection by this virus is not much of a problem. For patients whose health is compromised (cancer patients, in AIDS, unborn children, and so on), however, this virus may pose serious problems. Women who become infected while they are pregnant may deliver children with birth defects. For this reason, a previous infection with cytomegalovirus is checked for routinely with prenatal blood work.

There are some skin manifestations of cytomegalovirus (CMV) but these also are not very specific and can show up as ulcers, red bumps and nodules, bruising, skin ulcers, and hives. The diagnosis may be difficult to make but can be done with some skin biopsies and culture of body fluids.

Treatment consists of giving ganciclovir (Cytovene®) or foscarnet. Both have to be given intravenously and are expensive. Acyclovir and similar drugs are not very effective in persons with active infections. Interferon has also been used with some success.

Ichthyosis

The ichthyoses are a group of skin diseases characterized by dryness and scaling of the skin. The skin of affected persons may look like the scales of a fish. Some of these diseases are inherited but most arise by chance. Sometimes these disorders can be separated by the findings of a skin biopsy. Occasionally, more sophisticated diagnostic methods are required.

There are several different types of ichthyosis but the most common is called ichthyosis vulgaris. This may begin in childhood, but does not usually affect infants and children. It is believed to be inherited and may run in families. Persons with an atopic background of asthma, hay fever, and eczema are most commonly afflicted. The skin becomes dry and scaly and feels rough. The arms and legs are usually involved but the face and neck may also show some dry, scaling skin. The palms in affected persons may have an increased number of lines (hyperlinearity). Itching may occur but is usually not a major problem. The disease is lifelong; it is worsened by dry, cold weather and improves in the summer. Some persons have cleared their disease by relocating to a warm, humid environment. Other types of ichthyosis include X-linked ichthyosis (occurring only in males), lamellar ichthyosis, and epidermolytic hyperkeratosis (usually present at birth). These are uncommon and are occasionally associated with different physical defects. Ichthyosis may be a part of other, usually rare, conditions as well.

Treatment of ichthyosis vulgaris consists of increasing the amount of water or moisture in the skin. The same principles of moisturizing that apply to eczema also apply to ichthyosis. Using a humidifier as much as possible is recommended. Warm, humid environments are good for most patients. Application of moisturizers after bathing while the skin is still wet is helpful. Certain emollients, particularly those containing lactic acid and urea (Table 10) have proven useful. Emollients containing alpha hydroxy acid (glycolic acid) are helpful and are now available (Aqua Glycolic Lotion®, Eucerin Plus®). Some barrier creams have been produced (SBR-Lipocream®) and may help to seal in the skin's natural moisture. Emollients should be applied several times daily. This regimen of moisturizer application is tedious and expensive, but if followed religiously, may give considerable relief. Oral medications are not used to treat ichthyosis vulgaris.

Insect Bites

An insect bite or sting may cause more than just some momentary discomfort or pain. Some insects are capable of causing reactions in the body that involve the lungs, blood vessels, and gastrointestinal tract. The following insects are divided into several different families, each of which is capable of wreaking havoc on the human population in its own special way.

Scabies

Infestation by the scabies mite is one of the most common interactions that humans have with the insect world; it has been around for many thousands of years. These insects are very small and are rarely seen by humans. The infesting organism is called *Sarcoptes scabiei* and is usually spread by skin-to-skin contact. As a result, if one person has the disease then others, particularly bed partners, will commonly have it as well. Scabies may also be spread from contact with infested clothing and bedding.

Symptoms
Patients usually have small, raised red spots which ferociously itch. These typically occur on the wrists, abdomen, and webs of the fingers and toes. A "burrow" may be seen nearby and represents the female mite's tunneling through the skin. Since these areas are usually very itchy, many are scratched and picked. A bacterial infection is common as well. Some patients have larger nodular lesions affecting the groins and underarms. These typically occur in persons whose immune systems have reacted very vigorously to the insect's presence. Only the female scabies mite infests the patient and usually there are no more than thirty infesting mites at any given time. A variation of this disease, Norwegian scabies, occurs when persons with diseased immune systems such as in AIDS or cancer are infested by many thousands of insects. Such patients tend to shed a huge number of mites and may be responsible for infesting scores of others in nursing homes, emergency rooms, or hospitals. The diagnosis is made by scraping the skin and finding mites, eggs, or mite feces. This may be difficult and failing to diagnose scabies is not uncommon.

Treatment
Treatment of scabies is occasionally difficult. It is recommended that all persons living in the home be treated, since most will become infested at some point if they

are not already. A single infected person alone will allow the infestation to begin anew and spread back through the family. The traditional treatment is the use of lindane (Kwell®). This lotion is applied to the skin from the neck to the toes at bedtime and washed off the next morning. Repeating the process the next day is frequently recommended. The lotion must be applied between the toes and fingers, since that is a common hiding place for the insects. Application above the neck is not usually necessary. Lindane is usually well tolerated and inexpensive. In small children, however, there have been some reports of this drug causing seizures, presumably from the absorption of toxic amounts through the skin. There are also accounts of some scabies mites which have become resistant to lindane. Involvement of the head and neck is not common but may occasionally be seen; in such instances, 10% sulfur in petroleum gel is recommended.

The most popular treatment today is 5% permethrin cream (Elimite®). This is applied in the same manner as lindane but usually with better results. Crotamiton cream (Eurax®) is an older treatment and is not usually used today, since there are more effective medications. The importance of applying these medications thoroughly and appropriately can't be overemphasized. A newer method of treatment and one that will likely become much more popular in the future consists of giving the patient a single dose of ivermectin (Stromectol®). It is supplied both in a liquid and tablet form, but testing on children has not been done in the United States.

The clothing and bedding used by the treated patients should also be cleaned. It is not necessary to "go overboard" with this cleaning, but washing these items in hot water is recommended. Other personal items such as combs and brushes should also be cleaned. Finally, the house should be thoroughly vacuumed.

Killing the insect is the most important part of treatment and with the medications available today, this is relatively easy. However, the itch of scabies may take several weeks to subside. When patients no longer develop new "spots," then there is a good chance that the insects have been eradicated. Antihistamines and other medications may help control the itch. Some patients develop nodules where they were bitten. This is called nodular scabies and affects patients who have become particularly sensitive to the insect and its toxins. These nodules are very itchy and may take months to fully subside. The treatment for nodular lesions consists of topical steroids, topical tar preparations, and patience.

Demodex Mites

Demodex mites naturally inhabit the skin, and in most patients, cause no problems. These tiny insects are found in hair follicles and oil glands. They are most populous on the head and neck. Some patients, for reasons which are not clear, may become intolerant of these mites and develop an inflammation of the hair follicles, folliculitis (see section on folliculitis), which may appear as red, inflamed bumps on the face. These may have a small pustule as well. Acne rosacea is believed in some persons to be caused by demodex mites. Treating these patients with 5% permethrin cream as with scabies is often helpful, but many dermatologists do not believe that these mites play any role in skin disease.

Other Mites

Other mites found in the environment occasionally cause disease in humans. Probably the best known is the harvest mite or chigger. These mites live in grass and weeds and attack their human prey when they wear short pants. These insects leap up to the skin and attach themselves to it. They draw out a small amount of blood and then fall back to the ground. As a result, most bites occur below the knee. Chigger bites may take many forms, from small red bumps to large welts (urticaria), depending on the person's sensitivity to the mite. They itch ferociously but subside after a few days and, unless infected, uneventfully heal. Treatment consists of a topical corticosteroid for relief of the itching. Use of insect-repelling creams and sprays may help ward off these pests.

Some other mites such as the grain mite (*Pyemotes*), the fowl mite (*Dermanyssus*), and the *Cheyletiella* mite of cats and dogs may rarely infest persons who are around these sources. The eruption looks like small red bumps which have been scratched and traumatized. Treatment is as for chigger bites. Prevention is the most important aspect of therapy but may be difficult, since it is often hard to pin down where the patient may be coming into contact with the mites.

Tick Bites

Ticks may be acquired almost anywhere but they prefer wooded areas. They are most likely to bite in the spring and summer. Persons may be bitten when they go into this environment or when an animal, frequently a household pet, brings the tick to them. Most bites are painless, so affected persons may not know that they have been bitten. The local reaction to tick bites is an allergic response to the tick's saliva or mouthparts. If a reaction occurs at all, it is usually a small red bump. Some persons, however, react with a moderate amount of swelling or even blistering. Rarely, the skin may become so inflamed that the tissues break down and an erosion or ulceration occurs. Tick bites have taken on new importance over the past decade with the knowledge that these insects can pass on a number of diseases, the most worrisome being Lyme disease.

Associated Diseases

There are several diseases that occur in patients who have been bitten by a tick. One of the most well-known is Rocky Mountain spotted fever. While originally found in the Rocky Mountains of the United States, most cases today occur in the Carolinas and the southeast. The infection is caused by the bite of a tick infected with *Rickettsia rickettsii*. The rash usually begins on the hands and feet and gradually works up the extremities onto the trunk. Patients are usually sick, with high fevers and weakness. Treatment consists of hospitalization and the administration of tetracycline (Sumycin®) or clindamycin (Cleocin®). Colorado tick fever is caused by the transmission of a virus through a tick bite. This occurs in the Rocky Mountain and Sierra Mountain regions. Another disease called babesiosis occurs in persons who are bitten around Martha's Vineyard and Long Island. The tick bite transmits a parasite called *Babesia microti*. The symptoms are similar to those of malaria and include fever, sweats, and anemia. Another rare disorder, called tick paralysis, arises when the patient is extremely sensitive to the toxic features of the tick's saliva. The tick has usually been attached to the person for the better part of a week. An inability to move begins in the lower legs and gradually involves the arms and trunk. This problem goes away on its own but may take several days or weeks to do so.

The most common and most infamous tick-associated disease is Lyme disease, which occurs when a tick, usually of the Ixodes family, bites a person and transmits the bacteria *Borrelia burgdorferi*. Lyme disease was originally described in Lyme, Connecticut, but also occurs in the upper midwest United States. Most current cases come from the mid-Atlantic, northeast, and north central regions of the United States. There seems to be an increasing number of these infections with just under 20,000 of them reported in 1996. A similar disease called acrodermatitis chronica atrophicans arises from infection by the same bacteria and is seen in Europe. It is not clear why the symptoms of an infection by the same organism are so different on the two continents.

The infecting bacteria lives in ticks, commonly the deer tick. A bite from an infected tick allows the organism to invade the body and begin the infection. The skin disease begins several days to several weeks after the tick bite. Most infections occur in the late summer and fall.

There are three stages of Lyme disease. The first begins several weeks after the bite and is seen in about three-fourths of affected persons. An occasionally itchy red rash termed *erythema chronicum migrans* begins to develop on the skin. It forms around the bite and gradually enlarges. The center of the rash may clear and the eruption begins to look like a ring or target. This eruption may be no larger than a quarter or the size of a dinner plate. The second stage of Lyme disease involves the nervous system. Meningitis, paralysis of the nerves working the facial muscles (Bell's palsy), and poorly functioning nerves to the muscles may be seen. Perhaps most worrisome is an interruption of the normal flow of nerve impulses involving the heart. In such a condition, the proper functioning of the heart may be compromised. While not always dangerous, this is definitely a cause for concern. The final aspect of the disease is arthritis. The swelling and pain in the joints may be difficult to control and leads to loss of function.

Diagnosis of Lyme disease is accomplished with a simple and accurate blood test. Treatment consists of routine antibiotics such as tetracycline, doxycycline (Doryx®), penicillin (Pen-Vee K®), and erythromycin (ERYC®). These may have to be given for several weeks or a month. If the person is particularly sick, he or she may be admitted to the hospital for intravenous administration of penicillin or ceftriaxone (Rocephin®).

Tick-bite prevention is obviously very important. Routine use of insect repellents is suggested and protective clothing should be worn if a person will be in an area where ticks will be found. For a tick to transmit Lyme disease, it usually must be attached to the patient for twenty-four hours or longer. Inspecting the skin, particularly that of children, after an outing is a good idea. If ticks are found they should be removed. There are a number of methods suggested over the years for removing ticks. Applying fingernail polish remover (acetone), gasoline, or petrolatum are all likely to work. Slowly pulling the tick off the skin is also effective. If the tick's mouthparts remain in the skin, they may have to be removed surgically; they will act as a foreign body and cause inflammation.

Spider Bites

The majority of spiders in North America have no interest in or capacity to bite anyone. They are shy and reclusive creatures who prefer to be left alone and whose venom is only a problem for other insects. When they do on rare occasions bite someone, the mark they leave looks little different than a mosquito bite and causes no complications. There are, however, a few exceptions; the most notable is the black widow or *Latrodectus mactans*. This spider derives its name from its color and the fact that it consumes its much smaller partner shortly after mating. Black widows are dark black with a bright red hourglass figure on the abdomen. These spiders are found in woodpiles and brushy ground debris. Their bites are usually painless or at most mildly uncomfortable, and the bite site usually does little more than turn red. The toxin that they inject, however, is a neurotoxin and, as the name suggests, affects the nerves of the body. Abdominal pain, headaches, fatigue, shock, and even coma may ensue. Treatment is best given in a hospital setting.

The most common type of worrisome spider bite comes from the brown recluse spider or the *Loxosceles reclusa*. This spider is found throughout the midwest and southwest United States. It usually lives outdoors but has adapted well to living indoors, particularly in out-of-the-way areas. Attics, crawl spaces, and unused closets are particular favorites of this spider, but they are also found in abandoned buildings and sheds. These spiders are brown with a violin-shaped figure on the back and are up to an inch in length. They hibernate in the colder months so most bites occur in the spring and summer. The bite of the brown recluse spider can cause headaches, fever, nausea, and vomiting but the great damage done by this insect is in the area of the bite itself. The skin becomes red and may break down to form an ulcer. Frequently, a dark brown or black scab (an eschar) forms over the bite within a few days. The area may be painful and swollen. Treatment consists of rest, ice application, and certain antibiotics. The area should not be disturbed by trying to cut out the diseased tissue; this may cause the skin destruction to worsen. Additionally, applying heat to the area will cause the venom to spread into the surrounding skin. The drug dapsone has been shown to help inactivate the poison and is the preferred method of treatment. This drug has a number of side effects, including anemia, so frequent blood counts have to be done. Generally, dapsone has to be given for several weeks until the area begins to heal. It may take several months for the site to return to normal, and when it has healed completely, a scar usually remains.

Scorpion Bites

These insects are found in the southwestern United States and Mexico. They do not "bite" per se but usually sting with a stinger found in their tails. Most attacks occur on the extremities, particularly the hands and feet. The skin becomes painful with swelling and there are symptoms such as nausea, fever, and vomiting. Treatment consists of applying ice to the wound and sometimes the administration of corticosteroids either to the wound itself or by mouth. Antihistamines are also helpful. If other symptoms occur, such as increased blood pressure or convulsions, medications for these may have to be given.

Head Lice

Head lice is an infestation of the scalp hair with an insect called *Pediculus capitis*. This disorder is most common among children, particularly when there is over-crowding and poor hygiene. This infestation runs through schools and may affect even the most scrupulously clean children. As with scabies, there are few lice actually present on the scalp; usually less than twenty total. These insects lay their eggs along the hair shafts; these are the "nits" that are seen. The only symptom is mild itching. If the infestation has been present for a long time, a bacterial infection may occur on the scalp and can cause some swelling of the lymph nodes. These insects are spread by direct contact and the sharing of combs or brushes, earphones, hats, and bedding.

Treatment has traditionally been lindane shampoo. This shampoo is lathered into the scalp hair and allowed to sit for about five minutes. It is then rinsed out and the hair is carefully combed with a "nit comb" to remove any eggs that remain. Other children or adults in the home should be treated as well even if they have no symptoms. As in the treatment of scabies, there is some concern about the lindane being absorbed and causing toxicity. Over-the-counter treatments in shampoo, liquid, and gel form (Nix®, Tisit®, Barc®, Ambix®, A-200®) may help as well. These usually contain pyrethrin, however, and may cause wheezing in persons with seasonal allergies or asthma. Ivermectin as used for scabies may kill the lice as well and is very convenient.

The preferred method of treatment is with permethrin (Elimite®). This is a prescription cream; it is applied to hair which has been washed and dried. It should not be used on wet hair; it may not be as effective. Permethrin should stay in the hair for ten minutes and then be rinsed out. It may temporarily worsen the itching. A second application after one week is suggested. This drug remains active in the hair for up to two weeks and kills any hatching nits not destroyed with the initial treatment. During the two weeks following application, cream rinses and conditioning shampoos should not be used since they may coat the lice and protect them from the permethrin.

Since no therapy for head lice is 100 percent effective and any surviving nits can cause another infestation, getting rid of any residual nits should be considered. Two products, Clear Lice Egg Remover® and Step 2® are available over the counter. These come with nit combs to use on the hair. Bedding, clothing, and hair care items used by patients must be thoroughly cleaned or reinfestation will occur. Older treatments such as insecticides, kerosene, and alcohol are usually not effective and may be potentially dangerous.

Body Lice

Body lice are similar to those that cause head lice. They are called *Pediculus corporis* and usually only infest persons with poor hygiene, such as the homeless or persons subjected to overcrowding. These insects live off the blood of the infested person. Their bites initially cause a small red bump, but since there are usually a large number of insects infesting the victim, he scratches and causes the skin to look much worse. If the skin has been traumatized enough it may become infected, with swollen lymph glands and fever. The lice live on hairs or in the seams of clothing, where they lay their eggs.

Treatment includes improved hygiene. A change of clothing and environment will usually suffice. If the infestation is particularly bad, the same medications used for scabies are employed. Infestation with head lice and scabies in these patients may also occur. For the most part, these insects cause little more than discomfort; however, they are known to transmit certain bacterial diseases such as typhus.

Pubic Lice

This infestation is known as crab lice, or "the crabs." It affects the pubic hair and genitalia. These insects, known as *Phthirius pubis*, are transmitted by sexual contact. They cause a mild itching. The pubic hair is typically involved but they may also be seen in the eyelashes, eyebrows, and other body hair. They lay small nits on the hair shafts much as do head lice, and treatment is the same. The patient's sexual partner must be treated as well to avoid reinfestation, and bedding and clothing should be thoroughly washed.

Mosquitoes and Flies

Mosquitoes are probably the most common insect that bites humans. These are seen in the spring and summer and usually cause no problems aside from some mild itching. The only real danger with these insects is their capacity to transmit infections such as viral encephalitis (an inflammation of the brain which may be fatal or result in paralysis), malaria (much more common in Mexico and Central America), and some types of worm infestation. When these insects bite, they inject some of their saliva; this causes a reaction in the skin and the subsequent itching. This is an allergic reaction, and some persons are more allergic to the injected saliva than others. These patients may react very severely to such a bite with large red welts or nodules. If a large number of bites have occurred, the patient may feel sick and run a low-grade fever.

Topical corticosteroids are very useful for treating the itching and swelling. If the patient has a great many bites or is reacting very intensely, an injection of corticosteroid or oral prednisone (Deltasone®, Prelone®) for a few days is helpful. Oral antihistamines such as diphenydramine (Benadryl®) or hydroxyzine (Atarax®) are also useful. Prevention is the best medicine and over-the-counter insect repellents work well. Mosquitoes are attracted to bright clothing, so wearing darker clothes is recommended.

A number of different flies inhabit North America, but the majority of them do not bite or sting. The horsefly and deerfly are common in the early spring and summer. They are large and their bites may be painful. Some bites tend to bleed for an extended period and may leave large welts. Midges or "no seeums" are also biting flies which are seeking a blood meal. They are very small and are rarely seen. Their bites also leave small welts or red bumps. Topical corticosteroids, as for mosquito bites, are usually the most effective treatment. Insect repellents are also a good idea.

Bedbugs

These insects usually inhabit out-of-the-way areas in the house such as baseboards and unused closets. They are small and feed on blood at night. They are rarely seen. Their bites are not usually felt but may be itchy. Typically, the bites are present in groups of three or four and form a line. Treatment is best accomplished with topical corticosteroids, but prevention is better. A thorough housecleaning and extermination are the best methods.

Bees, Wasps, and Hornets

These insects sting with a special apparatus located in the back of their abdomens. Bees lose this stinger at the time of the attack, but wasps and hornets do not. Most persons react to these stings with mild to moderate discomfort. These produce either a red bump or a welt. Topical corticosteroids and antihistamines are useful to relieve pain. The swelling subsides in a few hours.

Some persons may have a more severe reaction, however, and from this group come the few people each year who die from these stings. Violent reactions may be accompanied by decreased blood pressure, swelling, and difficulty breathing. These are true emergencies and affected patients must be treated in hospitals. Persons who know they are allergic to such stings should take precautions by carrying special kits. These have a small amount of epinephrine to inject into the skin after a sting; the injecter should be kept at hand whenever in an area where a sting might happen. These kits may be purchased in most pharmacies.

Fire Ants

Fire ants are called *Solenopsis invicta* and are found primarily in the southeastern United States. These ants are particularly vicious, since they attack their victims as a group. They attach onto the skin with their mouthparts and pivot around while repeatedly stinging. The initial bite looks like a red bump and the individual stings later become small blisters. The blisters eventually become small pustules, crust over, and fall off. Applying topical corticosteroids will relieve the stinging and burning and if applied soon enough, may be able to prevent blistering. Patients occasionally experience feelings of faintness or fever and may need an injection of corticosteroids or oral administration of prednisone. Antihistamines can also help. Insect repellents are not very effective, so it is best to either avoid the area or use fire ant remover.

Fleas

These are small insects which infest and live off animals such as household pets. They only incidentally bite humans. Their bites are mildly irritating and may cause a small red bump or a welt. These insects are usually more of an irritation than a danger, but they are capable of transmitting bubonic plaque and typhus. Their bites are best treated with topical corticosteroids and antihistamines if necessary.

Insect Repellents

There are a number of different insect repellents on the market. The most common active ingredient in these is diethyltoluamide (DEET). This substance is effective in preventing the bites of mosquitoes, ticks, flies, and fleas. It is considered safe;

however, there is evidence that if it is in contact with children's skin for too long a time and at too great a concentration, absorption may occur and toxicity may result. Still, this is unquestionably the most effective substance currently on the market for avoiding insects. Permethrin spray is effective when used on clothing; it is most useful when combined with the topical application of DEET. The moisturizer Skin So Soft® by Avon has been touted as an effective insect repellent.

Itching

Pruritus is the medical name for itching. This symptom is usually associated with eczema, insect bites, dry skin, and so on which are covered elsewhere in this book. Most of the itching in these conditions can be controlled with corticosteroids (topical, injected, and oral), moisturizers, anti-itch medications containing menthol (Sarna® lotion, Aveeno Anti-Itch® cream), antihistamines and lifestyle changes. Unfortunately, there are conditions in which the skin appears completely normal, yet the patient itches to varying degrees. Control of this itching is best accomplished by treating the underlying condition causing it. The most common of these are discussed below.

Aquagenic Pruritus

This is an unusual but not rare condition; it is infrequently diagnosed since it is not well known outside of dermatology. Aquagenic pruritus occurs when persons itch after coming into contact with water. Temperature does not seem to play a role, since patients are affected by either cold or warm water. The itching usually lasts about an hour and a rash does not appear. Changing clothing and differences in temperature can also cause the itching, and it tends to run in families. Patients may have increased levels of histamine in their blood. Antihistamines do not seem to be very effective, but treatment with ultraviolet light B (UVB) may be useful. Baking soda baths have helped some patients.

Perianal Pruritus

This is a fairly common and frustrating disorder. Several conditions that occur around the anus may cause this itching, including psoriasis, fungal infections, seborrheic dermatitis, pinworm infection, hemorrhoids, and warts. Contact dermatitis from suppositories, spices and medications which have been consumed, and soaps and lotions also cause this problem. In some patients, the exact cause cannot be determined. Appropriate cleaning and skin care is important. The area should be cleaned with a mild soap (Dove®, Eucerin®, Purpose®) and a soft washcloth. This is particularly important after a bowel movement. Cleansing pads such as Tucks® are also helpful. Moisturizers such as used for atopic dermatitis may be applied as needed. Topical corticosteroid creams are beneficial if used in small amounts. Pramoxine-containing creams (Pramasone®, Pramagel®) may also control the itch. Finally, activated charcoal capsules may help and are available without a prescription. Contact dermatitis may be diagnosed with the use of patch tests (see section on contact dermatitis).

Pruritus Vulvae and Pruritus Scroti

Itching of the vulva and scrotum is often due to the same causes as perianal itching. Vaginitis from *Candida* and *Trichomonas* infection often causes itching of the female genitalia. Soaps, lotions, perfumes, and topical medications also can cause problems. Some patients scratch for psychiatric reasons as well. If the skin in this area is chronically rubbed, it will become thickened (lichenified), dark, and mildly scaly. Treatment is similar to that for perianal itching. The use of a good, thick moisturizer (Aveeno Cream®) is often very helpful. Topical corticosteroids may help but need to be applied in measured amounts, since chronic use may cause thinning of the skin.

Itching Conditions Caused by Underlying Diseases

Kidney Disease
Most patients with kidney disease, particularly those whose kidneys have failed or who are undergoing dialysis, will have some degree of itching. Often this is due to the dry skin which almost all these patients experience. Many feel better after dialysis; this suggests that something in the patient's blood is causing this problem. In some patients, their hormonal balance is altered and is causing the itching. In most persons, however, no definite cause is found. Aggressive moisturizing and use of an appropriate soap as for atopic dermatitis is helpful. Topical corticosteroids are also useful. Treatment with UVB has been effective in some patients.

Liver Disease
As with kidney disease, persons with certain types of liver problems may itch.. This occurs when the liver is having difficulty excreting one of the body's waste products, called bile. Since not all liver diseases result in this problem, not everyone itches. The best means of treating this situation is to correct the underlying liver disease. That failing, certain medications may be used to help "bind up" the bile in the colon and prevent it from being reabsorbed. An inexpensive and well-tolerated

medication for this use is activated charcoal (Charcoal Plus DS®). This substance is not absorbed but binds up numerous toxins within the gut. It must be taken several times per day and may cause some mild diarrhea and darkening of the stools. Some formulations are available without a prescription. Another option is cholestyramine (Questran®). This medication is used for lowering blood cholesterol levels but may also help with itching from liver disease.

Blood Diseases

Iron-deficiency anemia, the most common form of anemia in the United States, is associated in some instances with itching. This diagnosis is easy to make and may be confirmed with routine blood work. Treatment with iron replacement is effective.

A rare blood disease called polycythemia vera also causes itching. In this condition, the body's bone marrow is overly active and produces too many red blood cells, white blood cells, and platelets. Patients may particularly itch when they are taking a bath and for the next hour or so after leaving the water. The skin appears normal aside from some faint redness over the central face and extremities. Treatment consists of lowering some of the elevated blood counts with medications such as hydroxyurea (Hydrea®). The patient's platelet count is most important; when these counts are lowered the itching subsides.

Malignancy

Unfortunately, in some patients itching is related to a cancer about which the patient may or may not know. Hodgkin's disease and leukemia are probably the cancers best known for causing itching but other malignancies may do so as well.

Psychiatric Illness

Mental or emotional disorders may cause persons to either itch or to focus more attention on their itching. Treatment of these patients is difficult because it is hard to convince them that psychological or psychiatric care is needed. The most common scenario is a person with depression mixed with anxiety who is taking out their frustrations on their skin. They may have selected a particular site such as the groin, the lower legs, or the back to furiously scratch. They scratch until the skin breaks and infection sets in. The use of a scratching instrument such as a fork or comb is common. The surrounding skin becomes thickened, scaly, and darkened.

Treatment with moisturizers and topical corticosteroids is usually fruitless. Some patients endure long courses of oral or injected corticosteroids with the side effects that they cause. Such patients usually have some significant life stress; a failing marriage, financial difficulties, problems with a child, and so on. These patients may respond well to antidepressants such as fluoxetine (Prozac), nefazodone (Serzone), and sertraline (Zoloft®).

Leg Ulcers

Ulcerations of the lower legs are very common in the elderly and may be a source of considerable frustration as well as danger.

Venous (Stasis) Ulcer

The most common type of leg ulcer is a venous or stasis ulcer. These comprise about 90 percent of all leg ulcers. The typical patient is one who has had mild to moderate swelling of the lower legs and ankles for some time and is probably obese. In the beginning, the ankle swelling might have gone away overnight or with some minimal elevating of the feet. Over time, however, the swelling becomes more permanent and difficult to control. The overlying skin becomes mildly scaly and darkly pigmented. The deeper tissues of the skin may also become thickened and hardened. If this process is very extensive, the lower leg may have an "upside-down bowling pin" look. Varicose veins and spider veins are commonly present. This process is called stasis dermatitis; the veins that carry the blood from the lower leg back to the heart do not properly function. As a result, the skin and deeper tissues become more fragile with less capacity for repair if injured. When some minor trauma does occur, an ulcer results. The more swelling in the tissues, the worse the problem becomes and the less chance for timely healing. Most ulcerations arise around the ankle on the inside of the leg. They may be the size of a dime or as big as a dinner plate. Typically, they do not hurt. Since the tissues are wide open and oozing, they are often infected.

Treatment
The principal treatment for venous or stasis leg ulcers centers around controlling any infection which may be present, decreasing the swelling in the tissues, and keeping the wound covered so that the skin may heal. The key ingredient is leg elevation. The area of the ulcer should be kept *above the level of the heart* for several hours per day. This may be accomplished by propping up the ankle with several pillows. Proper and timely leg elevation cannot be overemphasized. This may take from an hour or two up to ten hours. Without a major decrease in swelling, healing will not take place. Wearing elastic leg supports (Jobst® stockings) is also helpful.

These may be custom fitted and help tremendously in getting rid of the tissue swelling. Avoiding prolonged sitting in the same position, as on a bus or airplane, and gentle walking exercise will help. Intermittent external pressure to the whole leg provided by an electric pump machine "drives" the fluid out of the leg and decreases swelling. This is an effective treatment for certain patients but is time consuming, cumbersome, and expensive. Patients must recline or lie down for the compression system to work. Sometimes surgical repair of the venous system is beneficial.

Antibiotics are often needed to combat a skin infection. These may be oral medications or topical antibiotic ointments (Bactroban®, Polysporin®). Neomycin-containing antibiotic ointments (Neosporin®) are not recommended; this ingredient often causes allergic contact dermatitis which can be disastrous in getting a leg wound healed. The use of antibiotic ointment also provides a moist environment for the skin cells in normal tissue to grow into the ulcer and begin to fill it in. Covering the leg ulcer is also vital. In the past decade, several occlusive dressings have come on the market (Duoderm®, Accuderm®, Vigilon®, Flexzan®). These allow the wound to remain covered for days at a time and provide a safe, moist environment for the skin to regrow. A common therapy involves applying an antibiotic ointment to the wound and placing an occlusive dressing on it for one to five days. The dressing is then removed, the wound cleaned, and the antibiotic ointment reapplied; then the cycle is repeated. The amount of regrowth of skin which will take place if the wound is simply covered is amazing. Obviously, if there is ongoing infection in an ulcer, this sort of occlusive treatment will not work.

Since leg ulcers are such a common problem and so difficult to control, it is not surprising that many different therapies exist. Phenytoin (Dilantin®) powder may be applied to the wound and then covered with occlusive dressings as above. This powder may not be easy to obtain as many pharmacies do not carry it. One of the older treatments is to apply to the wound a solution made of sugar and povidone-iodine (Betadine®). This treatment has not been scientifically tested but there is likely is some benefit to this therapy since it has many advocates.

One of the more noteworthy therapies involves the application of medical-grade maggots (purchased through a surgical supply store) to the wound bed and covering them with gauze. The gauze is taken off several days later and the maggots washed away. The maggots feed on the dead and decaying flesh but leave the healthy tissues alone. The dead tissue will be removed much more quickly and this allows for speedier healing. This is no doubt an effective therapy but one that requires a strong stomach on the part of the patient.

Unna boots (named for the dermatologist who invented them) function much as occlusive dressings do. They are essentially a "mini-cast"; when applied to the legs they allow the ulcer to remain occluded and healing. They are removed after about a week and if the ulcer is still a problem they are reapplied.

Some dermatologists believe that some of the building blocks for healthy tissues, certain vitamins and minerals, are lacking in these patients. Taking ascorbic acid (vitamin C) 250 mg/d and zinc sulfate 200 mg/d has been recommended. While this may help and is probably safe, it is not likely to cure the ulcer.

Finally, there are some persons who may do well with a skin graft. In this procedure a superficial section of skin from another healthy site, frequently the hip or buttock, is removed under local anesthesia. It is then applied to the ulcer bed, which has been appropriately debrided of dead tissue. The now-covered ulcer bed is then wrapped with gauze and left undisturbed for several days. The use of small sections of skin called pinch grafts is also effective and much better tolerated. These small pieces of tissue are put into the ulcer bed. As they grow they expand to cover the ulcer.

The most important aspect to treating this condition is improved care of the intact skin. Persons who have had stasis ulcers or who are at risk for them should realize that any sort of trauma to the skin, no matter how minor, may ultimately result in skin breakdown and the onset of an ulcer. Activities that may result in abrasions or nicks in the skin should be avoided. The legs should be washed only with a gentle soap and warm water. Gentle patting or very mild rubbing with a soft towel is advised and the areas between the toes should be thoroughly dried. A good moisturizer is also useful to prevent any cracking or drying of the skin. Lubricants that contain glycolic acid in moderate amounts may help strengthen the skin.

Other Types of Leg Ulcers

The next most common type of leg ulcer occurs when the blood vessels supplying a certain part of the leg become clogged. This usually happens in persons with high blood pressure and the ulcer typically is on the outside ankle. These lesions are very painful. The surrounding skin is usually cool and hairless. Treatment of these ulcers is very difficult; the therapies outlined for stasis ulcers are not helpful since the underlying problem is a diminished amount of blood flow. Surgical treatment is usually the most effective. This allows for increased blood flow to the leg and subsequent healing of the ulcer. Drugs that help the blood move more easily through the vessels, such as a baby aspirin daily or the use of pentoxifylline (Trental®) can be beneficial.

Another common leg and foot ulcer is caused by diabetes. Diabetic foot ulcers happen when the blood vessels become diseased and are no longer able to supply the appropriate amount of blood to the tissues of the skin. Since these patients also have damaged nerves in their feet and lower legs, they may traumatize their skin and not realize it. Infection may easily occur and the skin begins to break down. Ulcerations are more common on the feet than the lower legs or ankles. The presence of a long-standing ulcer is one of the most common reasons for having a foot, toe, or leg amputated. Because of the increased risk of infection, an ulcer cannot be ignored.

Treatment of diabetic ulcers is much the same as for stasis ulcers. Skin grafts are frequently used in treating the ulcers of diabetics. Many hospitals, clinics, and medical centers have specialized treatment plans for working with ulcer patients. In general, one of the best means for dealing with these ulcerations is better control of the patient's diabetes. This allows for some reversal of the blood vessel disease and more blood flow to the skin. Additionally, smokers should quit. Cigarettes worsen blood vessel disease and make it more difficult to get blood to the skin. Great attention should be paid to care of the skin of the feet. Shoes and socks should always be worn to protect against injury. The feet should be washed daily with a gentle soap and lukewarm water. Hot water or hot-water bottles and heating pads should be avoided since they may injure the skin. The feet should be gently dried with a towel (including between the toes) and a moisturizer should be applied to help soften the skin. Toenails should be cut straight across; they are easiest to cut when soft after bathing. If a person has vision difficulty and cannot focus on the nails appropriately, someone else should cut their nails. Shoes should be inspected weekly for sharp edges, foreign objects, or signs of wear. At the first sign of a cut or abrasion an antibiotic ointment should be applied under a dressing and the patient's doctor consulted.

There are a number of other causes of leg ulcers. Many of these are related to blood disorders or diseases of the blood vessels. Obviously, these are rare but many dermatologists will evaluate for these possibilities with blood work when the patient is first seen. Rarely, skin cancers such as basal cell carcinomas and squamous cell carcinomas will become so large as to look and act like a leg ulcer. In this condition a biopsy will be taken and usually surgery performed to remove the cancer. Some infections by fungus and unusual bacteria are also capable of causing leg ulcers. Evaluation for this possibility requires cultures, and treatment usually consists of a prolonged course of antibiotics.

Lichen Planus

This disease is an eruption of the skin that begins in later middle age for men and usually in the sixties for women. It is not common, affecting only about 1 percent of the population. Several different types of the disease, as well as an identical skin eruption that follows the ingesting of certain medications (lichenoid drug eruption), exist. It is unclear what causes this disease but it seems likely that a person's immune system becomes abnormal, allowing the skin to erupt as it does. The disease tends to run in families. Several of the medications used to treat lichen planus are antibiotics against bacteria or fungi. Despite great effort, however, no organism has ever been found to be infecting these patients.

Symptoms

Lichen planus occurs as lesions the size of a small pencil eraser with a particular lilac or dark color. They are found on the wrists and ankles and have a typical "flat-top" appearance. They are usually very itchy and when they heal they leave behind a dark discoloration to the skin that may take months to subside. The trunk and extremities may also be involved. There are rare variants of lichen planus with blisters and erosions. Lichen planus also affects the mouth. The most common feature is a lacy white eruption on the inside of the cheeks. This is symptomless and most patients are unaware that they even have the eruption. The more worrisome type of oral lichen planus also includes erosions or ulcerations. This may be particularly disabling since it prevents people from eating and drinking as they normally do. Lichen planus also affects the nails. There are several different types of involvement, but generally the nails become ridged, thinned, and prone to splitting. If severe enough, the nails may be shed and not regrow.

It is thought that persons with unusual forms of lichen planus may be more susceptible to having these areas form skin cancers. The risk is highest with oral lichen planus in persons who have been long-time tobacco smokers or chewers. This complication affects about 1 to 5 percent of persons with oral lichen planus overall. Lichen planus of the skin may also degenerate into skin cancer; however, it is much more rare. This disease may be associated with other disorders including high blood pressure, diabetes mellitus, and some unusual forms of immune diseases. In the past decade there has been increasing evidence that persons with hepatitis C, hepatitis B, or other types of liver disease are more susceptible to developing this condition. Persons who develop lichen planus should be evaluated for any signs or symptoms of other diseases.

A serious type of lichen planus is lichen planopilaris. This affects hair follicles, causing them to become permanently scarred and incapable of forming new hairs. It primarily affects women and may be devastating from a cosmetic standpoint. Other hairs besides those of the scalp may also be affected. The scalp is mildly to moderately itchy and may scale as well. Some patients show a slight purplish color to the skin but more commonly the skin appears normal. Treatment is difficult since the disease is relentless and progresses to significant hair loss.

Treatment

There are a great many different therapies for lichen planus since a single effective treatment does not exist. Good skin care is an absolute must since mild trauma (scratches and abrasions) may provoke lichen planus to erupt at the site of damage. This is called the Koebner phenomenon and is also seen in vitiligo and psoriasis. For some persons, treatment is not mandatory. Lichen planus will subside on its own without treatment in less than a year. For persons who are very uncomfortable and for those with more unusual types of disease, however, treatment is a must.

Corticosteroids are usually the first drugs tried for lichen planus. They may be applied to the skin as creams and ointments; these help the itching but are not usually strong enough to completely get rid of the rash. Since there are many spots, it is difficult to apply these to all the areas requiring treatment. Oral corticosteroids (prednisone [Deltasone®] and prednisolone [Prelone®]) are very effective in some persons and may be enough to solve the problem. These are good medicines with which to begin treatment but many patients require additional therapy. Additionally, corticosteroids are hard to give by mouth in persons with diabetes and many patients with lichen planus have this disease. Steroid inhalers, as for asthma, have been used to apply medicine to the mucous membranes of the mouth. Injecting triamcinolone (Kenalog®) into a lichen planus lesion is also usually effective, but not very practical if there are many areas of involvement.

The class of drugs known as the retinoids may help some persons with lichen planus and is often the next medication tried. Isotretinoin (Accutane®) is usually used at the same doses as for severe acne and acitretin (Soriatane®) at the same doses for psoriasis. Tretinoin (Retin-A®) is useful for oral lichen planus but must be applied several times a day.

PUVA (psoralens and UVA) is a helpful therapy. It is reasonably safe and often

Table 24 DRUGS KNOWN TO CAUSE LICHENOID DRUG ERUPTIONS

Antihypertensives	captopril (Capoten®)
	enalapril (Vasotec®)
	hydrochlorothiazide (Hydrodiuril®)
	propanolol (Inderal®)
Nonsteroidal Anti-inflammatory Drugs	acetylsalicylic acid (Bayer® Aspirin)
	naproxen (Aleve®, Naprosyn®)
	indomethacin (Indocin®)
	ibuprofen (Motrin®)
Miscellaneous	allopurinol (Zyloprim®)
	carbamazepine (Tegretol®)
	gold (Myochrisine®)
	penicillamine (Cuprimine®)
	pyrimethamine (Fansidar®)
	tolbutamide

very effective. PUVA is given the same way as for psoriasis. Unfortunately, there are few places to receive this therapy aside from a dermatologist's office or phototherapy center (usually associated with major medical centers). It is also expensive and time consuming.

Griseofulvin (Gris-PEG®) has been helpful in treating lichen planus. It is not very useful for oral disease. This drug kills certain types of fungus. It is considered safe but is not used much anymore since it is not as effective as other treatments. Other antifungal drugs such as amphotericin (Fungizone®) and fluconazole (Diflucan®) have also proven useful in certain patients with lichen planus. Antibacterial antibiotics such as sulfa drugs, penicillin, and tetracycline (Sumycin®) have been successfully used. Recently, a medication used to treat intestinal worm infections, levamisole (Ergamisol®), has proven useful for lichen planus.

Cyclosporine (Sandimmune®, Neoral®), dapsone, and hydroxychloroquine (Plaquenil®) are also effective but have to be carefully given. These drugs require blood work and may be expensive. Application of topical cyclosporine to the mucous membranes of the mouth and genitalia is safe and effective. Finally, some chemotherapy drugs such as azathioprine (Immuran®) and cyclophosphamide (Cytoxan®) have been effectively used in more severe cases of lichen planus.

Lichenoid Drug Eruption

A certain type of drug reaction may look identical to lichen planus and is called a lichenoid drug eruption, or lichen planuslike drug eruption (see Table 24). Certain medications are more likely to cause this eruption than others and the list of suspect drugs is almost endless. Persons taking these medicines who develop lichen planus should be evaluated for such a drug reaction. Lichenoid drug eruptions and lichen planus are similar but not identical under the microscope, and a skin biopsy is often helpful in distinguishing between the two. The treatment for these eruptions is to discontinue taking the offending medicines. This may not always be possible, however.

Lichen Sclerosus

This disorder has also been called *lichen sclerosus et atrophicus*. It primarily affects women but may also be seen in men and children. Most patients are white and the diagnosis is usually made in the third or fourth decade of life.

Symptoms

The disease typically begins around the vulva and anus. It starts as small white spots which group together to become a patch. Sometimes the areas may be slightly red or pink. As the disease progresses, the skin becomes thinned and scaly and loses its pigment. Some plugging of the hair follicles is seen and if trauma occurs there may be slight bleeding into the patch. In older lesions, the deeper skin becomes scarlike and thickened. Patients may have itching, burning, painful urination, bleeding, and vaginal discharge. Long-standing lesions may narrow the vaginal opening and cause difficulties with intercourse. Patches are also occasionally seen on the breasts, trunk, and arms. Involvement on the penis and foreskin may cause painful erections, itching, and discharge. Childhood lesions are usually seen in girls. At adolescence, lichen sclerosus may resolve but spontaneous healing in adults is uncommon. There is a risk in chronic lesions, particularly if they have been left untreated, of the spots becoming skin cancers. Treatment in such situations is similar to that for skin cancers elsewhere and the prognosis overall is favorable.

Causes

Causes of lichen sclerosus are not clear. Some dermatologists believe this is a type of morphea or scleroderma (see the sections on morphea and scleroderma). It almost surely has something to do with the hormonal or endocrine system. There is some evidence that infection by the same bacteria known to cause Lyme disease (*Borrelia burgdorferi*) causes lichen sclerosus. Other possibilities include chronic friction and ongoing irritation.

Treatment

Treatment of lichen sclerosus may be difficult. Topical corticosteroids are effective in many cases. Very potent medications may thin the skin, however, if used for too long. Topical corticosteroids help stop the itching and discomfort. They may be applied as creams and ointments. Application of potent formulations in two-week bursts has been useful for women and children. Topical estrogen (Premarin®) and progesterone creams have also been helpful. These hormones are usually mixed in petrolatum jelly and applied once or twice daily. Mixing hormone ointments with topical corticosteroids has also been used. Topical testosterone ointment is one of the preferred methods of therapy. This hormone may give very good results. Unfortunately, some of the testosterone is absorbed and if used for long enough may result in some male hormone effects (lowering of the voice, change in hair pattern, change in sex drive, and so on). This is a safe means of treatment but must be monitored very carefully. Alternating topical testosterone and topical corticosteroid application is also useful. Acitretin (Soriatane®) has been used with some success in persons with resistant and widespread disease. The dose is similar to that for psoriasis. Surgical excision is useful if the involvement is restricted to a single site such as the foreskin but otherwise doesn't play much of a role. Other less common treatments include vitamin B and D preparations, superficial x-ray, antimalarial drugs, crotamiton (Eurax®), doxycycline (Doryx®), penicillin, and wheat germ oil.

LICHEN SIMPLEX AND PRURIGO NODULARIS

Lichen Simplex

The full name of this disorder is lichen simplex chronicus or neurodermatitis circumscripta, meaning that the process is chronic or long standing. It may be considered a reaction by the skin to rubbing, scratching, picking, or other forms of trauma.

Symptoms
The most common scenario involves atopic dermatitis or eczema. Some dermatologists believe that anxiety or mental illness (depression, anger, psychoses, and so on) plays a large role in this disease. The skin is rubbed or scratched repeatedly, eventually becoming dark and thickened. The natural lines on the skin are exaggerated and mild scaling may occur. If the scratching has been recent there may be small spots of bleeding and scabbing. The wrists, ankles, arms, and sides of the neck are common sites of involvement.

There are some specialized types of lichen simplex. Lichen simplex nuchae involves the nape of the neck and back of the scalp. The skin is thickened and the hair may be thinned from scratching. Bleeding and excoriations are common. Anogenital lichen simplex is seen on the vulva, scrotum, and around the anus. This may occur after the skin becomes sensitive to some chemical, such as perfume, toiletries, or soap. There may also be a psychological need to scratch in some of these patients.

Treatment
Therapy is straightforward but often frustrating. Asking a person not to scratch is useless. People with lichen simplex scratch without knowing it and often in their sleep. Some of the same treatments suggested for atopic dermatitis are applicable here. Corticosteroids by mouth or injection are useful. Injecting corticosteroid suspensions into the skin may also provide considerable relief but obviously cannot be done if the disease is widespread. Topical corticosteroids are the mainstays of therapy and should be combined with very aggressive moisturization (five to six times per day). Use of a nondrying soap (see the section on moisturizers and soaps) is also important.

212

Over-the-counter topical anti-itch medications such as Sarna® lotion or Aveeno Anti-Itch® cream are useful and may be applied as often as desired. Oral antihistamines (hydroxyzine [Atarax®], diphenhydramine [Benadryl®]) work well, particularly at nighttime, but may be too sedating. Nonsedating antihistamines are usually not effective enough for significant use. Grenz-ray therapy as used for atopic dermatitis is very helpful but not widely available. PUVA therapy is also beneficial but has significant drawbacks when used for such a small area. Some treatment centers offer topical PUVA whereby the substance is "painted" on the skin or the skin is soaked in a psoralen-containing bath before being treated with ultraviolet light A. In some persons, there is a component of anxiety or depression causing them to scratch or rub their skin. These persons may do very well with antianxiety and antidepression treatment.

Prurigo Nodularis

Prurigo nodularis is similar to lichen simplex but arises as small pea- to grape-sized nodules and not as a patch. These are red to dark colored and typically involve the arms, legs, and trunk. They itch maddeningly and many show evidence of having been picked, dug, or otherwise traumatized. Persons with underlying kidney and liver disease commonly have prurigo nodularis because their skin has an increased tendency to dryness and itch. Insect bites and inflamed hair follicles (folliculitis) may also trigger an episode.

Treatment of prurigo nodularis is the same as for lichen simplex but generally more frustrating. All the lesions will completely subside if the patients will leave their skin alone. However, many persons do not realize they are responsible for the trauma. Corticosteroid suspension injections are probably the most effective means of therapy but are not useful if there are many lesions. Oral and intramuscular corticosteroids are initially very useful to get the condition under control. Since many of these have been scratched into infection, antibiotics are sometimes required. Treatment with liquid nitrogen (cryotherapy) has proven useful, as has surgically shaving off the tumor. Ultraviolet light therapy with UVB is helpful but time consuming and expensive. Thalidomide is useful in some cases but this drug is not available in the United States. Some patients have sought treatment in countries where this drug is still available. Antianxiety and antidepression medications have proven useful in certain patients.

Lumps and Bumps

One of the most common complaints or questions that people have is about a lump or bump on the skin. Almost all of these turn out to be benign growths. Biopsies occasionally are performed, however, to rule out a malignancy or to remove the lesion.

Angiokeratoma

Angiokeratomas are a collection of blood vessels which are covered by rough, dark overlying skin. There are several different types, including one that is seen in children. The most common one involves the scrotum and vulva of older persons (angiokeratoma of Fordyce). Most of these grow to the size of a pencil lead and have no symptoms. If they are numerous enough they may bleed with trauma and become infected. Angiokeratomas may be removed with a laser, by simple excision, or destroyed with electrical current (electrofulguration). They are not dangerous and do not become malignant.

Cherry Red Spots (Senile Angioma, Campbell de Morgan spot)

These are among the most common lesions that affect patients older than twenty-five years. They begin as pinpoint red dots and may enlarge to the size of a pencil eraser or more. They are usually found on the trunk but also occur on the head and neck. They may also be called "red moles" but actually have nothing to do with moles or nevi, since they are composed of blood vessels. They do not have symptoms. Treatment is the same as for angiokeratomas.

Cysts

There are a number of different types of cysts that the body produces on the skin. Almost all are related to the abnormal growth of some part of a hair follicle. None are capable of becoming malignant. The most common is called an epithelial, sebaceous, or infundibular cyst. These commonly occur on the head, neck, and trunk. Children may be affected, but most patients are past puberty. These cysts appear as pencil eraser- to egg-sized flesh-colored bumps. The overlying skin may be tight and occasionally shows a small pit in the center. If cysts are infected or inflamed, they may be very red, swollen, and painful. Typically, these cysts lie dormant in the skin until traumatized by attempts at "popping" them or bumping into something. At this point they rupture into the skin, begin to become inflamed, and start to grow in size. If they are allowed to drain on their own they produce foul-smelling pus and bits of solid material.

If the cyst is not inflamed, it will contain cheesy material with a sour odor. The production of cysts seems to run in families, with some persons more susceptible to forming these lesions. If the cyst is inflamed, it has to be removed. This can usually be done by simple surgical excision. Sometimes the overlying skin has become so damaged that allowing the area to drain and then heal is the only course of treatment. If the cyst is not too large, too objectionable, or too uncomfortable, it may be simply left alone. If removal is desired, the entire cyst, including the wall, may be excised. Extraction of the cyst contents and the majority of the cyst wall can also be done in some instances through a punch biopsy hole, which is then closed with stitches. It is usually best to remove all or most of the wall to prevent the cyst from reforming.

The second most common cyst is called a pilar cyst or wen. These are usually found on the scalp and have no symptoms. They have the same appearance as an epidermoid cyst but are rarely inflamed. Pilar cysts are easier to remove than epithelioid cysts and may generally be taken out through a small incision or punch biopsy hole.

A steatocystoma is a rare type of cyst which may be inherited. Most persons have a single cyst on the chest, head, or neck which is flesh colored and smooth. Multiple cysts occur in some persons. Steatocystomas contain an oily yellow to clear material. They rarely become inflamed. If only a single cyst is present, the simplest treatment is to surgically excise it. If there are multiple cysts, they may be drained with a needle but will usually reform. Some patients have been treated with isotretinoin (Accutane®) in doses similar to that for acne. These cysts are difficult to get rid of and their presence may be not only uncomfortable but embarrassing as well.

Dermatofibroma

This benign tumor goes by a number of different names (nodular subepidermal fibrosis, histiocytoma, sclerosing hemangioma, and so on) and is one of the most common benign growths. Dermatofibromas are believed to result from trauma (shaving, insect bites, and so on). They first begin to occur after puberty and usually affect the legs and arms. The trunk may have an isolated lesion or two, but the head and neck are rarely involved. Dermatofibromas are most often seen in women in their twenties and thirties. Tumors are pea-sized light brown to purple areas which are firm and usually even with the skin's surface. They "dimple" inward when squeezed from the sides. They are symptomless, and treatment is usually not necessary. They may be surgically excised, sometimes through a punch biopsy procedure. Injection of corticosteroid suspensions has also been helpful in some cases. A large dermatofibroma may become painful and require excision, but these are uncommon.

Dupuytren's Contracture

Dupuytren's contractures occur as thickening of the deep skin on the palms and soles. They begin in middle age and predominantly affect whites. They are more frequently seen among alcoholics, epileptics, and diabetics but may occur in otherwise healthy persons. These contractures begin as a thickening of the deep tissues on the palms. The tendons are involved and as the disease progresses, the fourth and fifth fingers are gradually drawn down. If left untreated, the fingers eventually cannot be extended and their use is lost. A similar situation occurs on the sole. While this condition is not life threatening, it may be very disabling. Treatment consists of surgical repair of the tendon and the surrounding fibrosis. If the disease is in the early stages, injecting corticosteroid suspensions may help.

Fibrous Papule of the Nose (Angiofibroma)

These small flesh-colored lesions occur on the nose (fibrous papules) or over the central face and forehead (angiofibromas). They begin in early adulthood and are symptomless. Multiple angiofibromas are also seen in a genetic disease called tuberous sclerosis. Most are the size of a pencil lead. They may be left alone without problems but some persons choose to have them shaved off under local anesthesia.

Keloid

These tumors are most common among dark-skinned people. Keloids are caused by scarring that has gone out of control. They arise in areas of trauma such as burns, cuts, scrapes, insect bites, ear piercing, and so on. Some begin spontaneously, particularly on the chest. Most are initially slightly tender but usually become symptomless. Keloids begin to appear following puberty. The tendency to their formation is inherited in some persons. These lesions look like very dark and enlarged scars. The skin is usually smooth and shiny.

Keloids are a frustrating problem because there is frequently not much patients can to do avoid them. Treatment is equally difficult. They may be surgically excised but, of course, can reform in the surgical scar. Injecting the site of excision with a corticosteroid-containing suspension will slow healing of the site but may also allow the wound to close without forming a second keloid. Injecting corticosteroid suspensions, usually in high concentrations, may help shrink and soften some lesions, but this is painful and requires multiple office visits. X-ray was used to shrink keloids in the past but this is no longer done. Compression of the excision site after surgery may help prevent the lesion from reforming. Special earrings are useful in this regard for women or men who want to have pierced ears but tend to form keloids. Application of tretinoin (Retin-A®) and injecting interferon (Intron-A®) has shown some promise.

Acne Nuchae Keloidalis

This is a very common pattern of hair loss and scarring which is present over the nape of the neck. It occurs almost exclusively in blacks when the hair is cut too short (usually flush with the surface of the skin) and the regrowing hair shaft, with a sharp point, curves around and begins to pierce the skin. This causes an inflammatory reaction which results in small keloids. The hairs may actually be "popped" out of the skin, but by this time the damage has been done and the keloids are forming. There is some evidence that the hair follicles themselves are inflamed (folliculitis).

The most important aspect of treatment consists of avoidance by not shaving the hairs so close to the skin but instead leaving them half an inch long or so. Antibiotics such as tetracycline (Sumycin®) and erythromycin (PCE®) have been helpful in controlling inflammation and infection. Topical antibiotics as used for acne have been useful as well. The keloids themselves are treated similar to keloids elsewhere.

Milia

Milia are small cysts similar to epidermoid cysts. These are usually found on the face and are called "whiteheads" by some people. As such, they may be confused with acne. Some patients attempt to express them by "popping" the cysts. This is impossible since unlike the lesions of acne, milia are completely beneath the skin with no connection to a hair follicle. Scarring and infection may then occur. Milia are common around the eyes and nose. They may arise in areas of trauma, after blistering diseases have subsided, and on skin which has had potent topical corticosteroids applied for too long. Most are not much bigger than a pencil lead. Treatment is relatively easy but not too pleasant. A sharp scalpel blade or syringe needle may be used to puncture the milia and the contents are removed. This may be done with minimal scarring but is uncomfortable. No topical medications are capable of treating these lesions.

Mucocele

These tumors arise in the mouth, usually on the lower lip or under the tongue. They are painless but may interfere with eating or speaking. Younger patients, particularly males, are more likely to be affected. Mucoceles result from rupture of small salivary glands. These glands then produce saliva which collects in the tissues. The tumors are flesh colored to clear and may drain fluid from time to time. Treatment consists of surgical excision of the mucocele along with the damaged minor salivary glands.

Leiomyoma

Numerous muscle cells exist in the skin associated with hair follicles and blood vessels. When they begin to grow out of control, they form leiomyomas. These benign tumors are red to brown and occur on the trunk or extremities. Some may arise in muscle around the nipples or scrotum. Leiomyomas commonly occur in small groups and are painful, particularly when they contact cold substances. Treatment consists of surgical excision. Some blood pressure medications which act on muscle within blood vessels (calcium channel blockers) may relieve the pain of leiomyomas.

Lipoma

Lipomas are collections of fatty tissue. They are benign and usually occur singly or as a few lesions. Some patients, particularly those with a family tendency to these tumors, may have many lesions. A variant of lipomas, angiolipomas, are more common in young patients and are typically painful. Lipomas appear as small pea to marble sized lumps under the skin that are soft and skin colored. Some lesions may grow to the size of a hen's egg but this is uncommon. They appear on the trunk and extremities. Alcoholics have a tendency to develop numerous lipomas. Unless the tumors are uncomfortable or particularly noticeable, they do not require treatment.

Surgical excision is the usual method of removal. Another approach is to do a punch biopsy over the lipoma and press the contents out. This results in less of a scar but is not always completely effective.

Lymphangioma

This is a collection of lymphatic vessels (very similar to blood vessels) that occurs in the uppermost portions of the skin. They appear like small blisters but have no symptoms and arise in childhood or shortly after birth. Lymphangiomas are clear to reddish brown. Some are slightly warty or scaly. Most are about the size of a dime but they may become very large. They are usually on the trunk, buttocks, and legs. While these lesions are benign, they are very difficult to get rid of. Surgical excision usually fails because these vessels are "fed" from deep in the skin so they reform after the surgery. Treatment with lasers may be helpful.

Metastases

Unfortunately, sometimes cancers of the internal organs metastasize to the skin. In some instances, this is the initial presentation of the malignancy. These lesions usually look like flesh-colored nodules from the size of a pea to a golf ball. They may be red or brown depending on the cancer but they are rarely painful. Some malignancies are more likely than others to metastasize to the skin. For men the most frequently metastatic tumors are malignant melanoma, lung cancer, colon cancer, and oral cancer. For women breast cancer, malignant melanoma, and ovarian carcinoma are the most common. Usually, involvement of the skin by a metastatic tumor is associated with a poor prognosis.

Neurofibroma

Neurofibromas are present in a disease called neurofibromatosis or Von Recklinghausen's disease. More often, however, these flesh-colored tumors occur on the trunk of middle age and older patients and have no association with any underlying abnormalities. These lesions tend to arise around the waist and buttocks, are usually solitary, and have no symptoms. They have a characteristic soft texture. They may be surgically removed either by snipping or shaving the neurofibroma off flush with the skin.

Pilomatricoma

Pilomatricomas are benign cystic growths which are most common in children. They usually arise on the head and neck but are frequently seen on the arms in older adults. They may be up to the size of a small marble and have normal-looking over-lying skin. They may also have a slightly blue or white color. Pilomatricomas often contain calcium or fragments of bone and as such are usually very firm to the touch. They are treated by surgical removal.

Pyogenic Granuloma (Lobular Capillary Hemangioma)

These lesions have also been called "proud flesh" and are rapidly growing nodules which ooze and bleed. They are usually about the size of a pea and have no symp-toms. If left alone they will eventually heal and form a dark spot on the skin. They are common in children on the hands, face, and arms. They also occur in the mouth during pregnancy. "Satellite" lesions may arise around the tumors and have the same features but are usually smaller. In adolescents and young adults they normally appear on the trunk, particularly the upper back. They arise following minor trauma such as scratches or insect bites. Pyogenic granulomas are usually treated by surgi-cal excision but a number recur. Coating them with silver nitrate will cause some to disappear; they also respond to laser therapy.

Sebaceous Hyperplasia

This is very common in persons past middle age. It appears as flesh-colored to slightly yellow-orange bumps about the size of a pencil lead. Sebaceous hyperplasia is seen almost exclusively on the forehead and central face. These lesions are symp-tomless but may be cosmetically objectionable. Treatment is not difficult but new lesions may form after a few have been removed. They may be taken off with sur-gical excision (usually shaved off after local anesthetic has been given). They also respond to application of topical acids and liquid nitrogen. Touching them with an electric needle will cause them to break down and bubble. A scab is then formed and falls off in a week or so. Sebaceous hyperplasia is completely benign.

Seborrheic Keratosis

These are the most common benign tumors affecting humans. They occur during middle age but may be seen in persons in their twenties. Seborrheic keratoses are usually brown but may be flesh colored, white, yellow, orange, or jet black. Some look like moles and are removed because they may mimic a malignant melanoma. Seborrheic keratoses are usually found on the head, neck, and trunk. Some persons may have thousands of these lesions. They do not have symptoms but may itch or become painful if they are irritated. They range from the size of a pencil lead to several inches in diameter. Some are scaly and warty. A condition known as Leser-Trelat may appear in persons with underlying cancers, particularly of the colon or bowel, in which many seborrheic keratoses suddenly occur on the skin. It is not clear what causes these lesions but they tend to occur in areas of sun exposure and chronic trauma.

A similar condition called dermatosis papulosa nigra occurs on the face and neck of blacks and Asians. These are small dark seborrheic keratoses which may protrude from the skin and are cosmetically disfiguring.

Treatment of seborrheic keratoses usually consists of simply destroying the lesions. This may be accomplished by freezing with liquid nitrogen (the most popular method), application of acids, or scraping them off. They may also be surgically excised or shaved off with a razor blade. Using an electric needle is another method of destruction. Dermatosis papulosa nigra responds to the same methods of therapy but in dark-skinned patients such treatment may result in a loss or increase of pigment.

Skin Tags (Acrochordons)

Skin tags are small lesions which are flesh colored to dark brown and occur on the sides of the neck, the eyelids, and under the arms. They are common in overweight persons. These tumors are usually just an annoyance but may become inflamed and painful. Clothing and jewelry occasionally catch on skin tags. Larger ones occur on the lower back, buttocks, and groin. These are usually flesh colored and may grow to the size of a small grape. Treatment consists of either snipping them off with scissors or freezing them with liquid nitrogen.

Syringoma

Syringomas are small flesh-colored bumps that occur on the central face, particularly around the eyes. These are benign and form when some of the sweat glands abnormally develop. They are more common in women, and in some people, may be inherited. Treatment consists of surgical removal; they may also be treated with lasers.

Lupus Erythematosus and Dermatomyositis

Lupus Erythematosus

This disorder is called a "collagen vascular" or "autoimmune" disease. For some reason, probably genetic, the body's immune system turns on itself and begins to attack healthy tissues. Most patients are women in their thirties and forties but almost anyone can be affected. There are several different types of lupus; the most pertinent to dermatology is chronic cutaneous lupus erythematosus or discoid lupus.

Discoid Lupus

As with all lupus, it is not clear what causes discoid lupus erythematosus (DLE). It is more common in the summer months, since it is worsened by sunlight. Some types of trauma to the skin may incite DLE but most often it arises for no apparent reason. Menstruation, fatigue, and illness may worsen the disease. The lesions of DLE begin as small, red, scaly patches, usually on the head and neck. They may also be seen on other sun-exposed sites such as the arms and legs, but sun-protected sites usually are not involved. The ears and nose are often involved. The mucous membranes in the mouth and nose may also be affected. The spots begin to expand and may become white in the center. Since DLE is a scarring process, the lesions may have a slightly sunken or atrophic appearance. They may sting or itch, but symptoms usually are not a major problem. In black skin they may be either excessively dark or light. There is a hyperkeratotic form in which the skin becomes very thick and scaly. The profundus form does not affect the overlying skin so much as the fat beneath it. These lesions are most often seen on the arms, legs, and trunk. They form deep sunken pockets of scarring with increased pigmentation and may be very disfiguring. DLE has typical findings on biopsy and this is the usual method of diagnosis. DLE usually stays confined to the skin with little likelihood of involving the internal organs.

Like almost all forms of lupus, DLE is aggravated by light exposure. Consequently, the use of a good broad-spectrum sunscreen is important. Sunscreens containing zinc oxide or titanium dioxide are useful as they block ultraviolet rays best. These should be applied frequently during the day, since even small amounts of sun exposure may make DLE worse. Appropriate protective clothing should be worn as well. Beta-carotene (Solatene®) is helpful for persons who are particularly sensitive to the sun. Topical corticosteroids are useful but remember, the lesions of DLE already have a tendency to be thinned and corticosteroids, if used improperly, make this problem worse. Injecting corticosteroids is an effective treatment option but oral prednisone is not very helpful. The mainstay of treatment for this disease are the antimalarial agents, specifically hydroxychloroquine (Plaquenil®). This is usually given as 200 to 400 mg per day. Other antimalarials such as chloroquine (Aralen®) or quinacrine may also be used, but are not as popular. If these drugs fail, the options for successful treatment are few and include isotretinoin (Accutane®), acitretin (Soriatane®), thalidomide, and azathioprine (Immuran®).

Systemic Lupus Erythematosus

Systemic lupus erythematosus (SLE) is the type of lupus familiar to most persons and is the form which poses the most health risks. It is fairly rare, occurring in only about 50 persons per 100,000 population. Like DLE, it principally affects women. This disorder seems to be inheritable to some extent, since persons with SLE may have close relatives with the disease. Some drugs (hydralazine [Apresoline®], procainamide [Procanbid®], isoniazide [Rifamate®]) and environmental exposures provoke SLE. The skin disease in SLE includes a rash over the upper face and bridge of the nose ("butterfly" rash), typical DLE-like lesions, puffiness of the fingers/toes, visible blood vessels around the cuticles, hair loss, and involvement of the mucous membranes. Arthritis with pain and swelling of the joints is common and resembles rheumatoid arthritis. Probably the most worrisome aspect of SLE is kidney involvement. This occurs in over half of affected patients and leads to total kidney failure in some. Seizures and mental illness are seen in unusual cases. Other features include an inflammation of the heart and surrounding tissues (pericarditis), nausea, vomiting, diarrhea, blood clotting, leg ulcers, hepatitis, decreased blood counts, and anemia. SLE is commonly diagnosed using blood tests. Biopsying skin lesions may be helpful but is not as useful as in DLE.

Since SLE is a serious condition, physicians may have to use potent medications to control the disease. Treatment initially centers around corticosteroids given intravenously or by mouth. These may have to be given in very high doses. Cyclophosphamide (Cytoxan®) is commonly administered, particularly when kidney involvement is present. Azathioprine is also used. Antimalarials are helpful for the skin, hair, and mucous membrane effects of SLE but don't do much for the other symptoms. They may allow the patient to decrease the dose of corticosteroids. Since most patients are sun sensitive, sunscreens are also useful.

Subacute Cutaneous Lupus Erythematosus

This is a recently designated category of patients whose lupus erythematosus falls somewhere between DLE and SLE. Again, most patients are white females between the ages of fifteen and forty. The skin eruption may look like psoriasis or large plaques of a scaly, red, raised rash. As the skin eruption resolves it tends to leave areas of increased pigmentation much as in DLE. Mild itching may occur. The trunk, arms, and other sun-exposed areas are most affected. Patients have joint pains and some blood count involvement but the serious effects seen with SLE are absent. Patients with subacute cutaneous lupus erythematosus (SCLE) usually have an unusual antibody in their blood called Ro or SSA. Blood analysis for this antibody and a skin biopsy are the most common means of making this diagnosis. Treatment is essentially the same as for DLE.

Dermatomyositis

The signs and symptoms of dermatomyositis (DM) overlap to a large extent with those of SLE and DLE. This is one of a group of diseases called inflammatory myopathies, meaning that the body's muscles become inflamed. DM is a connective tissue disease but is fairly uncommon. It is seen in several different groups. There is a childhood type; another type affects adults; and a third type is seen in persons, usually adults, who have an underlying cancer. Besides the kind associated with a malignancy, there is no known cause of DM. While most patients with this disease recover, there are a few who ultimately die of dermatomyositis.

The most common symptom is weakness of the muscles of the limbs and trunk. This typically causes difficulty with activities such as rising from a chair or toilet, combing hair, climbing stairs, brushing one's teeth, and so on. The weakness is progressive and some mild tenderness is seen in many patients. A red rash develops over the backs of the fingers and hands. A very distinctive red to lavender eruption around the eyes, called a heliotrope, is present in some patients. Dilated blood vessels around the cuticles, as seen in SLE, are also present. Pain in the joints may also be seen. The muscles and skin may become calcified, particularly in the childhood form of DM.

Diagnosis again rests on finding the appropriate constellation of symptoms and evaluating the blood. Most persons will have increased amounts of a protein called creatinine phosophokinase (CPK) in their blood. This enzyme is found in muscle cells and as these cells become inflamed and destroyed, their contents leak into the blood. Biopsying a person's muscle is very helpful in making the diagnosis but is both painful and difficult to do. An electromyogram tests the performance of muscles and is useful as well. Persons at risk for having an underlying cancer should be evaluated for that possibility. Such patients tend to improve significantly if such a malignancy is removed.

There are a number of treatments for dermatomyositis. Probably the preferred initial treatment is high doses of oral or intravenous corticosteroids. This is done until the CPK values in the blood begin to come down, indicating that the muscles have begun to heal themselves. Other useful medications are those that suppress the immune system such as azathioprine, cyclosporine (Sandimmune®, Neoral®), chlorambucil (Leukeran®), and methotrexate (Rheumatrex®). Intravenous administration of gamma globulin may also help. The skin findings usually respond to antimalarial medications such as hydroxychloroquine. Unfortunately, this class of medications does not benefit the muscle disease. Topical corticosteroids may also be used on the skin rash. Patients with DM are sensitive to the sun and must use sunscreens. Physical therapy is very important, particularly as the disease begins to subside. Patients usually take several months or years to regain their strength.

LYMPHOMA

Lymphomas are solid tumors of malignant inflammatory and immune cells. They arise in the bone marrow, spleen, and other internal organs but are seen in the skin as well. One specific type, cutaneous T cell lymphoma (CTCL; mycosis fungoides) arises in the skin and may remain there or may affect internal organs. Routine lymphomas which may affect the skin include Hodgkin's disease and non-Hodgkin's lymphomas. Skin lesions are usually seen as small to large nodules that are reddish to purple or "plum colored." They rarely have any other symptoms. These nodules may occur in patients who are known to have underlying lymphoma or may be the first signs of the disease. Treatment is usually the same as for the underlying lymphoma; either chemotherapy or radiation treatments. Occasionally, a lymphoma will be found only in the skin, in which case surgical excision may cure the problem. Unlike with metastases from other cancers, the presence of lymphoma in the skin does not necessarily imply a bad prognosis.

Cutaneous T Cell Lymphoma

Much more has become known about this disease in the past decade and it now appears that many more people have this disease than was previously thought. There are several different types of CTCL but the most common is termed mycosis fungoides. This name is inaccurate in that it implies that CTCL has something to do with a fungal disease; it clearly does not. Other rare types of CTCL include poikiloderma vasculare atrophicans, alopecia mucinosa, Sezary syndrome, granulomatous slack skin, and pagetoid reticulosis. What causes these disorders is not clear but it appears to be some chronic stimulation of the immune system. CTCL is a lymphoma formed by a group of immune cells called "T cells." These cells locate to the skin and form characteristic rashes. As time passes they may invade the bloodstream and the internal organs.

Symptoms

In the earliest stages, the skin shows a pink to flesh-colored rash which may come and go. It is mildly scaly and usually appears on the trunk and around the waist. Lesions are nickel to palm sized. It commonly responds well to topical corticosteroids and moisturizers. This rash has been termed parapsoriasis because it appears similar to psoriasis. As the disease progresses, the patches become thicker and better defined at the margins. They also are redder and scale more. Itching may become a problem. Sometimes dilated blood vessels are seen. Lesions become less likely to respond to treatments which previously were helpful. As more immune cells flow into the skin and mild fibrosis is seen, the plaques become thicker. Eventually, nodules in the skin may occur. These may break down and weep. Ulcerations and widespread redness of the skin (erythroderma) are also seen as the disease progresses. Unfortunately, by the time the disease has gotten to the stage of thick plaques and/or nodules, there is less of a chance for control or cure. CTCL may spread to the bone marrow, spleen, lymph nodes, lungs, and kidney. The diagnosis is made with skin biopsies. Specialized evaluation of these biopsies may be required to prove that the immune cells present in the skin are in fact malignant and not simply there because of some skin irritation or allergy. If there is a suggestion of internal involvement, the appropriate biopsies or x-rays will have to be done.

Treatment

Treatment is best begun when the disease is in its earliest stages. The patch stage may respond to potent corticosteroid creams and ointments. Applying chemotherapy drugs to the skin (topical chemotherapy) has long been used for CTCL. Nitrogen mustard or chloronitrosourea (BCNU) may be prepared in water or ointment and applied to the skin. This is very effective in some cases, but a large percentage of patients develop a contact allergy to these medications and are not able to use them. They are also somewhat messy, but relatively easy to use and can be applied at home. Radiation therapy is beneficial for some patients. Traditional radiotherapy may be used in certain patients, usually early in their disease. A newer type of radiation treatment called electron beam therapy penetrates the skin very little and concentrates in the areas of the body which need treatment the most. It is well tolerated and has a good success rate but is only given in specialized treatment centers and is expensive, and it takes a long time to complete a course. The typical side effects of radiotherapy include hair loss at the sites of treatment, dry and red skin, dilated blood vessels, and swelling.

Psoralens and ultraviolet light A (PUVA) is one of the most popular treatments. This therapy is given in the same manner as for psoriasis or lichen planus and is usually well tolerated. It is effective and comparatively inexpensive. It does take up a lot of time since treatments must be given three times a week for three months. Because of the increased amount of ultraviolet light exposure, treated patients are at an increased risk of skin cancer. However, in many cases PUVA is the preferred method of treatment.

Chemotherapy has been used for some patients with CTCL, particularly those with more advanced disease. The drugs used include chlorambucil (Leukeran®), cyclophosphamide (Cytoxan®), doxorubicin (Adriamycin®), vincristine (Oncovin®), and etoposide (Vepesid®), along with prednisone. While this is a helpful therapy, it is not always successful.

A newer therapy called photophoresis has been developed in the last decade. This treatment consists of the patient taking 8-methoxypsoralen (as in PUVA treatment), drawing off some of the body's blood, and treating it with ultraviolet light. The blood is then returned to the body. This may be very helpful for selected patients but is extremely expensive and time consuming and is available in only a few specialized treatment centers.

In the future, interferon drugs may be used for some cases of CTCL. In certain patients, it is helpful to combine different types of treatment to better control the disease. This has typically involved some form of chemotherapy and radiation treatment.

Mastocytosis (Urticaria Pigmentosa)

A group of skin cells called mast cells contain several different chemicals, one of which is histamine. Some parts of the body have more mast cells than others. When the skin has too many mast cells, a disease known as mastocytosis occurs.

Internal organ involvement is uncommon. If too much histamine is being produced, diarrhea and heart palpitations may result. Psychiatric symptoms such as depression, irritability, and memory loss are also seen. Flushing of the skin occurs when patients ingest aspirin, alcohol, or narcotics.

The diagnosis is usually made when the symptoms are put together with the findings on the skin and a skin biopsy. Measuring the amount of histamine present in the blood and urine is also done. Several types of mastocytosis are listed below.

Urticaria Pigmentosa

Urticaria pigmentosa (UP) is the most common form of mastocytosis and is seen in 90 percent of patients with this disorder. The skin develops small tan to brown bumps, usually about the size of a pencil eraser. These are composed of mast cells. They occur almost anywhere but do not usually involve the palms, soles, face, or scalp. They are usually without symptoms. When they are subjected to trauma such as scratching, however, the mast cells in the skin release histamine and itching begins. Because this process is similar to that for hives or urticaria, some of the same symptoms are seen. The surrounding skin becomes slightly swollen and may look like a welt. Patients usually have only a few lesions, but in some instances there may be many. This disorder is more common in children but may be found in adults as well. The skin may show evidence of scratching, and infection can occur. Some of the typical features of atopic dermatitis (eczema) may also be present. The itching of the skin may be provoked by temperature changes, medications, and the consumption of alcohol, hot beverages, and spicy foods.

Mastocytoma

Mastocytomas are similar to the small bumps seen in UP but tend to be bigger, usually about the size of a nickel or quarter. They are seen almost exclusively in children. The lesions itch and have a hivelike quality when traumatized, but are few in number and typically do not cause problems. They usually resolve on their own after a few months to years. If they contain a great number of mast cells they may actually form blisters (bullous mastocytosis).

Diffuse Cutaneous Mastocytosis

This is a very rare condition in which the skin has massive numbers of mast cells but they are evenly spread throughout the skin without forming small bumps or lumps. It occurs in children. The skin shows a diffuse yellowish brown color and is thickened. If large quantities of histamine are released, death may result.

Telangiectasia Macularis Eruptiva Perstans

This is a relatively rare form of mastocytosis in which the mast cells are present in the skin as small patches and not bumps. The skin shows small brown spots with a mildly red background. Dilated blood vessels are also present. It occurs almost exclusively in adults.

Therapy

For persons with just a few spots limited to the skin, potent topical corticosteroids are probably all that are needed. Mastocytomas usually subside on their own. Any trauma which will cause them to develop a hive should be avoided. Application of topical doxepin cream (Zonalon®) may also be useful.

Persons with diffuse cutaneous mastocytosis and telangiectasia macularis eruptiva perstans (TMEP) represent a difficult and more serious situation. These patients have a much greater number of mast cells in their bodies as a whole. As a result, if these cells all begin to release their histamine at the same time, symptoms such as drastically decreased blood pressure can result, which may be dangerous. Cromolyn sodium (Gastrochrom®) is a medication that stabilizes the mast cells so that they don't leak so much histamine. It has been useful in persons with asthma and may be of some help in mastocytosis patients. Ketotifen is a similar medication but is not available in the United States. PUVA therapy is useful in TMEP patients. Corticosteroids are usually reserved for emergency conditions, since they can't be given for long periods of time. Epinephrine likewise is used in emergencies to increase the patient's blood pressure. Severely affected patients may benefit from carrying a self-administration kit of epinephrine so that they can give themselves the drug if they are not near a medical facility. Antihistamines such as hydroxyzine (Atarax®), diphenhydramine (Benadryl®), and cimetidine (Tagamet®) are sometimes helpful if used on a regular basis.

The most important step to take with mastocytosis is avoiding histamine release. Sudden contact with hot water, such as jumping in a hot tub, can be very dangerous. Patients usually benefit most from short showers using lukewarm water. Certain medications cause mast cells to leak histamine. These include aspirin, alcohol, narcotics, and certain types of anesthetics. Patients should be monitored for evidence of internal involvement, such as that involving the bone marrow.

Moles and Other Dark Spots

The subject of moles has become a very hot topic in the past decade with the increase in melanoma incidence. Unfortunately, there is quite a bit of confusion about what moles are. Most people think of a mole as a flat to slightly raised bump which is tan to dark brown or black. These are called a nevus in dermatologic terms and are composed of cells called nevus cells; these are identical in almost all respects to the cells which give the skin its pigment (melanocytes). That is why some moles are dark. The worrisome aspect of moles is that some may become malignant (melanoma) and it may be difficult to tell just by looking at them which are cancerous and which are not.

Common Moles (Nevomelanocytic Nevi)

These are the most common moles that occur on the skin. They begin as early as six to twelve months of age, although some patients may be born with a nevus. These peak in the teens and then over the years gradually fade away. The number of moles a person develops is related to several factors. The more sun exposure a child and adolescent has, the more moles he or she will develop. How well a person handles that sun exposure may make a difference as well. Males develop more moles than females and whites have more than darker-skinned individuals. A person's genetic background also makes a difference; parents with lots of moles have children with lots of moles.

Moles may occur on almost any skin surface, including the beds of the fingernails and toenails, the inner eyelids, the genitalia, and the palms and soles. Moles begin as tan to brown discolorations of the skin. They are initially flat and as time passes they become larger, darker, and raised. They eventually may be every shade from flesh colored to jet black. Some may also have long dark hairs protruding from them. This may be cosmetically objectionable but does not indicate that the nevus is abnormal. Plucking these hairs is not dangerous.

Patients may wish to have a mole removed. Often this is for cosmetic reasons, but there are other instances which mandate that the mole be taken off. A change in shape or size is the most common reason for concern. These changes are usually not dangerous, but this may not be known until the nevus is removed and examined by a pathologist. A change in color is also a common complaint. Moles may become dark, particularly during times of hormonal changes such as puberty, pregnancy, or when beginning estrogen replacement or birth control pills. They may also change color when they are becoming malignant. Any shade of gray, blue, red, or white is particularly worrisome and should prompt evaluation by a dermatologist. Most moles never have any symptoms. They may become painful or sore, however, if they have been scratched or pulled. They may also develop symptoms if they become malignant. Moles which are bleeding, oozing, or scaling may be showing signs of a melanoma and should be examined. A good rule of thumb is to have a mole examined by a dermatologist whenever it changes. These changes are almost always from common conditions and not a cause for concern. This is not always the case, however, and it is better to be safe than sorry.

The treatment of moles should be entirely surgical, since this results in a biopsy specimen for evaluation. Shaving the mole off flat with the skin (a shave biopsy) is one of the preferred methods for removal. There is some degree of scarring, but usually this is minor and will be the same size as the original mole. This works particularly well on moles up to the size of a pencil eraser. Shave biopsies have the advantage of being quick and relatively inexpensive. If some of the nevus cells are left behind, however, the mole may regrow (a recurrent nevus) and have some splattered pigment which can look worrisome. Shave biopsies may not be appropriate if the mole actually turns out to be a melanoma. Since the prognosis of melanomas is based on their thickness, if some of the cancerous cells remain behind the pathologist evaluating the biopsy will not be able to give an accurate reading. Fortunately, this is a rare occurrence.

If moles are large or are suspected of being abnormal in any way, the preferred treatment is surgical excision. The dermatologist will excise around the entire mole, removing it all and some of the tissue underneath. This allows for adequate evaluation of the margins or edges of the mole. If the pathologist thinks the mole is worrisome or in fact is a melanoma, he will be able to tell the dermatologist if more of the area needs to be excised.

Perhaps most important are the ways not to remove a mole. Freezing with liquid nitrogen or dry ice or burning with an electric needle are inappropriate ways to get rid of a mole. Not only does this not usually take care of the problem; it leaves the patient with a scar and does not allow for evaluation of a surgical specimen. If the mole in fact was a melanoma, the patient will never know and the tumor will not have been removed. It is not uncommon to have patients turn up with metastatic melanoma for which no site of origin can be found, only to remember that at one time or another they had a mole burned off. This often has tragic consequences and is avoidable by proper removal of the mole. There has been some research recently into the use of lasers to destroy nevus cells and thus make the mole disappear.

The nevus cells are selectively abolished in the skin while the surrounding structures are left intact. This has the advantage of not deforming the skin so that it can be looked at later by a pathologist if necessary, but does not tell the dermatologist if any of the cells being destroyed are worrisome. Since not all the nevus cells will be destroyed, if some are malignant and remain behind an unsuspected melanoma may continue to develop.

The most common practice for dealing with moles is watching them. The dermatologist will note some of the larger lesions in the patient's chart and will have the patient return for future evaluations at regular intervals. If the patient has numerous moles and a personal or family history to suggest that they are at some risk for developing a melanoma, that interval will be brief (three months is common). If the patient represents a low risk, he or she may be instructed to simply return if a mole changes or becomes worrisome. There is now a new system (Nevus Scan®) of photographing these moles whereby dermatologists can keep a "map" of a person's moles in their computers and then compare those images with what they see on the patient. This way if a mole either changes or appears, it can be compared to what was previously present.

Dysplastic Moles

Dysplastic moles are the subject of some controversy. There are dermatologists who firmly believe that dysplastic moles exist, whereas others just as firmly believe these are common moles and not remarkable. These may occur as isolated moles or be the predominant type found on an individual. They also may run in families; these families usually have a greater incidence of melanoma. Patients with melanoma have an increased chance of having a dysplastic nevus. Dysplastic moles usually arise at about the same age as common moles and become most evident in adolescence or young adulthood. They do not tend to arise in persons with poor sunlight tolerance. They initially appear like normal moles but gradually enlarge. They have irregular coloration with shades of dark brown or black, light tan, and slight pink. Most are as big as a pencil eraser and some may grow to the size of a dime. The borders of the moles are usually irregular and difficult to see. They may have a "fried egg" appearance with the raised (and usually darker) part of the mole in the center and surrounding lighter, flat pigmentation. Most are oval to round but they may assume most any shape. Almost any skin site area can be involved but the trunk, buttocks, and breast are most common. The mole's surface is often somewhat pebbly or slightly rough.

As mentioned, the danger of dysplastic moles is that they may become melanomas. They are usually removed, therefore, either by shaving or excision. Under no conditions should they be destroyed with an electric needle, laser, or liquid nitrogen. In persons with many moles, it is obviously not feasible to remove each and every one. The dermatologist may remove just one or two of the most concern. If a person's moles are not very worrisome, the dermatologist will just observe even abnormal moles. On the other hand, if a mole is disturbing, the dermatologist may wish to take off more moles in the future. The only known medical treatment for dysplastic moles is tretinoin (Retin-A®, Renova®); this has shown to have some benefit when regularly applied.

The greater the number of moles and the more abnormal they are, the more often a dermatologist will need to see the patient. Mapping the moles with photographs or the Nevus Scan® is a common procedure, but somewhat controversial. Dermatologists are usually thorough in their examination of the skin, but there are places that they miss or for reasons of decorum choose not to look. If a patient has been diagnosed with dysplastic moles, it is a good idea to have a relative or friend look over areas that the dermatologist may have missed (groin, rectum, scalp, and so on). If a person must do this on his or her own, using a mirror is helpful as is a well-lit room. A hair dryer set on cool and "low" is useful for spreading the hair out over the scalp. Close relatives, particularly those with many moles, should be evaluated by a dermatologist as well. They may have dysplastic moles and, of course, are at an increased risk for melanoma.

It cannot be overemphasized that persons who have lots of moles or who have dysplastic moles must avoid the sun or sources of ultraviolet light (tanning booths). The use of a good sunscreen is encouraged not only for times of prolonged exposure but for routine daily use as well.

Halo Moles (Sutton's Nevus)

Like its name implies, these moles have the appearance of a halo. The mole itself is usually brown or pink but the skin around it loses its pigment so that it appears blanched or whitened. The halo extends about a pencil eraser's width around the mole. White hairs may be seen coming from the mole itself. The pigment-producing cells in the skin, the melanocytes, are being destroyed, accounting for the loss of color. The presence of a halo usually indicates that there is inflammation in the skin and that the mole is regressing. Most patients are adolescents or children, and these moles tend to arise on the trunk. If a halo nevus occurs in an adult, it may indicate a melanoma elsewhere and that the body is developing an immune reaction to other moles. Obviously, these patients should be thoroughly evaluated for the possibility of a melanoma at another site. If left alone, these moles will usually flatten out and lose their pigment. Most dermatologists choose to remove the mole so that it can be evaluated by a pathologist. Since the area of pigment loss is at increased risk for sunburn, application of sunscreen to the area is suggested.

Spitz Nevus (Spindle and Epithelioid Cell Nevus)

These moles were previously considered to be melanomas that arose in children. As might be imagined, they are capable of causing great concern unless accurately diagnosed. They are most commonly found in children and adolescents. Adults may develop them as well, but this is unusual. They do not look very worrisome. Most are pink to reddish brown and are single; they are usually found on the face and arms. Most Spitz nevi are about the size of a pencil eraser. The problem with these moles is that they may be very worrisome to the pathologist, with some of the features of a melanoma. It is not uncommon for a pathologist to show such biopsies to several colleagues to obtain a consensus diagnosis. Even with such measures, in some instances the pathologist may not be able to completely exclude the possibility that the mole is a melanoma. Treatment with surgical excision is usually best. This removes the entire mole and allows for adequate diagnosis.

Blue Mole

This is called a blue nevus and commonly occurs on the hands and scalp. It may be the size of a pencil lead to that of a pencil eraser or larger. These moles are blue in color due to the way the pigment in the skin reflects back the light that strikes it. They are not raised above the surface of the skin and rarely have any symptoms. Because of their dark color, they often cause concern and dermatologists may remove them with a punch biopsy or an excision. They can become melanomas but fortunately this is a very rare occurrence.

Nevus Spilus

This is a very unusual mole which may be present at birth or arise in early childhood. There is a background of tan skin very similar, if not identical to a cafe au lait spot. These moles are from the size of a nickel to that of a person's palm. Within this background develop raised dark moles from the size of a small pencil lead to slightly larger. Most nevus spilus occur on the trunk and arms or legs. They are usually stable throughout life and don't require treatment. If one of the dark moles in the lesion becomes inflamed or develops other worrisome characteristics, it must be biopsied. Removal of the entire nevus spilus is usually too big an undertaking. If the mole has to be taken out, a skin graft is generally needed to heal the wound.

Simple Lentigo (Lentigo Simplex)

This is a very common lesion. Simple lentigos are dark (sometimes jet black) and usually less than the size of a pencil eraser in diameter. They may arise on almost any skin surface, including the nail beds and mucous membranes. They begin to appear in childhood and may develop throughout adulthood. Sun exposure apparently has nothing to do with their appearance. They may be removed with liquid nitrogen or a shave excision, but the latter is preferred since this allows a pathological specimen to be obtained and examined. For the most part, the presence of simple lentigos is meaningless. Some persons appear to be particularly disposed to developing simple lentigos and have many lesions. When present on the nail beds or mucous membranes, they may resemble a melanoma and a biopsy is often necessary.

Solar Lentigo (Senile Lentigo)

Solar lentigos closely resemble simple lentigos but usually arise in sun-exposed (or sun-damaged) skin. They also go by such names as liver spots, sun-induced freckles, and senile lentigos. Solar lentigos are more common in persons who sunburn easily and less frequent in persons who tan well. They may also arise in persons who have had extensive ultraviolet light therapy such as PUVA or UVB treatment. They may begin in childhood, but commonly develop in middle age. They begin as small, often pinpoint dark spots and grow no larger than a pencil eraser. They are light brown to jet black. Most have well-defined borders but some are ragged. They do not scale or develop symptoms.

Treatment is usually not necessary but some lesions, particularly those on the face, may become cosmetically objectionable. Liquid nitrogen is the preferred method of therapy but laser treatments are also effective. Obviously, prevention with sun avoidance and use of a good broad-spectrum sunscreen is advised. Bleaching creams (Solaquin Forte®, Melanex®) provide some help but are not completely effective.

Ephilide (Freckle)

Freckles are small reddish-brown areas of discoloration that appear in sun-exposed skin. They are most often found on persons with red or blond hair and blue or green eyes. These persons tan poorly and easily burn. Freckles begin to appear in childhood. If a person refrains from additional light exposure, freckles may fade slightly or even disappear. Treatment is usually done only for cosmetic reasons and may be performed with light application of liquid nitrogen or trichloroacetic acid. Freckling can be prevented with appropriate use of sunscreen.

Becker's Nevus

Becker's nevus is a large area of increased pigment and dark hair that arises over the upper back around the shoulder blades. It begins around the time of puberty and is more common in males. It may first be noticed after an episode of intense sun exposure. The surface of the skin may be slightly rough or pebbly. As time passes the nevus may become more nodular. There is no treatment, although some types of lasers may be helpful. If the dark hair is objectionable, it may be bleached without any harmful side effects.

Lentigo Maligna (Hutchinson's Freckle)

This type of lentigo arises in sun-damaged skin in middle age or older patients and is a form of melanoma. Lentigo maligna often begins as a solar lentigo and then slowly expands. It begins with a tan color but gradually darkens and becomes irregular. The borders become notched and poorly defined. Lesions may be present for decades. The face and neck are the usual sites but other sun-exposed sites are susceptible as well. If left alone, the cancerous cells will eventually begin to invade the deeper parts of the skin. At this point, the tumor has usually become nodular and feels thickened. Surgical excision is the preferred treatment. Other methods of therapy including liquid nitrogen, laser, topical fluorouracil (Efudex®), dermabrasion, and radiation treatments have been useful in certain patients; however, these methods are uncommon.

Mongolian Spots

These dark blue to gray splotches over the trunk and buttocks are seen in infants. They sometimes occur in Caucasians but are much more common in children of Asian or Hispanic origin. The spots range in size from that of a penny to that of a small dinner plate. They are not usually disfiguring unless the face is involved. They do not have symptoms. The great danger with Mongolian spots is that they will be mistaken for signs of child abuse. In cases where this is a significant worry, parents can ask the dermatologist to write a letter stating what these lesions represent and that abuse or neglect is not taking place. Mongolian spots disappear after a few years and leave little or no trace. Until recently, there has been no treatment aside from using camouflage makeup (Covermark®, Dermablend®). Some of the newer lasers, however, are capable of treating these lesions if the need arises.

Nevus of Ota

This discoloration of the skin usually occurs in Asians and may be very disfiguring. It begins in childhood or around puberty and affects women much more often than men. Small gray to blue areas of discoloration begin around the eyelid, temple, side of the neck, forehead, and nose. The white part of the eyeball may also be involved, and some patients have spots on the inside of their mouths. Only one side of the body is affected. The spots tend to gradually enlarge and darken over time. Having one of these spots become malignant is extremely rare, but has occurred. Until recently, the only treatment was makeup application. Laser treatments, however, have shown good results in certain patients. Unfortunately, this form of therapy is expensive and most areas have to be treated several times to effectively get rid of the discoloration.

MOUTH ULCERS

Ulcerations in the mouth are common and can be due to various causes. Most are self-limited and go away in a few days or weeks, but some may be persistent and debilitating. If the ulcers are multiple and particularly uncomfortable, the patient may have difficulty eating and drinking.

Aphthous Ulcer (Canker Sore)

Aphthous ulcers are the most common cause of mouth ulcers. They are thought to be due to bacteria or viruses, but the exact cause is not clear. Most are small and occur as a single ulcer or perhaps a few lesions. Most resolve in about two weeks. Mucosal surfaces (the lips, tongue, cheeks, and so on) are more likely to develop ulcers. Interestingly, the higher the socioeconomic status of a person, the more likely they are to be affected by canker sores. These lesions are brought on by stress, menstruation, smoking, trauma, allergies, and menopause. Patients who have poorly functioning immune systems (in AIDS, cancer, organ transplant, and so on) are particularly susceptible to these ulcers. In some patients, there seems to be an inherited tendency to canker sores.

This disorder is divided into two groups—minor and major aphthous stomatitis. Minor aphthous stomatitis is present when the patient has one or a few lesions; these clear up in ten days or so. This condition is uncomfortable but usually manageable. Major aphthous stomatitis is pure misery. These patients have ulcers that may be the size of a nickel, are extremely painful, and can take up to a month to resolve. They may scar as they heal and can deform the mouth as they do so. It is unclear why either condition occurs. There seems to be some problem with the patient's immunity; the body's immune cells attack the skin of the mouth. A disorder known as Bechet's disease commonly has oral ulcers which are identical to canker sores. Patients with this disease also experience inflammation of the eye (uveitis), vasculitis, genital ulcerations, and neurologic symptoms similar to those of multiple sclerosis. Treatment is usually aimed at relieving the symptoms. The most common therapy is application of topical corticosteroids. These preparations are applied as gels, solutions, or sprays. Orabase® is a material in which triamcinolone (Kenalog®) is compounded; it adheres well to mucous membranes. Corticosteroids should be applied very frequently since saliva and eating will wipe away the medicine. Another very popular and effective treatment consists of mouthwashes. Most dermatologists and dentists have a recipe for a mouthwash that the pharmacist will compound for them. These usually contain a corticosteroid suspension and some type of numbing medicine, most commonly viscous lidocaine (Xylocaine®) or diphenydramine (Benadryl®). This will usually provide pain relief for thirty minutes or more. Other ingredients such as Kaopectate® may be added to help the other medicines stick to the ulcer bed. Liquid tetracycline (Sumycin®), triamcinolone (Kenalog®), and antifungal agents are also occasionally added. A tablespoon of these mouthwashes is swished around and held in the mouth for five minutes and then spit out. Swallowing the medication is not advised. Oral corticosteroids may be helpful but their use is generally limited to patients with major aphthous ulcers.

Thalidomide may be very effective in patients with serious ulcer problems but is difficult to obtain. As a result, this drug is usually given either as a last-ditch treatment or in cases of major aphthous stomatitis. The most serious side effect is damage to unborn children. Thalidomide seems to work extremely well, however, and is probably the most effective therapy today for this disease.

There are a host of other treatments. Mouthwashes containing chlorhexidine (Periogard®, Peridex®) are very beneficial. When used for prolonged periods, however, they may stain teeth and dental work. Tetracycline taken by mouth has helped some patients. Although there is no evidence that herpes viruses play a role in canker sores, some patients have been helped with acyclovir (Zovirax®) in high doses. Potassium iodide, colchicine (ColBENEMID®), cyclosporine (Sandimmune®, Neoral®), and pentoxifylline (Trental®) have been used with some success. The over-the-counter supplements lysine and niacinamide have been used as well. Application of the medication sucralfate (used for stomach ulcers) has been proposed as a treatment in some patients, but usually must be used for several years to provide any benefit.

Persons prone to develop canker sores can usually tell when they are about to occur. As a result, prevention may be possible in certain patients. If specific foods (spicy, salty, citrus, and so on) precipitate a course of disease, they should be avoided. Trauma from poor toothbrushing habits and gum or toothpick chewing should be avoided. Persons with persistent recurrent disease should keep a diary of what is going on in their lives when the outbreaks occur. They should especially note what foods they are consuming, since foods and food additives frequently cause canker sores.

Trauma

This is the second most common cause of mouth ulcers. There is no end to the number of things which may cause an ulcer in the mucous membranes of the mouth. Toothpicks, fingernails, pens and pencils, bites, dental work, and dental prosthetics such as braces or bridges can all precipitate a mouth ulcer. Burns from hot liquids and foods (particularly cheese among teenagers) will cause ulcerations. Some persons with a toothache will place an aspirin next to the painful tooth. Not only does this do very little for the pain, but as the tablet dissolves it may cause a chemical burn which will eventually become an ulcer. The use of whiskey and other alcoholic liquids for the same purpose may cause mouth ulcers. Radiation and chemotherapy treatments will also cause ulcers. The therapy for these ulcers is similar to that for canker sores.

Infections

There are a number of infections that cause mouth ulcers. Syphilis in several different stages and certain unusual fungal infections are known to cause ulcerations. Usually, these are without symptoms. Making the diagnosis almost always requires a biopsy or some type of blood work; some patients are more at risk for these infections than others. Antibiotics appropriate for the infecting bacteria or fungus are required. The most common infectious cause of mouth ulcers is Herpes simplex, usually type I. Unlike other herpes infections, this condition is rarely associated with sexual transmission. It is common in children, but may be seen in adults as well. Small ulcerations are found on the mucous membranes, including the back of the throat. Fortunately, in children the symptoms are not usually very severe. They may have some pain and discomfort from the ulcers as well as a low-grade fever and a mild headache. The diagnosis is not routinely made in children since many have such mild symptoms. Eating and drinking are uncomfortable and children may drool and refuse food or liquids. In adults, the disease is much more painful. Patients run fevers and may be incapacitated by the discomfort. The disease usually runs its course in about ten days. Treatment is with acyclovir. This drug is manufactured as a suspension for administration to children. Herpangina is a condition, usually seen in children, caused by infection with the coxsackie and echoviruses. Patients develop a fever and ulcerations in the back of the mouth and throat. These ulcerations are very painful and children wil not want to eat or drink. They may drool and be very fidgety and cranky. There is no treatment aside from antifever medications. The disease lasts about seven to ten days. Giving the child cool liquids and popsicles may help to prevent dehydration. Hand, foot, and mouth disease is a similar condition in which small blisters are found on the hands, feet, and mouth (see section on hand, foot, and mouth disease). There is no treatment for this condition.

Miscellaneous Causes

Several different diseases may cause the mucous membranes of the mouth to be fragile and either break down into ulcerations or form blisters. Bullous pemphigoid, cicatricial pemphigoid, and pemphigus vulgaris are the most common. These usually cause blisters or erosions on other parts of the body as well. They are considered autoimmune diseases, since the body is making antibodies that attack the skin. The mucous membranes, particularly over the gums, usually become red and show sloughing skin. They are uncomfortable and eating and drinking may be difficult. A diagnosis is made by biopsying other skin surfaces, but if only the mucous membranes are involved, a biopsy may have to be performed in the mouth.

The treatment for other parts of the body usually helps the oral involvement. Mouthwashes as used for canker sores, particularly when they contain corticosteroid suspensions, may be useful as well. Lichen planus of the mouth may also cause ulcerations; treatment is outlined in the section for that condition. Epidermolysis bullosa is a rare disease in which the skin is excessively fragile because of faulty development. This is an inherited condition. The skin is usually involved to a major extent with the mucous membranes of the mouth a secondary condition. Treatment is difficult and is centered around therapy for skin blisters elsewhere.

NAIL DISEASES

Fungus

Infection by fungus is the most common disease affecting the nails. These organisms are called dermatophytes and are the same ones responsible for jock itch, athlete's foot, and ringworm. Other fungi causing problems in the nails include yeasts such as *Candida.* Nail infections affect up to 20 percent of the population. Affected persons are usually somewhat older, but these conditions can also occur in children and adolescents. Toenails are more often involved than fingernails. Athlete's foot is very common in persons with nail fungus; unless the former is taken care of, any treated toenails will be reinfected. Because the elderly may have diseased or deformed nails, they are more susceptible to fungal infection. Men are more commonly affected than women. *Candida* infections are usually seen in persons whose hands are frequently wet; this is more typical for women.

Symptoms
The nail itself is usually thickened, yellow, and fragile with crumbling material under the free edge. It may be slow to grow. Not all nails that look this way are actually infected by fungus. Some may be malformed by aging or other processes. A diagnosis can be made by scraping some of the debris and looking for fungus under the microscope. This technique is inexpensive and easily performed, but fungus may be difficult to see and some patients may be misdiagnosed. The material may also be cultured and the infecting fungus grown and identified. This is reasonably accurate but takes a week or longer and is expensive. The most cost-effective method of diagnosis is to have a section of the diseased nail analyzed by a pathologist.

Treatment
Treatment options have improved remarkably in the past few years. Previously, griseofulvin (Gris Peg®, Grisactin®, Fulvicin®) was the only effective therapy. It remains the preferred treatment for children. This medicine sometimes worked to get rid of nail fungus but failed in up to half the patients. Griseofulvin has some interactions with other medications, may cause stomach upset, and makes some persons sensitive to the sun. The worst aspect of this treatment method, however, was that griseofulvin had to be taken twice a day for twelve to eighteen months! Recently, however, three new drugs—itraconazole (Sporanox®), fluconazole (Diflucan®), and

terbenafine (Lamisil®)—have been introduced to the market. These medications yield much higher cure rates (90 percent or better), are taken for only two to three months, and are better tolerated. Some are given as pulses: the patient takes several pills per day for one week out of the month and then repeats this weekly regimen for three or four months. These drugs tend to remain in the nails and prevent reinfection for months after the drug has been stopped. Some dermatologists give their patients a week's worth of treatment once or twice a year to prevent recurrence of the fungus. The different drugs are each effective against different fungi and itraconazole is probably the most popular of the three. The major drawback is that these medications are expensive; since they may affect liver function some blood work may be needed. Considering their success rate, the shortened length of treatment, and the low relapse rate, however, these drugs are clearly more cost effective than griseofulvin.

Topical antifungal drugs have been touted as helpful in some cases. Terbenafine and naftifine (Naftin®) are useful in certain instances but the nail must not be deeply affected and cure of more than one nail is rare. These creams may be applied after the nail is scraped and slightly thinned. Mixing fluconazole tablets with DMSO and applying this solution to diseased nails helps certain patients. There are a number of over-the-counter nail products that are supposedly effective. Most of these are supplied in a dropper bottle (Mycocide NS®) or as a lacquer that is painted on with a brush. These are not usually dangerous, but have never been proven to work. In some instances, it may be helpful to remove the nail completely and treat the patient with antifungal antibiotics as it regrows. This was done much more often in the past before the newer medications were available. There still is a role for this therapy, particularly if the nail is painful. Instead of antifungal medications by mouth, it may be feasible to use naftifine or terbenafine cream on the toe. Application of creams containing 40% urea will actually cause the nails to dissolve and slough off. This method of removing a nail is somewhat messy and requires a lot of the patient, but is relatively painless; it may be a safer alternative in persons with diseases such as diabetes.

Onycholysis

Onycholysis refers to a separation of the nail from the nail bed. This causes a whitish appearance under the nail which gradually expands back toward the cuticle. Onycholysis may be due to a number of disorders such as psoriasis, fungal infections, and reactions from medications such as tetracycline. Some persons develop onycholysis because of underlying conditions such as thyroid disease, pregnancy, and syphilis. In the majority of patients, however, the exact cause is not known. This disorder is more common in women. Trauma may play a role in onycholysis. Some nail cosmetic techniques put nails at an increased risk of onycholysis. Artificial nails and sculpted nails may form a bond tighter than that of the actual nail and nail bed. When they are pushed or pulled, this may cause the nail to separate from the nail bed. Onycholysis is not dangerous but is distressing, since it is cosmetically unappealing. Dirt, debris, and other materials may get under the nail and cause a bad odor. In persons who have onycholysis caused by fungal infections such as *Candida*, the smell may be very distinctive. The nails should be kept as dry as possible to avoid fungal infection. If the nails have been subjected to any undue trauma (for example, nail cosmetics) this should be discontinued. Unfortunately, in the great majority of cases not much can be done aside from the application of polish to hide the problem.

Skin Diseases

Many skin conditions involve the nails. The most prominent is psoriasis. Up to half of all patients with psoriasis have nail disease. The most common change is pitting. The nail looks as if someone has poked it with an icepick, leaving pinpoint indentations. The nail is usually thickened and may be yellow, gray, or brown. Under the end of the nail, crumbled skin becomes heaped up and may make using the nail more difficult. There may be some pain associated with nail psoriasis. Onycholysis and grooving of the nails are also seen. The surrounding skin may show the typical changes of psoriasis. In severe disease the nails may be shed altogether.

Nail changes in psoriasis are just about impossible to treat. Topical creams and ointments are generally of little help. Oral medications hold the most promise, but light therapy may be of some use. Soaking in tar baths is sometimes effective. Injecting corticosteroid suspensions into and around the cuticle is probably the most efficient means of treatment but is painful and not very popular. Since the nails are badly deformed they are more susceptible to fungal infections, particularly with *Candida*, and therapy with antifungal antibiotics is often useful. If the nail is particularly painful, it may be more merciful to remove it and treat the area with very potent topical corticosteroids as it regrows.

Alopecia areata and eczematous dermatitis also can cause pitting of the nails. This is usually not as prominent as with psoriasis. The only reasonable treatment is topical corticosteroids;however, these are not likely to be very helpful.

Lichen planus sometimes causes destruction of the nail such that it will not regrow normally. Finally, Darier's disease shows changes in the nail consisting of red and white lines with longitudinal ridges.

Pigmentation

Nails occasionally become discolored for a number of reasons. The most worrisome change is that associated with tan to black pigment. This begins as streaks from the cuticle to the end of the nail. Streaking is very common in blacks, Hispanics, and Asians. If this occurs in Caucasians it usually is a cause for concern since it is possible that a melanoma has developed under the nail or the cuticle. In such circumstances, a biopsy has to be done. Most often, however, this turns out to be either a benign mole or a collection of blood (hematoma). If the pigmentation is present as a brown to black spot extending over into the surrounding skin, a mole or melanoma is also suspected and a biopsy has to be performed. Some medications such as minocycline (Minocin®), zidovudine (Retrovir®), and antimalarials (hydroxychloroquine [Plaquenil®]) may turn the whole nail dark, but this is a harmless effect.

Just about every color has been found in nails at one time or another. Certain diseases or conditions may turn the nail white (tuberculosis, Hodgkin's disease), red (lupus erythematosus, rheumatoid arthritis), green (*Pseudomonas* infection), yellow (yellow nail syndrome), and blue (5-fluorouracil [Efudex®], antimalarials). *Pseudomonas* infections may be treated with gentamycin cream (Garamycin®) and arise in persons whose fingers are wet a lot. The purple to black color that comes from bleeding (hematomas) when the fingers are crushed is called purpura. These collections of blood may be painful and need to be removed. The dermatologist may take a heated wire loop and burn through the nail plate. The hole in the nail allows the blood to escape and relieves the painful pressure. Heating a paper clip to red hot in a flame may be used for the same purpose.

Tumors

The nail is an unfortunate place to get a tumor since removal may be difficult. Certain benign tumors are common. Warts, for example, are the most frequent growths around the nails. They seem to arise on the side and free edge of the nail. This makes them difficult to get rid of since freezing them is painful and often not effective. Other means of treatment tend to be equally unsuccessful. Pyogenic granulomas and moles may be present under the nail. An unusual tumor called a digital mucous cyst usually is found along the side of the fingers but may also arise under the nail. These tumors are painful and may leak a stringy, sticky fluid. They may be drained with a sharp instrument, excised, or injected with corticosteroid suspensions. A very painful tumor called a glomus tumor is also occasionally found under and alongside the nail. This benign tumor is a growth of blood vessels and must be excised.

Malignant tumors in the nail are uncommon. Squamous cell carcinomas and keratoacanthomas, a less worrisome type of skin cancer, may occasionally arise under the nail. They push the nail up and are usually very uncomfortable. If they have been present for enough time they may invade the bone. Treatment is difficult since it is hard to get around the tumor to cut it out. Recurrence of the tumor is common and in some instances the end of the finger has to be amputated. X-ray therapy has been helpful in some cases.

Paronychia

A paronychia is a swelling and inflammation of the skin around the nail (the nail folds and cuticle). These arise after infection with different bacteria and fungus. Paronychias are painful and red. Pus may be seen leaking out of the affected skin. Paronychias usually arise after the infection of a small cut or abrasion, such as a hangnail. If the process lingers for weeks and months, it is considered chronic. Chronic paronychia is usually caused by infection with *Candida* and is more common in persons whose fingers are continually wet (bartenders, homemakers, and so on). Those who traumatize the skin around their nails by workplace injuries or cutting and trimming the cuticles are susceptible to these infections.

Treatment of paronychia depends on what is causing the infection. Some dermatologists prefer to culture some of the pus before beginning therapy. If there is a lot of pus under the skin, it must be drained. Bacterial infections are usually caused by streptococci and staphylococci. These organisms are susceptible to antibiotics such as cephalexin (Keflex®) and dicloxacillin (Dycil®). Fungal (Candidal) infections must be treated with oral antifungals such as ketoconazole (Nizoral®) or itraconazole. Antifungal creams and ointments will not penetrate the skin enough to kill the fungus. If the tissues around the nails are being traumatized, this must be stopped. A good moisturizing program for the skin, the use of gloves at work or at home, and perhaps the use of a barrier cream to prevent water contact are all beneficial.

Ingrown Nail (Unguis Incarnatus)

This is one of the most common nail complaints. It is seen almost exclusively on the big toes and is more common in adolescents and young adults. Other nails may be affected as well, but this is uncommon. The nail itself is seen growing into the soft tissues at the side of the nail bed and acts like a foreign body. Ingrown nails are usually caused by poor nail grooming (cutting or tearing the nail at an angle) and wearing shoes that crowd the toes together. The toe is red, sore, and swollen. The skin at the side of the nail may show pus and crusting with a foul odor. If the ingrown nail has been present for some time, "proud flesh" may accumulate.

If there is extensive infection, oral antibiotics may be needed. In less severe cases, pushing small plugs of cotton or toilet paper under the edge of the nail may solve the problem. This lifts the nail up and away from the skin. This is somewhat uncomfortable, particularly when walking. Usually, however, ingrown nails have to be surgically treated. After the toe is numbed with local anesthesia, the entire nail or the ingrown portion of it are removed (avulsed). If the source of nail growth (called the matrix) is left alone, the nail will regrow; if properly cared for, it should not cause problems. Some dermatologists prefer to destroy part of the nail matrix with different chemicals such as phenol. This prevents a portion of the nail from regrowing but virtually eliminates the chance of that toe having an ingrown nail again. While all this sounds uncomfortable, the amount of pain relief achieved by removing the offending nail is amazing. After the nail has been removed it is a good idea to stay off your feet for the rest of the day and elevate the foot. Patients are usually able to get up and back to routine duties in twenty-four to forty-eight hours. If the skin alongside the nail is particularly swollen or affected with "proud flesh," surgically removing some of it may be helpful. Trimming the nail straight across (not at a curve as with fingernails) will prevent ingrown nails.

PITYRIASIS LICHENOIDES

This condition is divided into two forms—an acute and usually self-limited form (*Pityriasis Lichenoides et Varioliformis Acuta* [PLEVA]) and a more prolonged or chronic form (*Pityriasis Lichenoides Chronica* [PLC]). These conditions represent the same disease but have different time courses. There is no known cause for PLEVA or PLC, although some type of viral infection is suspected. These problems are more common in men and younger patients.

Pityriasis Lichenoides et Varioliformis Acuta (PLEVA)

In PLEVA there is an abrupt rash of small red bumps on the trunk and limbs. As the lesions become older, they form small blisters, crusts, and scabs. If the scabs and crusts are removed, a small ulcer may result. As this ulcer heals, the resulting scar has the appearance of chickenpox (varicella). Patients may have a low-grade fever, headache, and joint pains. The rash may burn or itch. More developed lesions are slightly purple to brown. The spots occur in waves. After several weeks, PLEVA begins to subside and eventually stops. Some patients continue to develop a few lesions and may progress to PLC. One form of PLEVA is more aggressive and occurs with larger lesions, higher fever, and more scarring. The diagnosis is usually confirmed with a biopsy.

No treatment is particularly effective. Traditionally, tetracycline (Sumycin®) has been used. This drug may be inappropriate for children, in which case erythromycin (Ery C®) may be helpful. Light therapy with ultraviolet light A (UVA), ultraviolet light B (UVA), or UVA and oral psoralens (PUVA) has been used with success. Other reportedly effective medications include small doses of methotrexate (Rheumatrex®), nonsteroidal anti-inflammatory agents such as ibuprofen (Motrin®) or indomethacin (Indocin®), pentoxifylline (Trental®), and dapsone. In some patients the disease simply has to run its course.

Pityriasis Lichenoides Chronica (PLC)

Pityriasis lichenoides chronica occurs as small spots and raised nodules on the trunk and limbs. These are slightly red, rarely have any symptoms, and eventually become brown and flat. Mild scaling is common but blisters, unlike with PLEVA, are rare. These areas rarely scar but may leave behind pigmentation. PLC tends to be very chronic. A skin biopsy is usually required to make the diagnosis. The treatments are essentially the same as for PLEVA, with an emphasis on light therapy such as UVB or PUVA. Tetracyclines have also been effective.

PITYRIASIS ROSEA

Pityriasis rosea (PR) is a common skin disorder. The disease strikes between adolescence and middle age but is more common in younger patients. Men and women are affected in equal numbers. In places such as North America, it is more frequent in the spring and fall. It may occur in epidemics.

Causes

The cause is not clear but since it is seen in families and school classrooms, some type of virus may be responsible. Persons are rarely infected more than once. Pityriasis rosea may be more common in pregnant women and persons with asthma, allergies, and eczema (an *atopic* background). Some dermatologists believe that wearing new or recently dry-cleaned clothing may provoke PR. Several different drugs such as barbiturates, high blood pressure medicines (captopril [Capoten®]), gold (Ridaura®), and isotretinoin (Accutane®) cause drug rashes identical to that seen in pityriasis rosea.

Symptoms

This disease usually begins with a single patch of slightly red skin called the "herald patch." The herald patch is slightly larger than the other areas of the rash and is about the size of a nickel to a quarter. It is mildly scaly but rarely itches. After the herald patch has been present for several days, the remainder of the skin becomes involved with similar spots rarely larger than a pencil eraser. They are salmon to brown colored and topped with mild scale. These appear on the trunk, neck, and arms. The face and legs are rarely involved. The patches are somewhat oval or oblong and fan out over the back in the vague pattern of a Christmas tree. Itching, if present at all, is usually mild. New lesions develop for several days to weeks. Without treatment they will remain for up to three months. Low-grade fever, headaches, nausea, and joint pain may rarely occur. Some patients have what is termed atypical pityriasis rosea. In such cases, the skin rash has fewer lesions, involves the face and legs (inverse pityriasis rosea), or forms as very small spots about the size of a pencil lead. Atypical PR is usually slower to resolve. A blistering form of PR is more common in dark-skinned races.

Treatment

Since PR will subside on its own, little treatment is required. The use of light cotton clothing will help with some of the discomfort. If itching is a problem, antihistamines such as diphenhydramine (Benadryl®) or hydroxyzine (Atarax®) are useful. Topical corticosteroids may be applied to very itchy spots. Mixing a corticosteroid cream in a moisturizing cream (quarter strength 0.1% triamcinolone [Kenalog®] in Eucerin® Cream) is a good method for applying a corticosteroid widely but not in too strong a dose. Anti-itch creams such as Sarna® lotion or Aveeno Anti-Itch® cream may be purchased over the counter and applied as often as desired. If itching is a problem, an injection of corticosteroids may be useful. The best and probably safest therapy is ultraviolet light B treatment. Only a few treatments are necessary and may be very effective in controlling the itching. If a light treatment center is not available, mild sun exposure (twenty minutes between 10:00 A.M. and 3:00 P.M.) several times weekly is often helpful.

Pregnancy and Oral Contraceptives

Women experience many physiological changes when they are pregnant or begin taking oral contraceptives. Since these are of a hormonal nature, different organ systems of the body are affected, including the skin. Some of these effects return to normal once the pregnancy is completed or the patient no longer is taking birth control pills; however, in other cases they are more prolonged.

Pregnancy

There are several different skin conditions unique to women who are pregnant or who have recently given birth. While some are annoying, others may be life threatening to both the mother and the child. Unfortunately, treatment may be hampered by the fact that whatever is done to the mother may also affect the fetus.

Skin Changes of Pregnancy

Because of changes in the hormone status of pregnant women, the skin may be affected. These changes are thought to be produced by progesterone, estrogen, or some of the hormones produced by the placenta.

The most noticeable effect of pregnancy is pigmentary changes. The nipples and genitalia may become darker as may moles, freckles, and other sun spots. Most of these changes are of no consequence and may disappear after the pregnancy is over. As moles grow, darken, and change configuration, they may concern the patient and physician. Any woman with a question about one of her moles is advised to consult a dermatologist. Melasma (the mask of pregnancy) develops during pregnancy in about half of women. This condition consists of darkening of the central face and neck. It is covered later in this section.

Since the blood flow in pregnant women is increased, their skin may take on a slightly pinker or redder color. This is most noticeable on the face and palms. These so-called "pregnancy palms" will subside after delivery. Tumors composed of blood vessels, such as hemangiomas may enlarge during pregnancy as well.

One of the most common and aggravating conditions of pregnancy is striae or stretch marks. These arise to one degree or another on almost every pregnant woman. They are usually found on the breasts, abdomen, and thighs. They begin as red to purple bands and may occasionally itch. In the months and years following delivery they become slightly pink to flesh colored. The exact cause of stretch marks is unclear but is believed to be related to the increased steroids that are present during pregnancy. These may also arise during puberty, with significant obesity, and after taking corticosteroids for extended periods. There is no complete treatment for stretch marks but topical tretinoin (Retin-A®, Renova®), if applied while they are still "fresh," may be useful. Since tretinoin is a retinoid it should not be used until after delivery. Some recent research has also reported that laser treatments with the pulsed-dye laser may be useful.

During pregnancy the blood vessels of the body are affected. Some veins of the lower legs may become more prominent under the skin's surface. These are often called spider veins. They are technically a form of varicose veins but are not typically large or uncomfortable. They are, however, unsightly and many women elect to have them removed after pregnancy. They may be injected with a solution, causing them to collapse, but a newer form of therapy is laser treatment. While this may eliminate a particular spider vein, other veins may develop as a part of aging or with future pregnancies. There is a familial tendency to develop spider veins. Varicose veins arise when the veins of the pelvis become choked off from the weight of the pregnant uterus pressing on them. The tendency to develop these also seems to run in families. They can be painful. If the varicose vein is small enough, it may be injected with the same material used for spider veins. The most effective treatment, however, is surgical stripping of the veins. This is done in an operating room but has become less popular in recent years; such veins may be later needed for heart bypass surgery and patients have become reluctant to destroy them for primarily cosmetic purposes. Laser treatments have not been useful. Elastic stockings provide pressure to the veins and may be of some help (Jobst® stockings).

Spider angiomas are different from spider veins. These red spots may arise on the head and upper trunk during pregnancy or when birth control pills are taken. They are not much bigger than an ink spot but may grow to the size of a pencil eraser. Usually, there is a central portion which is redder than the rest and may be slightly raised. This is the central blood vessel, or arteriole which is supplying blood to the lesion. When pressed on, the whole spot will blanch and become much less noticeable. Destroying this vessel with a fine electric needle or laser will cause the smaller vessels to disappear. Spider angiomas are not dangerous but may be somewhat disfiguring.

While a woman is pregnant the hair on her scalp often takes on a more lustrous and thicker appearance. This occurs because fewer scalp hairs are lost. Hair and nails may grow faster during pregnancy. Unfortunately, after pregnancy this process reverses itself, and hair begins to be lost at an increased rate. This hair loss is called telogen effluvium and begins about two to six months after delivery. This may be very disturbing to women who believe that they are going bald. While the scalp hair may become thin, there is no need to worry. Baldness will not develop. Over a twelve-month period the hair cycles will straighten themselves out and assume a normal growth and loss pattern.

Certain other skin conditions may change during pregnancy. Psoriasis, for example, commonly subsides significantly during pregnancy only to worsen after delivery. Other diseases such as acne, eczema, lupus erythematosus, sarcoidosis, and alopecia areata are known to improve. Unfortunately, some conditions tend to worsen during pregnancy (see Table 25). To make matters worse, treatment may be limited for fear of affecting the unborn child.

Pruritic Urticarial Papules and Plaques of Pregnancy (PUPPP)

This is one of the most common conditions that occur during pregnancy and is the source of considerable misery. It typically affects women during their first pregnancy and usually in the last trimester. Beginning on the abdomen (particularly in the stretch marks), the skin develops small red bumps and hives. These may itch furiously and tend to come and go. The itching is worse at night and with the usual difficulty sleeping at this stage of pregnancy, these patients may be truly miserable. Over a few days the rash spreads to the thighs and buttocks. Some bumps may appear blisterlike. The rash fades shortly after birth but it may return with subsequent pregnancies.

Fortunately, PUPPP tends to respond well to topical corticosteroids. Usually, a very potent cream or ointment will stop the itching and redness, but it may have to be used four or more times per day. Baths containing oatmeal or baking soda may help. Getting into a cooler environment may also be beneficial. Although PUPPP is aggravating and uncomfortable, it does not harm the unborn child or pregnant mother.

Melasma

Melasma is also called "the mask of pregnancy." It may also occur when a woman takes birth control pills or hormone replacements. It arises over the cheeks, forehead, nose, and around the mouth. The sides of the neck may also be involved. The skin becomes gradually darker. There are no symptoms. Melasma may occur in men, but this is unusual. This condition is more common in Latinos, Asians, and persons of Caribbean origin. The sun seems to provoke or worsen the disorder. Persons with poor nutrition seem to be more susceptible to developing melasma.

Treatment is centered around avoiding sun exposure. Sunscreens must be used and frequently applied. Opaque sunscreens, such as those containing titanium dioxide or zinc oxide work best. Bleaching creams containing hydroquinones (Solaquin

Table 25 CONDITIONS THAT WORSEN DURING PREGNANCY

Canker sores (aphthae)

Dermatomyositis

Erythema nodosum

Genital warts (condyloma accuminata)

Increased sweating

Keloids

Lupus erythematosus

Melasma

Neurofibromatosis

Porphyria

Pustular psoriasis

Pyogenic granuloma ("proud flesh")

Spider angiomas

Sweet's syndrome

Telangiectasias

Tinea versicolor

Warts

Forte®, Melanex®, Benoquin®, Eldopaque®, Melquin®) are used to gradually bring the skin back to its original color. These creams may contain sunscreens; if they do not, sunscreens should be applied at the same time. They are used once or twice daily. Some dermatologists have their patients apply low-strength tretinoin at bedtime and hydroquinone in the morning. It may take several months or up to a year for the condition to clear. If possible, stopping the birth control pills or other hormones will usually help. A good diet and a multivitamin supplement may also be beneficial.

Herpes Gestationis
This disease is discussed in the section on blistering diseases.

Impetigo Herpetiformis

Like herpes gestationis, this disorder is misnamed, since it has nothing to do with infection by the *Herpes simplex* virus. Most dermatologists consider this to be pustular psoriasis occurring during pregnancy. It is a rare condition and usually arises late in the pregnancy. Small pustules develop on the trunk. There is little itching, but patients generally have fever, chills, nausea, vomiting, diarrhea, and decreased blood levels of calcium. In short, these women are usually very sick. Treatment consists of hospitalization and oral or intravenous corticosteroids. Children born to affected mothers may themselves be affected.

Oral Contraceptives

Birth control pills (BCPs) simulate a state of pregnancy in the body and suppress ovulation. As a result, some of the same things affecting the skin when a woman is pregnant may be present in those taking oral contraceptives. Spider angiomas, mild hair thinning, red palms, melasma, and vaginal yeast infections are all more common while taking BCPs. The most frequent response to these drugs is acne. Both improvement and worsening of acne have been described after beginning BCPs. It is more common for a person to find that beginning oral contraceptives worsened their acne (or brought it on) than improved it. In other words, for women with acne, starting to take BCPs is not likely to provide them the improvement they desire. However, some BCPs are more likely to provoke acne than others. Oral contraceptives containing norgestrel (Ovrette®, Lo/Ovral®, Ovral®) and norethindrone (Brevicon®, Modicon®, Norinyl®, Ortho-Novum®, Ovcon®, Tri-Norinyl®, Necon®) may be associated with a worsening of acne. Those containing ethynodiol (Demulin®, Zovia®) tend either to slightly improve acne or at least not make it worse. Certain disorders such as erythema nodosum, herpes gestationis, porphyria cutanea tarda, and lupus erythematosus may be provoked by BCPs.

Psoriasis, Psoriatic Arthritis, and Pityriasis Rubra Pilaris

Psoriasis Vulgaris

Psoriasis (psoriasis vulgaris) is classified as a papulosquamous disease, meaning that if you run your finger over a spot of psoriasis it will feel raised and scaly. It is one of the oldest known skin diseases and afflicts millions of people. What was called leprosy in the Bible is now believed to have been psoriasis; it differs from what is known as leprosy today. Some patients with this disease also have a form of arthritis called psoriatic arthritis.

Almost anyone can develop psoriasis. This condition affects about 1 percent of the population but is more common among certain ethnic groups. Men and women are equally afflicted and it can involve almost any age group. It is not a transmissible disease, but it does run in families. Smoking, excessive alcohol consumption, and poor dietary habits are commonly seen in patients with psoriasis and make the disease difficult to treat. Certain medications such as antimalarial antibiotics, high blood pressure medicines, lithium, and especially corticosteroids may provoke and worsen psoriasis. A phenomenon known as the "Koebner" reaction involves the development of psoriasis in areas of skin subjected to trauma. Sunburns may similarly traumatize the skin and result in rapid development of widespread disease.

Psoriasis can involve almost every skin surface in a variety of ways. The classic patch of psoriasis is sharp at the edges with overlying scale. The spots are usually no larger than a quarter or half-dollar but may be up to the size of a dinner plate, and some patients have almost total body involvement. The lesions themselves are pink to dark purple/brown. The scale may be all but absent or extremely thick. It is usually white but may be gray or yellow/brown. Classically, lesions develop over the elbows and knees. The scalp is similarly involved, particularly behind the ears. Psoriasis on the face is rare but usually means that the patient's disease is severe and difficult to control. The palms and soles may become very thickened, scaly, or cracked. Most patients do not complain of itching. This may help distinguish psoriasis from other skin diseases. There are several different types of psoriasis, each with unique features.

- *Guttate psoriasis* is a common way for this disease to begin. It usually affects children or adolescents, but all age groups are at risk. Small spots of psoriasis appear suddenly on the trunk and limbs. There is little scaling and itching is slight. The spots look as if they have been splattered on the skin. Guttate psoriasis typically follows an upper respiratory infection such as strep throat, an ear infection, or sinusitis. Treating the infection elsewhere may help the skin considerably but will not completely eliminate the psoriasis.

• *Erythrodermic (exfoliative) psoriasis* involves almost the entire skin surface. The patients are usually red, uncomfortable, sensitive to sunlight, and chilled. These people have usually had psoriasis for many years but are no longer able to control it. This type of psoriasis may be seen with an underlying illness, alcoholism or drug abuse, or a change of medication for high blood pressure or diabetes. It also occurs after receiving corticosteroids by mouth or injection. Persons with erythrodermic psoriasis may have fevers, decreased blood pressure, severe itching, loss of fluids, anemia, and shortness of breath. Some patients require hospitalization.

• *Pustular psoriasis* is similar to erythrodermic psoriasis in that some of the same symptoms are present. The skin shows numerous pustules on a red background. There are different subtypes of pustular psoriasis, including one restricted to the palms and soles. Patients with pustular psoriasis are also ill and are often hospitalized.

• *Psoriasis* involves the nails in most patients. Usually many nails are involved; fingernails are more common. Almost all psoriatics will have small pinpoint indentations of the nail plate called pitting. This may be so subtle that patients are unaware of the pits, or be so noticeable that the nail looks like it has been stabbed with an icepick. Ridges and grooves are also seen. The "oil drop" sign is yellow-brown discoloration of the nail bed. A phenomenon called onycholysis is also commonplace. The nail plate begins to lift off the nail bed and, in severe cases, the nail can actually separate completely. Nails frequently accumulate debris under the free edge. Infection of diseased nails by yeast and bacteria may occur.

• *Psoriatic arthritis* is called a seronegative arthritis, meaning that the blood tests positive in other arthritics (for example, rheumatoid arthritis) but tests negative in psoriatics. Fortunately, not everyone with psoriasis develops psoriatic arthritis. There is about a 5 to 8 percent incidence overall, but this figure is closer to 10 percent in persons with severe psoriasis. The likelihood of developing psoriatic arthritis increases with worsening disease. Women are more often affected than men and patients are usually over the age of thirty-five before they develop the disease. There are five principal types of psoriatic arthritis, but the most common affects the hands and feet. The joints are swollen and tender. Routine tasks are difficult and with time, the fingers and toes may become deformed (arthritis mutilans). The joint disease often parallels the skin disease. Persons with severe psoriatic arthritis should consult a rheumatologist for care.

The cause of psoriasis is unclear. It is known that a patient's immune system is somehow involved. Worsening of a person's psoriasis when he develops AIDS or cancer may occur. Additionally, many of the drugs used in psoriasis therapy affect the immune system. There is an inherited component to psoriasis; this disease runs in families and persons with two afflicted parents are much more likely to develop it themselves. Skin cells proliferate faster than normal in this disease, and various theories have been advanced as to why. Many believe that diet plays a role in susceptibility to psoriasis, but there is no scientific evidence to support such a claim. Finally, some dermatologists believe that psoriasis results from infection with bacteria, fungus, and/or viruses.

Psoriasis tends to wax and wane. It is usually worse in the winter and better in the summer. Sunlight exposure probably has a great deal to do with this phenomenon. Persons with this disease are very adept at figuring out what will improve or worsen their skin. While there is no cure for psoriasis, there is control. Almost all patients may improve if appropriately treated and are appropriately compliant. This disease causes significant embarrassment and shame in some persons. Patients, particularly young ones, are often reluctant to go out in public when their skin is flaring. A negative self-image is common and suicides have occurred. Parents need to assist their children with psoriasis in making a healthy adjustment to the disease. Self-help and information groups are available and many patients find these useful.

There are a great many treatment options available. The important part of any therapy regimen is to adjust it to the patient and the type of disease with which they are afflicted. The number of medicines used in psoriasis has grown steadily, so almost every patient may be helped to some degree. It must be kept in mind that this is, in most cases, a relatively benign disease; powerful and potentially dangerous drugs should be given only to the most stubborn cases.

Self-Care

It is important for psoriatics to take good care of their skin to prevent worsening of their disease. The Koebner phenomenon may provoke lesions after a sunburn or other skin trauma. A healthy lifestyle and diet will help a person to more effectively manage their psoriasis. The easiest treatment for psoriasis is applying moisturizing creams, lotions, and ointments to the skin. These are available over the counter and are usually without side effects. There is some benefit to this type of therapy but for severe disease more aggressive treatments are needed. Applying moisturizers with ammonium lactate (Lac Hydrin®, Amlactin®), is effective, but these medications require a prescription and are expensive. Urea-containing compounds (see Table 3) may be similarly effective and are available over the counter. There are sauna suits available to use with moisturizers or some of the topical medicines to be discussed. This clothing allows the applied medications to better lubricate and/or treat the skin. While it is very effective in some persons, it is expensive and uncomfortable. The use of bathing treatments such as Dead Sea salts and other salts has been advertised as effective for psoriasis and may be helpful in some patients, particularly to get rid of the scaling. While these will not cure most psoriatics, there is no evidence that they cause any long-term harm. Most affected patients are aware that sunlight helps their disease and a mild exposure (twenty minutes) to the sun several times a week is an inexpensive and effective means of controlling mild disease. Prolonged sunbathing or going to tanning salons, however, is not recommended and may worsen the disease.

Topical Corticosteroids

Topical corticosteroids are among the most popular treatments for psoriasis (see section on topical steroids). They are relatively inexpensive, easy to apply, cosmetically acceptable, and safe if properly used. Disadvantages include limited potency, ineffectiveness in stubborn disease, cost (mostly for brand-name medications), and a limited time for application. In patients with large plaques of psoriasis, topical preparations will be expensive, limited in effectiveness, time consuming, and potentially dangerous if too much of the drug is absorbed. Applying potent steroids to the skin for excessive periods of time can cause thinning of the skin (steroid atrophy), acne (steroid acne), and can lead to psoriasis becoming resistant to topical treatment. In short, if a person has disease limited to a few areas, intermittent therapy with topical corticosteroids is an effective and cost-efficient means of treatment. Many preparations prescribed by dermatologists have to be mixed up by the pharmacist and contain corticosteroids. The same benefits and drawbacks apply to these medicines as well. Wrapping the affected area with a waterproof film (Saran Wrap®) after applying the topical cream or ointment is a useful method for treating small resistant areas. Usually this wrapping is left on for a few hours or overnight. Taking oral corticosteroids (prednisone [Deltasone®], triamcinolone [Kenalog®], methyprednisolone [Medrol®], and so on) is an unacceptable treatment option for psoriasis. The same is true of steroid injections. Although these initially make the disease better, it will always rebound and sometimes does so with such fury that the patient's psoriasis becomes pustular or erythrodermic. Deaths have resulted from the administration of these drugs.

Topical Tar

Tar preparations have been widely used in dermatology for decades, especially for psoriasis. They may also be used in eczema and other inflammatory skin conditions. Coal tars are derivatives of bituminous coal. A similar medication, ichthammol, is derived from shale. Oil of cade, an older topical medicine, comes from distilling woods such as juniper and beech. Ichthammol is useful but is cosmetically unacceptable. It is available in 10 and 20% ointments. Oil of cade is now almost solely restricted to bar soap.

Coal tars are actually a mixture of over 10,000 different chemicals. They are believed to slow the growth of the skin cells and act as anti-inflammatory agents. The application of tar to the lesions after therapy with ultraviolet light is known as the Goeckerman regimen. This treatment method is helpful but is fading in popularity due to cost. Tars are effective, safe, and relatively inexpensive. Unfortunately, they are also messy and smelly. They may make the skin excessively sun sensitive. Most patients do not readily accept the use of these medications. Pharmacists may mix up preparations containing crude coal tar (usually in 2 to 5% concentrations), but this is rarely used since it is so cosmetically unappealing. Liquor carbonis detergens (LCD) is a distillate of crude coal tar and is much more elegant. It is used in 5 to 15% concentrations. Concentrations above 15% are likely to be irritating to the skin without being more effective. LCD may be mixed into almost every proprietary cream and lotion currently marketed. Adding 1 to 5% salicylic acid will promote shedding of some of the thick scale. Over-the-counter tar products include bath oils, topical lotions and creams, shampoos, soaps, and conditioners (see Table 26). Some tar products also contain salicylic acid. Generally, these products may be safely used unless the skin is so irritable that they cause further inflammation. Not every patient responds well to tars. If they are helpful, however, most dermatologists will make every effort to continue their use since they are believed to be much safer in the long term than other therapies (for example, topical corticosteroids). Tar lotions are usually applied to the skin at bedtime and washed off in the morning. Some patients prefer to treat their skin for three to four hours in the evening after work and wash the tar off before going to bed. Some preparations may be rubbed into the skin with no remaining residue and are more compatible for daytime use. The number of potential regimens is endless. Shampoos are most effective if left on the scalp for five to ten minutes before rinsing. Bath oils containing tar are useful for treating large surface areas but are not very cosmetically acceptable. An unrelated shampoo containing the antifungal antibiotic ketoconazole (Nizoral®) is also very useful.

Table 26 OVER-THE-COUNTER TAR PRODUCTS

Brand Name	Active Ingredients	Form
Alphosyl®	coal tar, allantoin	cream, lotion
AquaTar®	coal tar	gel
Balnetar® oil	coal tar	bath oil
Denorex®	coal tar	shampoo
DHS®	coal tar	shampoo
Doak Tar®	coal tar	shampoo, bath oil, lotion
Doctar®	coal tar	shampoo
Elta® Lite Tar	coal tar	lotion
Estar®	coal tar	gel
Fototar®	coal tar	cream
Iocon®	coal tar	shampoo
Ionil T®	coal tar	shampoo
Ionil T® Plus	coal tar, salicylic acid	shampoo
Levatar®	coal tar	bath oil
MG217®	coal tar, sulfur, salicylic acid	ointment, lotion, conditioner
Medotar®	coal tar	ointment
Neutrogena® T/Derm	coal tar	lotion
Neutrogena® T/Gel	coal tar	shampoo
P&S Plus®	coal tar, salicylic acid	gel
Pentrax®	coal tar	shampoo
Polytar®	coal tar	soap, bath oil
Pragmatar®	coal tar, sulfur, salicylic acid	ointment
Protar®	coal tar	shampoo
Psorigel®	coal tar	gel
Sebutone®	coal tar, sulfur, salicylic acid	shampoo
Tarlene®	coal tar	lotion
Tarsum®	coal tar, salicylic acid	shampoo
Tegrin®	coal tarl	otion, shampoo
X Seb T®	coal tar, salicylic acid	shampoo
X Seb T® Plus	coal tar, salicylic acid, menthol	shampoo
Zetar®	coal tar	shampoo

For reasons that are unclear, the use of this drug on the scalp is helpful in controlling psoriasis.

Anthralin

Anthralin is a chemical somewhat similar to coal tar. It was initially manufactured from a tree found in South America but is now synthetically made. Like tar, its method of action is not clear but probably involves slowing the growth rate of the skin's cells. It may be mixed into creams, ointments, and pastes but most dermatologists prefer to use commercially available compounds (Dritho-Creme®, Anthra-Derm®, Dritho-Scalp®). A program for psoriasis care using anthralin and light therapy is called the Ingram regimen and is similar to Goeckerman treatment. This is very specialized therapy, popular in Europe, and is available in only a handful of medical centers. Anthralin works best in patients with a few large, noninflamed plaques of psoriasis. Most applications of anthralin are done in what is called "short contact." The medication is applied for twenty to thirty minutes and then washed off. The anthralin is applied *only* to the plaques, being careful not to get any on surrounding normal skin (it is irritating to uninvolved skin). If there is no stinging, redness, or other signs of irritation after several days of therapy, the length of application is gradually increased by several minutes. An increase in the strength of anthralin preparation is also effective. A similar regimen is used on scalp psoriasis. These compounds stain the plaques of psoriasis but discoloration will fade after the medication is discontinued. Anthralin is safe for long-term use, reasonably helpful with properly selected patients, and cost effective. This therapy suffers from poor patient compliance, however, because it is messy, stains clothing, and may occasionally inflame the psoriasis. Anthralin may be combined with topical tar use. While this drug is an older treatment option, it is still very effective and useful for certain patients.

Vitamin D

Calcipotriene (Dovonex®) is a vitamin D derivative topically applied. Its usefulness was noted when oral doses were found to be effective in treating psoriasis. It is relatively new but is believed to be safe for short- and long-term therapy. It is applied twice daily to involved areas. Mild skin irritation may develop in some patients. It is best reserved for those with limited disease, since application over large areas is time consuming and expensive. Taking large oral doses of vitamin D is not comparable to using topical calcipotriene. Not only is this unlikely to improve a person's psoriasis, but it may be very dangerous as well.

Sulfa Drugs

Sulfasalazine is a sulfa medication that has been available for many years. It is effective in less than half the patients who try the medication. It is inexpensive but has to be taken four times daily. Also, it usually causes a mild degree of anemia and modest fatigue. As a result, regular blood counts must be performed. Sulfasalazine has been used in persons with widespread disease who have failed with other therapies.

Zinc Pyrithione

One of the newest and hottest treatments for psoriasis is zinc pyrithione. This drug kills yeasts called *Pityrosporum*, thought by some dermatologists to play a role in psoriasis. This product is available as a pump spray, bar soap, and scalp solution (DermaZinc®, 1-800-753-0047). It has become quite popular and is effective in certain patients. DermaZinc® is not known to have any worrisome side effects and appears to be safe. It is expensive, however. A similar product, Skin-Cap®, was recently discovered to contain a powerful corticosteroid, clobetasol; this may have accounted for its success. It has since been taken off the market.

Light Therapy

One of the oldest and most effective therapies for psoriasis is ultraviolet light. It has been known for centuries that sunlight has a beneficial effect on this disease. Today, light therapy is given using machines that dispense ultraviolet light B (UVB) and ultraviolet light A (UVA). Many dermatologists have a UVB machine in their office or access to one at a local hospital. Certain medical centers have offices dedicated solely to light therapy with staff who are well trained in its administration. Patients are usually treated two to three times per week with gradually increasing amounts of light. The total number of treatments and dose are carefully recorded. After the disease is better under control, the frequency of dosing is decreased. Treatments are designed by a patient's tolerance to sunlight. Patients with very light skin who do not tan well are given smaller doses, whereas darker skinned patients (Hispanics, African Americans) are given more. This is *not* the same as going to a tanning salon. Tanning beds use UVA and may worsen psoriasis. UVB treatments are a central part of Goeckerman therapy. UVB has been combined with almost all the topical therapies including tars, anthralin, corticosteroids, and calcipotriene as well as oral medications such as methotrexate and retinoids. Some treatment centers give UVB with UVA together. Light treatments are designed to control a patient's disease with the idea that more conservative therapies, such as tars or corticosteroids will be gradually substituted for longer term maintenance. Some companies manufacture UVB and UVA units for use at home. These are very expensive and require that patients be able to appropriately use them. Patients whose psoriasis is very inflammatory (erythrodermic) or who have a light-sensitive disease are not candidates for light therapy. Disadvantages are expense and time consumption. Too much light may produce a burn similar to a sunburn; this can worsen the disease. Long-term effects are essentially the same as from prolonged sun exposure and include increased skin wrinkling, precancerous spots, and skin cancer. However, these side effects are unusual since most patients do not receive treatments for extended periods.

PUVA Therapy

Another effective means of psoriasis therapy is called PUVA. This stands for *Psoralens* plus *UVA* light. This treatment is about twenty years old and involves ingesting a drug called psoralen followed by treatment with UVA light. Patients who cannot or should not take psoralen may have it applied to their skin, either in a bath or painted on the affected areas. The treatment regimen is essentially the same as for UVB. Treatments are given two to three times per week and gradually reduced as the disease comes under control. The total doses are tabulated and periodically reviewed. Patients who ingest psoralens are required to wear UVA-blocking sunglasses for twenty-four hours after their treatments to prevent ill effects of sunlight on the eyes. Occasional checkups by an ophthalmologist are suggested. This is a very effective therapy, particularly for widespread disease, and like UVB is designed to control a patient's psoriasis so more conservative treatments may be implemented. PUVA therapy is expensive, time consuming, and not tolerated by all patients. The psoralens make the skin more sensitive to light and despite small doses of UVA, some patients do not tolerate it. Mild nausea is an occasional problem, as is skin itching. Evaluations of liver, kidney, and bone marrow function by means of blood tests are done regularly. Long-term effects include cataracts and an increased incidence of skin cancers. PUVA suppresses the immune system to some degree as well. While rarely a problem in healthy patients, this may not be tolerated in persons with impaired immune systems (in AIDS, cancer, and so on).

Retinoids

Retinoids are vitamin A derivatives and may be very effective in psoriasis patients. The most common medication used is acitretin (Soriatane®). Isotretinoin (Accutane®) is rarely used for psoriasis. Retinoids are occasionally used in combination with UVB and PUVA therapy. Acitretin is most commonly given to patients with severe disease, particularly those with erythroderma or pustular psoriasis. It may also be effective for large-plaque disease. The medication is taken orally once or twice daily. Kidney, liver, and blood tests are intermittently done. Acitretin is very harmful to unborn children, so most dermatologists restrict its use to men or women who are no longer fertile. The side effects from acitretin are essentially identical to those found in persons taking large doses of vitamin A. These include chapped lips, dry skin, mild hair thinning, dry eyes, sticky/clammy skin, and nosebleeds. Less common side effects are bone/joint/muscle pain and diminished night vision. Every person given acitretin will develop increased blood fats (cholesterol and triglycerides). While these will return to normal following discontinuation of the drug and are rarely of significance to the patient, in rare cases the drug has to be stopped. The drug is expensive but is designed to be a crutch to get the patient's disease under better control so more conservative therapies may be implemented.

A new topical retinoid, tazarotene (Tazorac®) has recently come on the U.S. market. It is a gel and is applied once daily to psoriasis plaques. Early tests have shown it to be very effective; it has the additional benefit of keeping psoriasis under good control for several months after stopping its use. Tazarotene may be applied to almost any area, but folds of skin are best avoided since mild irritation may occur. It is applied at night and washed off in the morning. The major side effect of this medication is mild skin irritation. Moisturizers should not be used at the same time as the tazarotene; they may inactivate the drug. Treated skin may become slightly red (retinoid erythema). Although there is no evidence that this medication is harmful to unborn children, it is not recommended for use in pregnancy or while breast-feeding. For the most part, tretinoin (Retin-A®, Renova®) has limited effects on psoriasis.

Chemotherapy Drugs

Methotrexate (Rheumatrex®) is an anticancer medication which has become popular for severe psoriasis. It may also be used in conjunction with UVB and PUVA. It is usually given once weekly and may be administered as an injection if needed. Doses are initially small and gradually increased. Laboratory evaluation of the patient's blood is performed similar to that with acitretin (Soriatane®), but methotrexate more often diminishes the patient's blood counts or is toxic to the liver. There is a limit to the total amount of this drug that may be given so it must be carefully tabulated. Careless use of methotrexate has resulted in liver damage severe enough to require liver transplantation and cause death. Overall, it is well tolerated by most patients. Fatigue for forty-eight hours after ingestion and mild nausea may be experienced. Persons with a previous history of liver disease, certain types of anemic states, alcoholism, or who are unreliable are not candidates for methotrexate therapy. Despite the expense of methotrexate, it is one of the most cost-effective means of psoriasis therapy and one that has become a favorite of patients and dermatologists. It is very toxic to unborn children and the same precautions apply for its administration as for acitretin (Soriatane®). Methotrexate interacts adversely with some medications, so it is a good idea to inform the prescribing physician that methotrexate is being taken before any new drugs are begun.

Hydroxyurea (Hydrea®) is a chemotherapeutic agent used for certain blood diseases. It is also effective for some patients with psoriasis. Psoriatics with unstable disease or who have widespread involvement don't benefit much from this drug; it is primarily indicated for patients with mild to moderate psoriasis who are not candidates for other treatments. It is given in capsules twice daily and side effects are few. Blood evaluations are done intermittently to check for anemia. Since better medications are available today, this drug is not used as much as in years past.

Thioguanine (Tabloid®) is another anticancer drug that has been effective in some patients with severe disease, usually those with kidney or liver problems who cannot use other medications. The side effects are similar to those of hydroxyurea.

Immune System Suppression

The newest drug for use with psoriasis is cyclosporine (Sandimmune®, Neoral®). This medication is given to patients who have received organ transplants. It suppresses the immune system and is very effective in widespread psoriasis. Because of its side effects, it is usually reserved for severe and/or life-threatening disease. It is administered based on the patient's weight. Laboratory evaluation of kidney function is vital; this drug may result in kidney failure if not appropriately monitored. Cyclosporine causes and worsens high blood pressure. It also interacts negatively with numerous drugs. Finally, cyclosporine is very expensive. There is some benefit to topical use of this drug, but absorption through the skin may still result in measurable blood levels. While there are a great many negatives to using this drug, in some patients it is the only medication that will control their disease. Results after administering cyclosporine have been spectacular in certain patients. Unfortunately, the psoriasis tends to relapse within a few months after discontinuing the drug. Like most other powerful drugs used to treat psoriasis, it is used to control severe disease as more conservative therapies are begun.

Pityriasis Rubra Pilaris

Pityriasis rubra pilaris (PRP) is a skin disease much like psoriasis. There are several different types; some involve adults and another affects children. Adult disease usually affects those middle aged and older. A genetic inheritance to pityriasis rubra pilaris is likely. The skin around the ears and upper neck are initially involved, and the disease spreads to the trunk and extremities. The palms and soles become very thick with an orange color. The rest of the skin is also somewhat orange colored but may appear red and various shades in between. There are patches of uninvolved skin called skip areas. The affected skin has a rough texture like that of the surface of a nutmeg grater. This is particularly noticeable over the backs of the hands and fingers. There is considerable scaling associated with pityriasis rubra pilaris, particularly on the face and scalp. Itching is usually seen and may be severe in some cases. With the large body surfaces involved and so much of the body's blood flow directed to the skin, patients are often chilled and uncomfortable. The internal organs are not involved, and unlike in psoriasis, arthritis does not occur. Patients with PRP are usually sensitive to the sun and particularly to heat.

If left alone, the disease will usually run its course in a matter of months, but it may take years. Since patients are usually incapacitated to a certain degree, treatment is almost always indicated. Most therapies are similar to those used in psoriasis. Creams and lotions can help with scaling and discomfort but don't cure the illness. Tars and anthralin aren't helpful and may worsen the disease. The most commonly used drugs are the retinoids such as isotretinoin. They are effective but usually take several months to begin working. Methotrexate has been used successfully but is also slow in taking effect. Drugs which suppress the immune system have been used in difficult cases. Topical steroids are effective for small surface areas such as the face and scalp, but applying them all over the body is impractical. UVB and PUVA are not used, since patients are sensitive to light.

SCLERODERMA AND MORPHEA

Scleroderma is considered an autoimmune or connective tissue disease and is in the same general category as lupus erythematosus or dermatomyositis. It is not seen very often but is by no means rare. Morphea is believed by most dermatologists to be a category of scleroderma. These disorders have several different manifestations, but all involve a thickening or hardening of the skin. In most instances, this is little more than an inconvenience or a matter of an unpleasant appearance, but in others the disease may be life threatening. All types appear to be more common in women. In some patients, the thickened skin is due to contact with a chemical or other substance. The precise cause of scleroderma is not clear, but for some reason the cells in the skin and other body organs producing fibrous tissue become more active and productive.

Localized morphea is the most common form of the disease. It begins as a small dime-sized area, commonly on the trunk, which is slightly pink or lilac colored. The overlying skin is normal but the deeper tissues are hard and thickened. As the area expands, the coloration is lost and it becomes very white or slightly yellow. In patients with dark skin, the loss of pigment may be very disfiguring. Usually only a single spot is present, but multiple lesions may arise. There are no symptoms aside from some occasional mild itching. Generalized morphea involves similar lesions but there are usually numerous spots all over the body. Guttate morphea is similar to generalized morphea but the spots are smaller (pencil-eraser sized) and very numerous. The prognosis overall is good since the disease tends to subside after several years. There is no involvement of other body organs. There is some evidence that infection with the same bacteria that causes Lyme disease, *Borrelia burgdorferi*, is responsible for some cases of morphea. This is a controversial point, however, and most persons who have been treated with antibiotics have not improved.

Linear scleroderma is present as a linear area of skin which is thickened and hardened and dark colored. It most commonly affects the lower legs. A very peculiar form called *coup de sabre* ("cut of the sword") affects the forehead and scalp. It begins in childhood and forms a groove of thick, hairless skin. As it grows it may extend to the back regions of the scalp or down the face, causing significant disfigurement. In some cases, this process may go so deep as to involve the muscles and bone.

Systemic scleroderma has some of the same changes as morphea, but there are other symptoms as well. These include pain and/or stiffness of the joints, particularly the hands and knees. The skin over the hands and fingers becomes very tight and bound down. It may later ulcerate and is slow to heal. As the process worsens, movement becomes limited and eventually the fingers are frozen and useless. Raynaud's phenomenon may also affect the fingers. They are blanched and moderately painful, particularly when exposed to cold weather. The skin of the trunk, face, and arms are involved with thickened, cold skin. When the face is affected, it may make facial expression difficult. The ability to open the mouth is hindered and chewing becomes a problem. Small blood vessels (telangiectasias) are found on the cuticles and cheeks, and some hair loss is common. Internal involvement is perhaps the most worrisome. The esophagus may gradually narrow and swallowed food often causes a sticking sensation in the midchest. Heartburn with reflux follows. If the intestines become involved, they may function poorly with decreased absorbtion of food, diarrhea, bloating, and constipation. Thickening of the lungs also occurs and makes it more difficult to breath. Probably the most dangerous effect is kidney involvement. About half of patients with systemic scleroderma eventually experience this complication. Kidney failure may develop. A variant of systemic scleroderma is called CREST. This stands for *C*alcinosis cutis (deposits of calcium in the skin), *R*aynaud's phenomenon, *E*sophageal disease, *S*cleroderma, and *T*elangiectasias.

Treatment

Treatment of these disorders is often difficult. In the more benign forms no treatment at all may be the best course, since morphea commonly "burns out" on its own. Corticosteroids either applied, injected, or taken by mouth have not usually proven helpful. Some patients have gotten good results from using very potent topical corticosteroids under occlusion with plastic wrap (Saran Wrap®) or occlusive wound dressings (Duoderm®, Vigilon®). This requires a lot from patients, however, and is only helpful if there is a single or very few involved areas. Penicillamine (Cuprimine®) has been a traditional treatment in many cases. This drug is believed to influence the cells making the fibrous material in the skin. Overall, it is only partially effective and has some worrisome side effects on the patient's blood counts. Other sometimes successful medications include isotretinoin (Accutane®), griseofulvin (Gris-PEG®), kantaserin, phenytoin (Dilantin®), colchicine (ColBENEMID®), ketotifen, and cyclosporine (Sandimmune®, Neoral®). The anticancer agents cyclophosphamide (Cytoxan®), chlorambucil (Melphelan®), and azathioprine (Immuran®) have also been helpful in some patients. Since the blood vessels are frequently involved, blood pressure–lowering drugs may be effective for persons with Raynaud's phenomenon. Useful medicines include captopril (Capoten®), prazosin (Minipress®), nifedipine (Procardia®), verapamil (Calan®), and al-phamethyldopa (Aldomet®).

Commonsense skin care measures may be the most important therapy. Keeping the skin well moisturized will help prevent cracking or peeling; this may be slow to heal in affected skin. Smoking and prolonged exposure to cold weather are absolutely prohibited since these activities cause blood vessels to constrict, making it more difficult to promote blood flow. Some patients believe that soaking the ulcerated skin in dimethyl sulfoxide (DMSO) is useful. There is no scientific evidence to support this practice, but it seems harmless.

Sexually Transmitted Diseases (STDs)

Infectious diseases transmitted by sexual contact have been present in one form or another for centuries. The recent AIDS epidemic has focused people's attention on what had been a somewhat fading interest in sexually transmitted diseases (STDs). Considerable resources are now used for treating and preventing STDs. Certain risk factors for acquiring an STD have been established and include young age, smoking, alcohol use, drug abuse, the presence of other STDs, and the type of contraception used.

Syphilis

This is the prototype of STDs and until recently was believed to be under control. Evidence of syphilis infection has been found in numerous bony fossils. It was believed to be carried back to the Old World by sailors with Columbus who contracted it from the natives on the island of Haiti. Subsequently, it spread rapidly throughout Europe and settled into a stable pattern of infection until after World War II. Then penicillin, to which the organism causing syphilis, *Treponema pallidum*, was extremely sensitive, became widely available. The number of cases dropped almost twentyfold and continued to do so until the mid-1980s. After 1985, however, the number of patients with syphilis began to increase again. The reasons for such an increase are not completely clear but appear to be related to the greater number of HIV infections, changing sexual practices, and the widespread use of crack cocaine. Currently, the persons most at risk for this disease are young black men and women, particularly those from the inner city. Unfortunately, when young women are infected they may transmit the infection to unborn children.

Syphilis has several different phases or stages. The first or primary stage consists of a skin ulcer, usually occurring on the genitals. It is painless and arises about three weeks after infection. The ulcer heals on its own in about two weeks. About half of infected patients go on to the second stage. This is characterized by a rash on the skin and mucous membranes. The rash is small, about the size of a pencil lead, slightly brown in color, and has no symptoms. The patient may also have fever and swollen lymph nodes. The final, or third stage of this disease is rare. It consists of large swollen areas of skin that break down to ulcers. Involvement of the brain and nerves (neurosyphilis) and blood vessels (cardiovascular syphilis) also occurs and may cause severe symptoms. A different form of syphilis occurs in children born to infected mothers and is called neonatal syphilis. These children may be born with different types of birth defects, some of which will emerge as the child grows older.

The diagnosis of syphilis may be made with the skin changes as mentioned, but commonly there are no skin changes or they may have happened years ago and the person no longer remembers them. He or she continues to be infected but does not realize it. In these instances, blood testing for donation or an insurance physical may initiate the diagnosis.

Treatment

Fortunately, the bacteria which causes syphilis has remained sensitive to penicillin. While other organisms have developed resistance to antibiotics over the years, *Treponema pallidum* has not. The preferred drug for treatment is penicillin but tetracycline (Sumycin®), erythromycin (E-Mycin®), and ceftriaxone (Rocephin®) are also used. The treatment regimen depends on the stage of infection. In some instances, particularly in persons with AIDS, it may be necessary to receive penicillin intravenously for several weeks to cure the infection. Infection does not provide any immunity and once the condition is cleared reinfection may occur.

Gonorrhea

This disease is caused by the bacteria *Neisseria gonorrhoeae*. During the 1960s and 1970s, the number of reported cases of gonorrhea increased to over one million annually. Part of this was from an increased reporting of the disease and part was from changing sexual practices in the United States. Today, between 500,000 and a million cases are reported each year and this probably represents only a third of the actual cases. Treatment is relatively easy, but unfortunately there has been a great increase in the number of infections with resistant bacteria. This makes therapy much more difficult and expensive.

Gonorrhea is transmitted almost exclusively through sexual activity, although children may rarely contract the disease by being born through an infected birth canal. From a few days to a week after exposure, most men will develop painful urination (dysuria) and a white- to yellow-colored discharge. Some men never have symptoms, don't realize that they are infected, and spread the infection to others. Gonorrhea, if left untreated, may infect other organs in the genitourinary system and cause significant damage.

Infected women may have some of the same symptoms, such as painful urination and discharge, but may also have vaginal bleeding. The most dangerous complication is infection of the fallopian tubes and its spread into the pelvis and abdomen; this results in pelvic inflammatory disease (PID). PID may be caused by several different organisms but gonorrhea is the most common. Pain, fever, and cramping are usual and life-threatening infection may occur if the disorder is not treated. Disseminated gonorrhea is rare and results from bacteria entering the bloodstream and spreading to other organs. Small skin blisters and arthritis occur.

Diagnosing gonorrhea involves evaluating the discharge and occasionally the blood. It is important to remember that organisms besides *N. gonorrhoeae* may be responsible for very similar symptoms but will require different antibiotics.

Treatment

This bacteria has traditionally been very sensitive to penicillin and penicillinlike drugs. As mentioned, some strains now are resistant but may be treated with other antibiotics. The typical treatment consists of an injection of penicillin, tetracycline, or ampicillin (Omnipen®), or amoxicillin (Amoxil®) by mouth. With the increasing number of resistant infections, ceftriaxone (Rocephin®) injections are more likely to be effective. Giving a course of doxycycline (Doryx®) for a week will also kill other organisms causing the infection. Other treatments using spectinomycin, trimethoprim-sulfamethoxazole (Bactrim®, Septra®), ciprofloxacin (Cipro®), ceftizoxime (Cefizox®), and cefuroxime (Ceftin®, Zinacef®) have been used. Use of a condom for prevention is extremely effective.

Venereal Warts (Condyloma Accuminatum)

Venereal warts are small growths occurring on the genitalia after contact with an infected person. Like all warts, condyloma acuminatum are caused by infection with the human papillomavirus (HPV). HPV is divided into more than seventy different types; types 6 and 11 are the most usual cause of genital warts. These warts are extremely common, and over thirty million Americans are infected with them. A million new infections begin each year; that number has been steadily rising for the past decade. The infection is almost universally contracted by sexual activity but children may become infected if they are born to mothers with active disease. These warts are small, flesh-colored to dark brown growths. They may be flat or have a warty appearance. Very large lesions become the size of a pencil eraser or greater. Almost any part of the genitalia can be affected. Some dermatologists apply a weakened formulation of acetic acid (vinegar) by a washcloth or gauze to the infected skin. The infected area will usually turn a whitish color and allow for a better estimation of how much involvement is present. This virus is considered a risk factor for developing malignancies of the reproductive organs, such as cervical cancer.

Treatment

The treatment for condyloma is not much different than for warts elsewhere on the body. Liquid nitrogen is the most popular therapy. This is useful if the warts are small and there are not a great number of them. Multiple treatments may be required. This does not necessarily get rid of all the wart virus in the skin, but destroys the obviously infected tissues. Unfortunately, liquid nitrogen treatment is uncomfortable. Carbon dioxide laser therapy similarly destroys the wart. This method is not very popular since it is uncomfortable and expensive. Podophyllin resin is a substance derived from the root of a plant. It may be mixed in solution and applied to venereal warts in different concentrations. Depending on the podophyllin concentration, it may have to be washed off the skin in a few hours. Podophyllin is similar to chemotherapy drugs; it prevents the infected cells from multiplying. This treatment may be very effective but it is inconvenient and if not removed appropriately may cause burning and blisters. Application of podophyllin after liquid nitrogen treatment is a popular combination therapy. Podofilox (Condylox®) is a derivative of podophyllin manufactured for home use. It is applied twice daily for three days followed by four days off. This weekly cycle may be repeated as necessary. This is a convenient method for treatment since patients can do it on their own, but the drug is moderately expensive and works best for smaller warts. Neither of these drugs are recommended if the patient is pregnant. A new medication, imiquimod cream (Aldara®), has been approved for use in the United States for genital warts. This cream stimulates the body to kill the warts. It is applied overnight three nights per week and then washed off in the morning. It seems to be more effective in women than in men. Applying acids such as trichloroacetic or bichloroacetic acid is helpful in some patients. These acids may be very destructive if applied in too high a concentration or not removed after the appropriate time. Surgically excising warts is useful if there are not too many, but this is painful and may require some time for healing. The use of 5-fluorouracil cream (Efudex®, Fluoroplex®) helps some patients. It is applied either daily for several days or once per week. It may cause significant irritation and discomfort. Injection of interferon in the area of wart infection is useful in certain patients. This must be done two to three times per week, is expensive, and can cause flulike symptoms. As a result, it is generally used as a last-ditch effort for wart control. A new treatment on the horizon is the injection of a gel containing fluorouracil and epinephrine (adrenaline) into the skin just under the wart. This method allows the medication to slowly leak out of the gel and gradually destroy the wart. The injections may have to be repeated at regular intervals. Treatment is likely to be expensive but this may be a good option for particularly stubborn warts.

The problem with most, if not all, of these therapies is that in many instances the warts come back. This may result from reinfection but usually occurs because the wart virus has not been completely removed from the skin. It is almost certain that normal-looking skin around the warts harbors the virus. As a result, after the wart has been removed new warts can arise from the residual virus. Persons with active warts are able to spread the virus. What is not clear is whether persons with normal-appearing infected skin shed the virus. If so, this is of considerable concern; many persons likely presume that when they are free of warts they are virus free and not able to infect their partners. Infected men with active warts should always use a condom. The use of a condom should continue even after the wart is removed, since they may still be able to infect their sexual partners.

Molluscum Contagiosum

This condition has been covered in the section on warts and molluscum contagiosum.

Chancroid

Chancroid is caused by infection with the bacteria *Haemophilus ducreyi*. It had been declining until the past decade. It is most often present in prostitutes and their customers but is also seen in drug addicts and is common in central Africa. A red to dark ulceration arises on the genitalia; it is painful and bleeds easily. It may grow to the size of a nickel. Lymph glands in the groin are swollen and may actually break down and ulcerate through the skin. Chancroid is treated with erythromycin, ciprofloxacin, and ceftriaxone. One of the great risk factors with chancroid is that through the ulcerated area of skin the virus causing AIDS (HIV) can enter the body.

Herpes Simplex

This infection has been covered in the section on herpesvirus infections.

Pubic Lice

This condition has been covered in the section on insect bites.

SUN-SENSITIVITY DISEASES

Skin Diseases Worsened by Light

This group of diseases are termed photoexacerbated or photosensitive dermatoses (see Table 27). In some affected patients, UV light worsens the disease; the disorder spreads more widely, is more resistant to treatment, is associated with worsening symptoms, or is more visible. In persons with any of these conditions, avoiding excessive sunlight and using a good sunscreen is necessary.

Table 27 SKIN CONDITIONS WORSENED BY LIGHT

Acne

Atopic dermatitis (Eczema)

Dermatomyositis

Erythema multiforme

Familial benign pemphigus (Hailey-Hailey disease)

Keratosis follicularis (Darier's disease)

Lichen planus

Lupus erythematosus

Mycosis fungoides (Cutaneous T-cell lymphoma)

Pemphigus

Pityriasis rubra pilaris

Porokeratosis

Psoriasis

Rosacea

Seborrheic dermatitis

Transient acantholytic dermatosis (Grover's disease)

Viral infections (for example, varicella [chickenpox])

Porphyria

The porphyrias are a group of diseases resulting from enzyme deficiencies in the red blood cells or liver. There are more than a dozen such disorders, but the only one occurring with any frequency is porphyria cutanea tarda (PCT). In this condition, an enzyme in red blood cells called uroporphyrinogen decarboxylase is either absent or poorly functioning. PCT is incited by drugs such as estrogens (including birth control pills), iron supplements, barbiturates, furosemide (Lasix®), naldixic acid (Negram®), naproxen (Anaprox®, Naprosyn®), and tetracycline (Sumycin®). Infections from the human immunodeficiency virus (HIV) or hepatitis C virus may also cause this condition. The most frequent cause of PCT is alcohol, however, and this condition is most commonly present in middle-aged to older men who drink heavily or steadily. About 25 percent of affected patients are diabetics.

Symptoms

The skin becomes fragile and sensitive to the sun. Blisters and ulcers appear on the backs of the hands and forearms. Similar changes may be seen on the face. There may be an increased growth of facial hair. Small cysts (milia) arise in the affected skin. Over time, the skin becomes thickened and scarred. Most patients are only vaguely aware that the sun makes their skin condition worse, but sunlight makes their skin more painful. Naturally, the disease tends to be worse in warmer months and improves in the winter. The diagnosis is usually made by an evaluation of urine collected over twenty-four hours for the presence of porphyrins. It is now possible to make the diagnosis using a blood test.

Treatment

Control of PCT is usually not difficult but may be unpleasant. Since the most common cause of PCT is overindulgence with alcohol, the best treatment is abstinence. Many patients are alcoholics, however, so this is not always easy to do. If the PCT is caused by other medications or substances, they should be avoided as well. One of the oldest therapies involves drawing off a unit or two of blood (phlebotomy) every few weeks. This helps take away some of the iron that builds up in the patient's body and allows the damaged enzyme to work more normally. The patient's blood counts and serum iron stores are watched carefully as this process proceeds. After a series of blood draws, the patient may be put into a remission lasting for several months to several years. If a relapse occurs, the phlebotomies can be performed again. The antimalarial drugs hydroxychloroquine (Plaquenil®) and chloroquine (Aralen®) are useful for persons who cannot tolerate blood loss. These are given once or twice per week. Some dermatologists give these medications along with a regular schedule of blood removal. Finally, use of a good sunscreen may help avoid some of the sun sensitivity that occurs in these patients.

Polymorphous Light Eruption

There are a number of different light eruptions that occur for unknown reasons. In the past, they have all been lumped under the heading of "sun poisoning." They go by many different names and some are more common in Europe. The most common in the United States is polymorphous light eruption (PMLE). This condition begins in the spring. After several exposures to the sun and several eruptions the skin tends to "harden" and becomes less susceptible to the sun's rays, at least for that sunny season. Over the winter the body again becomes susceptible and the whole cycle begins anew in the spring. There is an inherited tendency to develop PMLE. Native Americans and Hispanics are commonly affected, and it tends to be a disease of younger patients and women. With the initial sun exposure in the spring, it may take as little as thirty minutes to provoke the disease. The skin changes begin within a few hours to a few days. Small to large red bumps arise in the areas exposed to the sun, particularly on the face and arms. If there are a large number of lesions, they may merge together to form plaques. Blisters may arise but these are not common. The bumps of PMLE tend to be mildly painful and itchy. Some persons have fever, chills, and headaches. If kept out of the sun, the skin clears in a week or so. As mentioned, as the spring and summer progress, patients gradually become immune to the sun so that sunlight either causes no rash at all or causes only minimal problems. Certain diseases such as lupus erythematosus may also begin with sun exposure and may look very much like PMLE. Consequently, it is important to consider this condition in persons who appear to have PMLE. Sunscreens help prevent PMLE but only if they block out UVA, since this is the disease-provoking form of ultraviolet light.

Polymorphous light eruption may be controlled by allowing gradual exposure to the sun or use of light therapy. UVB light therapy is somewhat effective but PUVA, as done for psoriasis, is more helpful. Oral prednisone (Deltasone®) or an injection of triamcinolone (Kenalog®) controls the disease in its acute state. Topical corticosteroids are also beneficial. Persons with more severe disease may respond to hydroxychloroquine and beta-carotene (Solatene®). Very stubborn PMLE may be treated with thalidomide and nicotinamide, but the use of these medications is unusual. Finally, azathioprine (Immuran®) has been helpful in severe disease.

Diseases similar to PMLE are called actinic prurigo and hydroa vacciniforme. These are rare but have skin changes similar to PMLE; they arise in children prior to puberty.

Solar Urticaria

This unusual disease shows the same skin changes seen in urticaria or hives. It is more common in females between the ages of twenty and forty. Over time it may improve, stay the same, or worsen. When susceptible persons are exposed to the sun they develop itching, redness, and hives within five to ten minutes. Most lesions subside within an hour or so after getting out of the sun. If an attack is severe enough, headache, nausea, wheezing, and fainting may occur. These symptoms may arise if a person is taking certain photosensitizing medications or has one of the rare photosensitive diseases such as porphyria.

Treatment is difficult. Giving corticosteroids by mouth or injection will help in the short term but do nothing to control the disease. Antihistamines such as hydroxyzine (Atarax®) and diphenhydramine (Benadryl®) may help. Nonsedating antihistamines such as terfenadine (Seldane®), astemizole (Hismanal®), cetirizine (Zyrtec®), and loratadine (Claritin®) are also useful but expensive. Antihistamines designed to prevent stomach acid buildup, such as ranitidine (Zantac®) and cimetidine (Tagamet®) have helped some patients. If the condition is severe enough, PUVA or UVA treatment as for psoriasis may be used. This obviously must be done with care since too much light will worsen the hives. Sunscreen use may help prevent solar urticaria.

Chronic Actinic Dermatitis

Chronic actinic dermatitis (CAD) is an uncommon disease, but one that can make a person truly miserable. CAD is also called photosensitive eczema or photosensitive dermatitis. This condition has the features of eczema or atopic dermatitis. However, the disease differs in that the use of light provokes and aggravates the problem rather than improving it. Both UVA and UVB are thought to be responsible for CAD. This disorder is almost solely restricted to middle-aged or older adults, usually men. The problem is worse in the summer but never really subsides even in the winter.

Sun-exposed areas such as the face, forehead, arms, and hands are most affected. The skin becomes red, scaly, and thickened. Itching is a problem at best and at worst is maddening. Eventually, the patients may become so uncomfortable that they take night jobs and rarely venture out during the day. Many become recluses or hermits with dark plastic taped over their windows and lights rarely turned on. Treatment is difficult and frustrating. Topical sunscreens may help a little but many persons with CAD are aggravated by visible light; this is not blocked by routine sunscreens. Topical and oral corticosteroids are only partially effective. More aggressive treatments such as with azathioprine (Immuran®) or cyclophosphamide (Cytoxan®) are almost always required. If these fail, cyclosporine (Sandimmune®, Neoral®) may be tried. Some patients respond to PUVA as used for psoriasis but this has to be very carefully done. Additionally, most persons with CAD are leery of any therapy that has to do with more light being applied to their skin.

Nodular Cysts and Comedones (Favre-Racouchot Disease)

This is a skin condition that most people have seen but can't identify. Favre-Racouchot disease is seen in older patients and almost exclusively in men. It occurs after years of sun exposure. There is a tendency for this condition to run in families. In the beginning blackheads (comedones) develop on the upper cheeks, temples, and to the sides of the eyes. As time passes these blackheads rupture under the skin, forming scars and small- to moderate-sized cysts. They are not usually uncomfortable but may grow to the size of a large marble and can be very disfiguring.

Treatment is difficult. If the problem is in the early stages, the use of sunscreens (with a physical blocking agent), topical tretinoin (Retin-A®), or isotretinoin (Accutane®) may be helpful. If the condition is well developed there is little effective therapy aside from surgical removal. Prevention and early intervention are most effective.

Sweating Disorders

The production of perspiration or sweat is a well-known phenomenon that causes problems in few persons. Two types of sweat glands are present in the body: apocrine sweat glands, which produce very little of what we know as perspiration, and eccrine sweat glands, which produce almost all of the body's perspiration. The body makes sweat in response to several different stimuli, such as heat, exertion, emotional changes (nervousness), medications, internal diseases, and so on.

Excessive Sweating (Hyperhidrosis)

Some persons sweat excessively. While this is usually noticed in the armpits, it may also occur on the forehead, hands, feet, and other body sites. The reasons for this are not understood, but whatever controls the rate of sweating has gone awry. These patients have a higher baseline of sweating than normal. This condition, termed hyperhidrosis, may occur in families. The skin of the armpits, soles, and palms is essentially normal. This may interfere with normal daily functioning. The skin tends to sweat in response to emotions such as fear or nervousness; however, some patients sweat continually for no apparent reason. Oddly, these patients do not usually suffer with much odor; the sweating proceeds so quickly that the perspiration washes away any of the odor-causing sweat from apocrine glands.

Treatment

Most therapies involve pills and topical treatment. It was thought that making these patients less nervous would make them sweat less, but antidepressants and antianxiety drugs such as benzodiazepines (Valium®, Xanax®, and so on) have been used with little success. Another class of drugs designed to stop the stimulation of the sweat glands themselves is called anticholinergics (Robinul®). This type of medication is usually only partially effective and may have intolerable side effects. Another reported successful treatment is the use of the high blood pressure medication clonidine (Catapres®). The most common topical therapy is the use of aluminum chloride (Drysol®, Xerac AC®). This chemical is a common ingredient in most antiperspirants. It works by decreasing the amount of sweat that an eccrine sweat gland can produce. It is applied at night to the skin and then washed off in the morning. This is done for several days in a row each week until the problem is brought under control. It may take a month to appropriately reduce the rate of perspiration. For persons with severe armpit sweating, the medication may be applied to very dry skin and then covered with plastic wrap. Putting on a T-shirt over the plastic wrap will keep it in place for the rest of the night. In the morning, the aluminum chloride can be washed off. This should be done for three to five consecutive nights initially and then several times per week for control. A similar regimen may be used for palms and soles with a sock or glove.

Aluminum chloride, aluminum chlorohydrate, and aluminum sulfate are the most common chemicals used in antiperspirants. Zirconium is also effective but may cause some skin irritation. Antiperspirants may be applied in several different ways. Roll-ons, lotions, and creams are the most effective and sprays and sticks the least. The most common problem with these products is skin irritation and/or discoloration of clothing. If redness and irritation develop, changing the brand of antiperspirant or trying a less irritating method of application such as a cream or roll-on may be helpful. Deodorants do not diminish sweating but mask the odor produced in the armpit by using antibacterial chemicals and perfuming agents.

One of the most effective methods of treatment is iontophoresis. This program uses tap water and an iontophoretic unit (Drionic® unit). The foot or hand is placed on a water-soaked pad or the pad is applied to the armpit for several minutes per day and a very low electric current is run through the pad. This is not dangerous or uncomfortable and most patients feel nothing. It is most effective for persons with excessive sweating of the palms. These units are manufactured by the General Medical Corporation and may be purchased without a prescription (1935 Armacost Avenue, Los Angeles, CA, 90025-9937; 1-800-432-5362). It is not clear how or why this method of therapy works but it seems to stop the sweat glands from forming perspiration.

Topical solutions of formaldehyde and glutaraldehyde will also diminish sweating. These medications were much more popular several years ago. They are not used much anymore because so many persons are allergic to these chemicals They also tend to stain the skin an unpleasant yellowish orange and have an unpleasant odor.

There is a surgical approach to excessive sweating. Cutting the nerves supplying the sweat glands (sympathectomy) has been used in severe cases. This has some serious side effects and is rarely done anymore. Removing the sweat glands from the armpits has also been successful. This is a major surgery with the potential for complications but certainly solves the problem. It too is usually reserved for severe cases.

Anhidrosis

More severe from the standpoint of health is a person who is unable to sweat to an appropriate degree (hypohidrosis). Persons who do not perspire adequately may be suffering from certain diseases, have tumors or lesions in the brain, be taking medication suppressing the sweat glands, or be dehydrated. Some genetic diseases (anhidrotic ectodermal dysplasia) result in few or no sweat glands being present in the skin of affected persons. Since perspiration is the body's means of eliminating excessive heat, an inability to sweat may turn into a dangerous situation. Patients experience light-headedness, fatigue, weakness, and fever. If they are not moved to a cooler environment they may eventually die. Treatment is largely environmental. Most patients must stay in air-conditioned environments (moving to a cooler climate is helpful), wear light clothing, and avoid strenuous activity.

Miliaria

The formation of miliaria arises when the sweat is unable to get from the gland where it is produced to the surface of the skin. There are several different types of miliaria depending on where in the skin the blockage occurs. The most common type is called *miliaria crystallina*. These form as small clear blisterlike areas usually no bigger than a pencil lead when the most superficial aspect of the skin blocks the sweat gland. They arise quickly, are without symptoms, and may conglomerate to form larger blister pools. Miliaria crystallina are very common after a fever has broken and sweating has occurred. They may also occur when a person sweats several days after being sunburned and before peeling. Aside from being unsightly, there is no danger to this form of miliaria. As the small blisters pop, the skin will slough off and no longer be a problem.

Miliaria rubra (also known as prickly heat) occurs when the sweat gland is obstructed a little deeper in the skin. These red bumps may itch and sting. Miliaria rubra is seen in infants and adults after sweating in a very humid environment. This condition usually resolves after the person moves to a cooler environment. There is some evidence that 1 gram per day of vitamin C or applying lanolin-containing moisturizers may help.

Miliaria pustulosa consists of miliaria rubra that has become a pustule. *Miliaria profunda* is not common but is uncomfortable. Persons who are not accustomed to heat and humidity (as in the jungle) may experience considerable sweating when they are in such environments. If there is a block deep in the sweat glands, a gooseflesh appearance may arise in the skin. The only treatment is moving to a cooler environment.

Body Odor (Bromhidrosis)

This is technically called bromhidrosis and occurs from sweat produced by the apocrine sweat glands. Some persons have bad-smelling body odor because of the foods they eat or the medications they take. Others may have certain diseases, many genetic, causing them to excrete odorous chemical substances onto their skin. Bromhidrosis may also be due to excessive sweating of the feet and the thick, sodden skin resulting from it.

Bromhidrosis rarely occurs prior to puberty, since the apocrine sweat glands function very little before that time. Since most apocrine sweat glands are found in the armpits, this is where most of the odor arises. It is more of a problem in the warmer months but usually present year-round. Blacks tend to be affected more since they have greater numbers of apocrine sweat glands. Asians are affected the least. Frequent body washing tends to make the problem less severe. Significant sweating of the feet is more common in younger persons, particularly males. The elderly are rarely affected.

As the sweat arrives on the skin's surface, it is invaded by bacteria; these proliferate and form the chemicals producing the odor. If the sweat is not frequently washed off, odor-causing substances remain and the smell worsens. Sweat-soaked clothing may also result in odor. Bromhidrosis from the feet results from the thick mass of soggy skin that soon becomes infested with numerous bacteria. This is worsened by the feet being contained in both socks and shoes.

Treatment

Treatment of bromhidrosis of the armpits involves keeping the area as clean as possible with frequent washing. Antibacterial soaps are best and are usually marketed as deodorant soaps. These products kill off bacteria that cause the odor. Liquid soaps containing chlorhexidine (Hibiclens®, Hibistat®, Betasept®) and povidone-iodine (Betadine®) are useful for thorough cleaning of the skin. Both are very safe for long-term use but chlorhexidine may cause a very irritating reaction if accidentally gotten in the eye. These should be used on a daily or twice-daily basis. Hibistat Towelettes® may be used without water, so they are helpful for use during the day. Most antiperspirant products inhibit bacterial growth as well. Deodorants strictly attempt to mask the odor of the skin and are usually not very effective. Absorbent powders and perfumes are also usually of limited help. Shaving the armpits may be beneficial. Reducing the amount of sweat produced is also helpful. This may be accomplished to some degree by using the methods previously listed.

Excessive foot sweating and odor may be treated with aluminum chloride solutions and iontophoresis, as described earlier. Some formaldehyde-containing medications are available for use on the feet (Lazerformalyde®, Formalyde-10® Spray). These are applied once or twice daily to diminish the amount of perspiration produced. Frequent washing with antibacterial soaps, use of dusting powders, and frequent sock changes are also helpful. Soaking the feet daily in Burrow's solution (Domeboro®) at 1 to 40 concentration will help reduce the number of bacteria on the feet.

Tongue Disorders

Geographic Tongue

The most common tongue condition is called geographic tongue. This condition is named for the configuration that the tongue takes when affected. The surface becomes slick in some areas and almost fuzzy in others; this picture changes even from hour to hour. As a result, the tongue looks like a map or a geographic formation. Geographic tongue is thought by some dermatologists to be a form of psoriasis or eczema. It is more common in persons who have allergies and asthma in their families. It may be seen in any age group but tends to affect younger patients. It causes some mild discomfort and changes in taste but is usually well tolerated. It tends to subside but may later recur. Treatment consists of topical corticosteroids or perhaps a corticosteroid injection. Corticosteroid preparations such as gels and solutions work best. Kenalog in Orabase® is a formulation that adheres to moist mucous membranes and may be useful. Mouthwashes containing corticosteroids may be mixed up by a pharmacist and often help. The antibiotic suspension cephalexin (Keflex®) may be applied to a cotton ball and held onto the tongue for a few minutes. This is done several times daily. Applying topical tretinoin (Retin-A®) in the liquid form can also be used. This has a bad taste, however, and use of the liquid form is expensive.

Hairy Tongue (Black Hairy Tongue, Lingua Villosa Nigra)

This is a frightening condition. The tongue looks furry or hairy and may have a black color. This occurs predominantly in smoking patients who have been taking antibiotics or corticosteroids. The surface of the tongue becomes thick and has a foul taste. Bad breath (halitosis) usually accompanies this disorder. There is bacterial and fungal overgrowth on the tongue. The most effective treatment is elimination of the cause (smoking, antibiotics, and so on). Brushing the tongue with a toothbrush and toothpaste is helpful. Topical tretinoin gel (Retin-A®) may also be used.

Hairy Leukoplakia

Hairy leukoplakia is different from hairy tongue. Hairy leukoplakia is found almost exclusively in patients with AIDS but can also be seen in patients who are taking chemotherapy. It is found on the lateral borders of the tongue and appears slightly white and wispy. There are no symptoms. It is thought to result from infection of the tissues with the Epstein-Barr virus (the cause of infectious mononucleosis). It has been successfully treated with zidovudine (Retrovir®) and antifungal medicines.

Fissured (Scrotal) Tongue

Fissured (scrotal) tongue results in the tongue having mild to deep fissures on its surface. It gets its name from its similar appearance to the skin surface of the scrotum. It occurs for unknown reasons most of the time but may be seen in a condition called Melkersson-Rosenthal syndrome. It is also seen in patients with geographic tongue. There usually are no symptoms but food may become trapped in the furrows, resulting in an offensive odor. There is no good way to improve the appearance of the tongue. Brushing with a toothbrush is a good means of keeping the odor and foul taste under control. Frequent use of mouthwashes is also helpful. Application of topical tretinoin gel (Retin-A®, Retin-A Micro®) may also be tried but is unlikely to be of much benefit.

Squamous Cell Carcinoma

The most worrisome of the tongue lesions is squamous cell carcinoma. This usually occurs in men beginning in their fifties. While there may be some pain associated with this tumor, it is usually minimal and some patients are completely unaware of the cancer. Persons who smoke, drink alcohol, and chew tobacco are at greatest risk. The tumors appear as ulcers with heaped-up borders that are white to red colored. They are usually thick and hard. Cancers on the back of the tongue have a worse prognosis than those on the front. The best therapy is surgical excision but tumors commonly have spread before much can be done. Radiation therapy may be useful, but chemotherapy is rarely helpful.

Urticaria and Angioedema

Commonly known as hives, welts, nettle rash, and cnidosis, these lesions appear suddenly on the skin and mucous membranes and, in most cases, disappear within twenty-four hours but may be replaced by other hives. Their size ranges from that of a pencil lead to a dinner plate. They are usually light red to pink and slightly raised above the surface of the skin. The skin may resume its normal color in the center of the lesions. There may be a red to pink halo on the surrounding flat skin. Hives usually itch but a stinging or burning sensation may also occur. The trunk and extremities are the usual sites. Swelling of the palms and soles occurs and may be disabling. Involvement of areas with loose tissue such as around the eyes or on the genitalia may lead to massive swelling and disfigurement. While this condition is not usually dangerous, if the airways are involved they may become swollen and close off. Wheezing and abdominal cramping also occur but are rare. Some patients with widespread involvement complain of feeling very tired and listless, particularly if their disease has been present for some time. Urticaria is usually divided into acute and chronic stages. Acute urticaria has been present for less than six weeks and chronic urticaria for longer than six weeks. Another subset are the physical urticarias.

Causes

This skin eruption is an allergic reaction to something with which the patient comes in contact, either externally or internally. Medications are the most common cause. This may be due to drugs usually associated with allergy such as penicillin, aspirin, and narcotics, but virtually any medication may cause urticaria. Food and drug additives are also a problem. These include preservatives, dyes, and yeast. Different foods themselves, such as strawberries, chocolate, shellfish, nuts, tomatoes, pork, and onions cause about a third of the cases. Another large category is infections. These include routine illnesses such as colds and flu but also more uncommon infections such as intestinal worms, diseased teeth, and infected sinuses. Virtually every chemical and infection at one time or another has been associated with urticaria.

Less common causes include diseases such as lupus erythematosus and underlying cancers, insect bites, and inhalants. Stress is not likely to cause urticaria but as in many skin diseases, it certainly worsens it. It may be real detective work figuring out which chemical is causing a person's urticaria, and in a large number of cases this remains a mystery. In chronic urticaria, only about half the patients eventually find out what is causing their disease. Often it is more important to alleviate the patient's symptoms, because in the majority of cases the hives will appear, will be treated, will go away, and the reason for them will remain unknown.

If the cause of the hives is known, the therapy becomes fairly simple—avoid the offending agent. Almost all patients, however, need some form of treatment. Topical corticosteroids, particularly potent preparations, are very effective. Corticosteroids by mouth or injection are the most popular treatment; they require little of the patient and in the case of an injection, may gradually leach out of the injected muscle into the bloodstream for the next two to three weeks, allowing for continued benefit. Sedating antihistamines such as hydroxyzine (Atarax®), diphenhydramine (Benadryl®), doxepin (Sinequan®), and chlorpromazine (Thorazine®) have been popular for years but may make patients so drowsy that they have difficulty functioning. Antihistamines such as terfenadine (Seldane®), astemizole (Hismanal®), cetirizine (Zyrtec®), and loratadine (Claritin®) are easy to take and don't cause drowsiness. They tend to be more expensive, however, and interact with various antibiotics. The antihistamines used for control of gastritis and stomach ulcers, ranitidine (Zantac®) and cimetidine (Tagamet®), have also been successfully used in urticaria. Soaking in oatmeal baths is soothing. Some dermatologists give patients a course of antibiotic therapy under the premise that an infection is present but causing few or no symptoms aside from the urticaria. Other less common therapies include sulfasalazine (Azulfidine®), dapsone, colchicine (Col-BENEMID®), anabolic steroids, anti-inflammatory drugs (Nuprin®, Motrin®, Aleve®), calcium channel blocking antihypertension agents (Procardia®, Cardizem®), cromolyn sodium (Gastrochrom®), and cyclosporine. Most dermatologists will evaluate the patient for underlying disease if the urticaria persists. This may consist of x-rays, skin tests, a skin biopsy, blood work, and so on. The results of these tests will hopefully reveal what is causing the hives as well as what is *not* causing them.

Physical urticarias are a collection of diseases in which the skin breaks out in hives due to contact with unusual agents. The treatment consists of avoidance if possible and the use of the medications mentioned above.

Uncommon Disorders

These are uncommon disorders and may be very difficult to manage:

DERMATOGRAPHISM　　This is also called factitious urticaria. Patients show a tendency to break out in hives when the skin is scratched or stroked. This disease may be associated with underlying hormonal imbalances or infections. Pressure urticaria is a subset of dermatographism in which persons get hives on the skin following applied pressure.

AQUAGENIC URTICARIA   Patients with aquagenic urticaria break out in hives upon contact with water. While this is rare, aquagenic pruritus, a similar condition with itching after water contact, is not. Some types of light therapy may be helpful.

COLD URTICARIA   The hands and face are common sites for involvement. The lesions don't actually appear until the skin begins rewarming.

CHOLINERGIC URTICARIA   This is also called exercise urticaria, since it usually occurs while exercising. The hives are usually very small and surround hair follicles. This may also occur with emotional stress or hot weather.

PAPULAR URTICARIA   Papular urticaria occurs most commonly in children. The hives are very small and present on the arms and legs. These are believed to arise in persons who are sensitive to insect bites.

HEAT URTICARIA   This may be what some persons call "sun poisoning." Persons develop hives soon after exposure to the sun. It usually is simply an annoyance but can be dangerous for some patients.

Angioedema

Angioedema is a more severe form of urticaria. It is also known as giant urticaria or Quincke's edema. Attacks of angioedema may be sudden and usually involve severe swelling of the soft tissues such as the eyelids, lips, and face. Distortion of facial features may be so severe that the affected person is unrecognizable. Mucous membranes, including the genitalia, are commonly affected. Attacks sometimes occur in the night with lesions found on awakening. These lesions may itch but patients commonly complain of pain and burning. Patients also may feel very tired and weak, with wheezing and decreased blood pressure (hypotension). Between attacks patients feel relatively normal. The same triggers that cause urticaria cause angioedema. Additionally, there is a hereditary form called *hereditary angioneurotic edema*.

Management of angioedema is difficult. The evaluation for underlying disease is essentially the same as for urticaria. Almost all persons will improve if given oral corticosteroids, but these can't be given for prolonged periods. Topical medicines are not very effective. Since angioedema is a state of exaggerated reactivity by the immune system, medicines designed to suppress the immune system such as aza-thioprine (Immuran®) or methotrexate (Rheumatrex®) are often used. Epinephrine may also be employed, particularly if the patient is wheezing or has diminished blood pressure. Dapsone is helpful in some cases. Hereditary angioneurotic edema is best treated with an anabolic steroid, danazol (Danacrine®), which stimulates the body to produce more of this protein. Unfortunately, danazol causes unwanted side effects in women and cannot be used during pregnancy.

VASCULITIS

The word *vasculitis* literally means inflammation of the blood vessels. Since the body contains a number of different types of blood vessels and the list of things which may inflame them is almost endless, there are several different categories of this disease. Categorizing these conditions is difficult, but for the most part they are divided according to what size blood vessel has been affected.

Leukocytoclastic Vasculitis (Necrotizing Vasculitis)

The more common term for leukocytoclastic vasculitis (LCV) is palpable purpura. This means that the rash that arises on the skin can be felt by passing a finger over the surface of the skin (palpable) and that the color derives from red blood cells which have escaped the confines of a blood vessel and are now free in the tissues (purpura). When this occurs on the lower legs, the most common site of involvement, a diagnosis may be easy. The skin may also show hives (urticaria), blisters, ulcerations, and swelling, however. Unfortunately, these are not specific changes in the skin and a biopsy will usually have to be performed. While the lower legs are most commonly affected, almost any skin surface can be involved. The rash may burn or sting but usually is not uncomfortable. If the LCV is quick in onset it may be accompanied by fever, chills, stomach pain, joint aches, and joint swelling. An episode usually lasts several days and the lesions take up to a month to eventually subside.

Causes
The causes of LCV are practically endless. The most common etiologies are "drugs and bugs," meaning medications (prescription and otherwise) and infections. The number of drugs causing LCV is also endless. The more common causes include antibiotics (especially penicillin and penicillinlike drugs), sulfa drugs, high blood pressure medications, and anti-inflammatory drugs such as ibuprofen (Motrin®) or naproxen (Aleve®). Virtually any medication, however, is capable of causing this reaction. Infections such as staph and strep and different types of hepatitis are also common, although any infection is theoretically capable of causing vasculitis. The next most frequent cause of LCV is underlying diseases such as lupus erythematosus and rheumatoid arthritis. Again, almost any chronic disease can cause this rash. Table 28 lists the more common causes of LCV.

Table 28 **COMMON CAUSES OF LEUKOCYTOCLASTIC VASCULITIS (PALPABLE PURPURA)**

Drugs and Chemicals	Allopurinol (Zyloprim®)
	Aspirin and Aspirin-Containing Medications
	Diuretics (particularly Thiazides)
	Herbicides
	Insecticides
	Iodine-Containing Medications
	Nonsteroidal Anti-Inflammatory Drugs (Phenactin, Ibuprofen, and so on)
	Penicillin and Penicillinlike Antibiotics
	Sulfa Drugs
Infections	Candida
	Hepatitis B and Hepatitis C
	Influenza
	Mononucleosis (Epstein-Barr Virus)
	Staphylococcal
	Streptococcal
	Tuberculosis
Malignancies	Hodgkin's Disease
	Leukemia
	Lymphoma
Internal Diseases	Cryoglobulinemia
	Lupus Erythematosus
	Rheumatoid Arthritis
	Sjogren's Syndrome
	Ulcerative Colitis

There are several different subtypes of LCV, most of which are rare. These include erythema elevatum diutinum, livedoid vasculitis, urticarial vasculitis, and cryoglobulinemia. Henoch-Schonlein purpura is a condition that may be seen in children and adolescents or young adults. It begins with a sore throat or other upper respiratory disease. Several days to weeks later these bruiselike areas arise on the lower back, buttocks, and legs. Unfortunately, these may look like areas of child abuse, causing some confusion. There may be blood in the urine and kidney involvement as well. Treatment consists of watching for the urinary changes to normalize and the skin lesions to resolve.

Treatment

The treatment of LCV is usually fairly simple if a cause is known. The inciting drug is discontinued or the underlying disease is treated. This is obviously most effective in cases of LCV caused by medications. A course of oral prednisone (Deltasone®) or an injection of triamcinolone (Kenalog®) will usually make any discomfort disappear and the skin rash clear up sooner. Colchicine (Col-BENEMID®) and dapsone are also used if steroids are not effective. Suppressing the immune system with medications such as azathioprine (Immuran®) or cyclophosphamide (Cytoxan®) may also be required if more conservative treatments fail. Antihistamines such as hydroxyzine (Atarax®) and diphenhydramine (Benadryl®) are also useful but will not completely clear the eruption. Unfortunately, in a certain number of patients a cause is not found and treatment has to be continued until the problem subsides. If the LCV involves other organs such as the kidneys, liver, or brain these patients will have symptoms from these systems as well.

Giant Cell Arteritis

In elderly patients, an artery (the temporal artery) which lies over the temple and extends onto the forehead may become inflamed. This is called giant cell arteritis because this blood vessel will develop large inflammatory cells in the artery's wall. This condition is also closely related to another disease called polymyalgia rheumatica. Patients usually develop GCA in their seventies or eighties. The first symptoms are a headache or pain in the temple. Sometimes the pain is sharp. The skin over this area usually does not change, but if the problem is severe there may be redness or even ulceration. The most worrisome aspect of GCA is the risk of affecting some of the blood vessels leading to the eye and causing eventual blindness. Patients with GCA are usually put on prednisone with good results. Many patients have to remain indefinitely on this drug.

Kawasaki Syndrome (Mucocutaneous Lymph Node Syndrome)

This condition has become better known in the past decade. It is not commonly thought of as an inflammatory condition of the blood vessels and largely affects children under the age of five. It is most common in Japan but does occur in the United States, more often in the winter and spring. It may occur in epidemics. Most patients are between twelve and twenty-four months of age. It's not clear if Kawasaki syndrome occurs in adults. Girls are more commonly affected than boys. For unknown reasons, families of higher socioeconomic status are affected more often.

The cause of this condition is not clear but it may be due to a virus. Patients typically develop a fever which is difficult or impossible to control. Temperatures routinely climb to 104°F. The fever usually continues for one to two weeks. The skin rash is red and raised and affects the trunk, arms, and legs. There are no symptoms with this rash. Sometimes the skin around the groin becomes red and begins to scale. The eyes are red and swollen and the lips become fiery red. One of the most noticeable features of Kawasaki syndrome is the "strawberry" tongue; in this condition, the tongue becomes very red. The skin of the fingers usually turns red to pink and begins to scale after a week or so. Swelling of the lymph glands in the neck occurs. Some mild joint and muscle pains may also be present. The most worrisome aspect of this disorder are changes affecting the heart. Abnormal muscle function and electrical impulses may be noticed but when the blood vessels around the heart are affected the situation becomes dangerous. Up to a fourth of patients have some dilations of the coronary arteries called aneurysms. With the small aneurysms, the majority will disappear on their own in the following months. Larger lesions may require surgical repair, however. Most patients are followed by a pediatric cardiologist.

Treatment consists of aspirin in measured doses during the early phases of Kawasaki disease. This helps cut down on the inflammatory response and prevents the body from damaging the heart and other organs. Corticosteroids have been used but seem to make the problem worse. The newest treatment, and probably the most effective, is giving children high doses of immunoglobulin by vein. This has to be done in the hospital and is expensive.

Other Vascular Disorders

There are other diseases in which inflammation of the blood vessels plays a significant role. Fortunately, most of these conditions are uncommon and do not affect very many people. Patients with these conditions are taken care of at major medical institutions since they are frequently very sick. The usual therapies involve either corticosteroids or suppression of the immune system with drugs such as azathioprine or cyclophosphamide. Polyarteritis nodosa is an inflammation of the larger arteries. The internal organs such as the kidneys and nerves are commonly affected. The skin is involved in about half the cases and shows nodules in the deeper tissues, particularly over the lower legs. These may be tender. Fever and muscle aches may also occur. Patients are usually infected with hepatitis B or other virus infections. Wegener's granulomatosis and Churg-Strauss disease are conditions that also affect the larger blood vessels. Middle-aged persons are most commonly affected and not all patients have skin changes. When the skin is affected, it usually displays ulcerations and nodules.

VIRAL INFECTIONS

Viruses are a collection of chemicals and proteins that infect a human (or animal or plant) cell and force it to produce more viruses. As the cell becomes full, these viruses may infect surrounding cells or cause the cell to burst. In other conditions and with the appropriate virus, the cell may become cancerous and a malignancy begins. Most infected persons eventually manage to destroy the infecting viruses. The body develops antibodies and is able to prevent an infection. Unfortunately, in some instances the patient is not able to fight off the infection before immunity can be developed. Antibiotics against viruses are very different from those used to treat bacterial infections. In the first place, there are fewer of them. In the second place, they don't work quite as well. As with bacterial infections, avoidance or immunization is the best rule.

Measles (Rubeola)

About thirty-five years ago, the first immunizations for measles were produced and what was once a potentially fatal disease was conquered. Persons are immunized at fifteen months of age with the MMR (measles, mumps, and rubella) shot and are immune from the disease for at least a decade. Not everyone receives this immunization, however, and about ten years ago small epidemics of this disease once again began to occur in the United States. Measles is most common in the spring. Current measles outbreaks tend to occur in poorer neighborhoods among black and Hispanic children.

It takes about a week and a half after exposure for children to become ill. The first symptoms are fever with a cough, runny nose, and inflamed eyes (conjunctivitis). The rash comes after a day or two while the patient is still ill. It begins on the head and neck and extends to the trunk and extremities. The fever and rash peak at about the same time. The skin is slightly red and swollen but without any symptoms such as pain or itching. As the rash subsides, mild scaling begins. Bright red spots about the size of pencil erasers are found in the mouth and are called Koplik's spots. Measles itself rarely causes any problems. It is the secondary bacterial infections that may come with it that pose a danger. Ear infections and pneumonia are the most common. Younger, malnourished, and dehydrated children are at greatest risk. Infection of the brain by measles (encephalitis) is a rare occurrence but the one most feared. Most patients recover from this event but some do not; they either die or are mentally disabled.

There is no specific treatment for measles infection. Patients should be given plenty of fluids to prevent dehydration and their fever controlled with acetaminophen (Tylenol®) or ibuprofen (Motrin®). If a secondary bacterial infection occurs, they should be placed on antibiotic therapy as soon as possible. If a child has been exposed to measles, immune globulin may prevent the disease if given within six days of exposure.

Rubella (German Measles)

This viral infection usually affects older children and young adults. Worldwide epidemics are noted every five to seven years. It is present in all countries and is spread by secretions from coughs, sneezes, and runny nose. The symptoms begin two to three weeks after infection and include runny nose, cough, congestion, fever, sore throat, headache, and swollen glands. The rash begins after one to four days but unlike measles, peaks as the other symptoms are fading. It is initially pink to red. The head and neck are involved first, followed by the trunk and extremities. The skin clears in less than three days (faster than with measles) and mild scaling may follow. Small, pinpoint red spots are found in the mouth. Swelling of the lymph glands may be very prominent and usually affects the neck and behind the ears. Pain in the joints may be present and is more of a problem in adults. Treatment is usually symptomatic with fluids and antifever medications.

For the most part, rubella is little more than an inconvenience to patients and their families. Serious complications are rare and are much less common than with measles. The real danger with this infection is in pregnant women. The earlier in the pregnancy rubella occurs, the greater the danger. Affected babies may have deafness, heart defects, mental retardation, and cataracts. For this reason, immunization is important. The MMR given at age fifteen months contains a rubella vaccine. Revaccination at five to eleven years is recommended. Women should wait three months after vaccination before becoming pregnant.

Hand, Foot, and Mouth Disease

This oddly named disease is most common in children. As the name suggests, it involves the hands, feet, and mouth. It is caused by a virus named coxsackievirus A16. Hand, foot, and mouth disease occurs in epidemics in the late summer and early fall.

The virus is spread among children and then to adults. It is highly contagious. It takes about three to six days after infection for the symptoms to begin. A low-grade fever develops, along with mild runny nose and cough. Painful mouth ulcers arise early. Children may refuse to eat, are very fussy, and if the pain is great enough, will drool. Five to ten ulcerations develop; they are red with a grayish base and rarely become larger than a pencil eraser. Shortly after the mouth ulcers arise, small blisters on the hands and feet are seen. They are somewhat red and only slightly bigger than the width of a pencil lead. They may be football shaped. Most are slightly tender. All the lesions resolve in a week to ten days. Treatment consists of fever control and mouthwashes with numbing medications.

Herpangina

Despite its name, this condition has no relation to infection by the herpes simplex virus. Herpangina is an infectious condition that affects children in epidemics in the late summer and early fall. Adults are rarely susceptible. The initial symptoms are low to moderate fever, headache, and muscle aches. Stomachache and nausea may also be present. After a day or so, a sore throat begins to develop. This may be only mildly uncomfortable, but usually is very painful. Small ulcers arise at the back of the throat and around the tonsils. The surrounding skin is also somewhat reddened. The glands in the neck are swollen and uncomfortable. The disease lasts five to seven days.

Treatment is directed at making the patient more comfortable. Acetaminophen and ibuprofen are useful for controlling the fevers and some of the discomfort. Because these ulcers may be very painful, some physicians prescribe a solution containing codeine. Children may go several days without eating without any serious complications. Many are so uncomfortable, however, that they stop drinking and become dehydrated. Cool drinks, Popsicles, and ice cream help children take in fluids. A solution containing viscous lidocaine (Xylocaine®) to numb the ulcers may be prescribed and is beneficial. Since this condition is contagious, an infected child should be kept away from other children.

Erythema Infectiosum (Fifth Disease)

Erythema infectiosum got the name "Fifth Disease" from a classification of several diseases of childhood that was common many years ago. It is caused by a virus known as parvovirus B19. This virus is found worldwide and epidemics occur in the late winter and spring. It usually occurs in children. The first symptoms are headache, runny nose, and low-grade fever. A sore throat and cough occur in some patients, but for the most part the symptoms of erythema infectiosum are mild. The most characteristic feature of this disease is a rash occurring on the cheeks. It is slightly red and has a "slapped cheek" appearance. The rash lasts one to four days and then gradually fades. A similar rash may be seen on the trunk, neck, and upper arms. Even after it has gone away it may return in the following days with heat, exercise, or emotional stress. Infected adults usually have worse symptoms. Arthritis is a common complaint. Erythema infectiosum is a self-limited condition that causes few problems in most patients. It may be dangerous, however, in patients with sickle cell anemia. Under these circumstances, the patient's bone marrow may stop producing blood cells. Severe anemia, bleeding, and a susceptibility to infection then occur. This is considered a medical emergency and patients must be evaluated by a hematologist. Infection of pregnant women may also be dangerous; unborn children are affected to different degrees.

Treatment consists of controlling the fever and discomfort with acetaminophen or ibuprofen. The rash will fade with time and requires no therapy. There is no vaccine for this disease. Infected children and adults should be kept away from pregnant women.

Infectious Mononucleosis

Infectious mononucleosis (or "mono" as it is commonly called) occurs after infection with the Epstein-Barr virus (EBV). EBV is a member of the herpesvirus family and is known to cause several different conditions, including a type of lymphoma typically found in Africa and cancer of the nasal structures. Infection is very common. In undeveloped countries, most infections have occurred by early childhood. In more affluent societies such as the United States, infection is usually delayed until adolescence or young adulthood. Mono is unusual in that the time between infection and the development of symptoms is long, between thirty and fifty days. Over a three to five day period the patient begins to develop headache and fatigue. Sore throat, fever, and swollen neck glands appear. The throat becomes red with pus on the tonsils. The glands in the neck may become very large. A skin rash is present in about 15 percent of patients. This consists of a reddish to pink eruption on the trunk and arms. It usually appears in the first several days of the infection. If patients are given ampicillin (Omnipen®) or amoxicillin (Amoxil®), the skin may develop a very intense dark red rash. Small red spots may be present in the mouth. Swelling of the eyelids is seen in about a third of patients. Symptoms last from two to three weeks and most patients are fully recovered by four to six weeks.

Treatment is usually symptomatic. Acetaminophen or ibuprofen are useful for controlling the fevers and headaches. Although EBV is a member of the herpesvirus family, acyclovir (Zovirax®) and related drugs are not helpful. In about 20 percent of patients, an infection with streptococcus also takes place, in which case antibiotics will be required.

The worst aspects of mono are the sore throat and crushing fatigue. If the pain becomes too intense, narcotics such as codeine may be required to control the discomfort. Mouthwash rinses containing lidocaine are also useful for pain control. In some instances, the swelling of the tonsils and surrounding tissues may be so severe as to restrict breathing. If this happens, a short course of corticosteroids (Deltasone®) may be needed. After the acute symptoms have passed, the fatigue may require several months to subside. The so-called "chronic fatigue syndrome" may be linked to chronic infection with EBV. Persons with mono usually have some degree of swelling of the spleen and liver. It is therefore usually suggested that the patient restrict all contact sports and activities which could result in trauma to the abdomen.

Exanthem Subitum (Roseola)

Roseola is one of the best known of the viral infections causing skin rashes in children. It is present in children under two years of age. There is no seasonal pattern for this condition and it occurs worldwide. The incubation period is five to fifteen days. Boys and girls are equally affected. The virus causing this infection is the human herpesvirus 6 (HHV-6); it is chemically similar to other herpesviruses but does not cause the same type of symptoms. The patient initially runs a high fever for three to five days. There are few other symptoms and usually the child does not appear particularly ill. As the fever breaks, the rash appears on the trunk and neck. It is red to pink and some of the spots may have a halo of white skin around them. The rash lasts several days and then fades. Giving the patients acetaminophen or ibuprofen is helpful for fever control. Complications are few.

Orf and Milker's Nodules

These two conditions together are called "barnyard pox," since they arise in farm animals and then are spread to humans. Orf is found on the mouths of lambs, sheep, and goats. Milker's nodules are found as sores and weeping wounds on the udders of infected cows. Persons who have contact with these animals (ranchers, veterinarians, and so on) may touch these lesions and become infected. In both diseases the animals are not particularly uncomfortable and the sores heal in several weeks. In orf and milker's nodule the initial lesions look like red bumps; these break down to form sores. They may blister but usually form nontender ulcers. They take several weeks to heal and during that time the patient is infectious. There is no treatment for barnyard pox since it subsides on its own.

Vitiligo and Albinism

Vitiligo

Vitiligo is a condition in which the pigment in the skin is lost and a white or near white color is formed. It is noticeable but not necessarily disfiguring among whites. In blacks and Native Americans, however, it may be devastating. It is an ancient disease and one that has probably been confused with leprosy in the past. Some of the oldest writings from Egypt and the Middle East discuss vitiligo and different treatments for it. In some cultures it may mark the person for life and make him unacceptable for association with others.

This disease begins at any age but usually arises in adolescents and young adults. One to 2 percent of the population is affected. It is more common in dark-skinned persons. Vitiligo is inherited to some extent, meaning that it runs in families. It is not clear what precipitates this condition, but many persons relate it to stress or illness including accidents, trauma, family sickness, and sunburn. In vitiligo, the pigment-producing cells in the skin called melanocytes begin to die. This results from some abnormality of the immune system, and may explain why vitiligo is sometimes associated with other diseases involving the immune system.

Vitiligo begins as small patches of white discoloration or pigment loss. Essentially any skin may be affected, but some areas are more typically involved than others. The central face is commonly affected as are the fingers, hands, and wrists. The trunk and upper extremities may also be involved but this is less common. Involvement of the genitalia is particularly upsetting. The small patches gradually enlarge as the disease progresses. Mucous membranes may show pigment loss as may hair. Halo nevi are moles that have lost the surrounding pigment in vitiligo and now appear to possess a halo. Skin trauma (cuts and abrasions) may provoke vitiligo in the damaged skin. Consequently, it is important for persons with vitiligo to be careful with their skin. This condition is associated with other disorders such as alopecia areata, thyroid disease, diabetes, Addison's disease, and some types of anemia. Occasionally, the skin may begin to repigment on its own. Since the pigment-producing cells, the melanocytes, are no longer present in the skin, they must migrate in from normal skin or from deep in the hair follicles. Recovering skin will show small dots of repigmentation centered around hair follicles. These areas merge together as the skin repigments.

The most important point for persons with vitiligo to remember is that their skin no longer has any protective pigment; therefore, it is easy to sunburn. Not only is this painful, but it is dangerous over the long run since such skin is more prone to develop skin cancer. Potent sunscreens, preferably those containing zinc oxide and titanium dioxide, should be used if the patient will be out in the sun. These should be frequently reapplied. Sunscreens should also be used for routine daily wear even if no sun exposure is anticipated (see the section on sun exposure).

Treatment

Covering the areas with dyes and makeup is a popular method of treatment. Vitadye® and dihydroxyacetone-containing compounds will stain the skin and make the vitiligo less visible. These stains usually have to wear off and provide no protection from sun exposure. They may be applied repeatedly until the desired skin stain is achieved. Covermark® and Dermablend® are two makeups available for purchase in upscale department stores. When properly applied, they almost completely cover the changes of vitiligo. They wash or rub off, however, and have to be frequently reapplied. They are also expensive and learning how to use them takes some skill. Most makeup counters selling these products have someone trained to teach customers how to apply them.

Since vitiligo involves the immune system, the use of corticosteroids both topically and internally is popular. Creams and ointments may be useful for children but rarely are very effective for adults. A very potent preparation applied frequently for several days will usually indicate whether these drugs will help. The same is true for oral corticosteroids. Prednisone (Deltasone®) taken for a week or two will usually show some effectiveness; if not, it should be stopped.

One of the most effective and popular therapies is PUVA, particularly topical PUVA. With topical PUVA a solution of 8-methoxypsoralen is painted on the spots and subjected to UVA light after thirty minutes. The psoralen is then washed off. Although the psoralen is no longer in contact with the skin, the area may remain photosensitive and care must be taken for the next seventy-two hours not to expose these sites to unwarranted amounts of sun.

Transplanting small sections of pigmented skin into the areas of depigmentation is called minigrafting. The skin with vitiligo is removed by creating small blisters with a suctioning device. Then small sections of normal skin are placed into the diseased portions. The pigmenting cells from the transplanted tissue gradually spread out to repigment the entire area. The risks with minigrafting include scarring and infection, but most worrisome is that the vitiligo will begin in the area of donated skin. Minigrafting is usually reserved for very stubborn cases. In addition to being uncomfortable, it is also expensive. A similar process is the transplanting of skin grown in a laboratory culture and then placed onto the diseased skin. The recipient site has to be prepared as with minigrafting, but there is no donor site. This therapy is largely experimental and is not widely available.

In some persons, either the treatment fails or the vitiligo is too widespread and disfiguring. These patients may choose to completely remove the pigment from the surrounding normal skin to improve their appearance. Monobenzylether of hydroquinone (MBEH) is applied as a 20% cream and destroys the remaining pigment-producing melanocytes. This may take up to a year and the drug has to be applied twice daily. The pigment removal is permanent. The major side effect to this product is skin irritation. Obviously, it is very important that these patients use sunscreens, since they will be completely without protective pigment.

Albinism

Albinism is a collection of about twelve different diseases, almost all of which are genetic conditions. Albinos are born with a defect in the way their melanocytes function; they do not produce a normal amount of pigment. This applies not only to the skin but to other areas of the body, such as the hair and eyes. Since the pigment of the eyes is critical to their proper functioning, albinos have light sensitivity, poor vision, and watering of the eyes. They also have essentially no protection from the sun and easily develop skin cancers and precancerous changes. Obviously, albinos prefer to stay indoors in poorly lit areas. The skin is not completely white but is very light. The hair is blond to dirty white and the eyes are pink to red.

There is essentially no therapy for this condition aside from avoidance of the sun and treatment for the eye disorders. Patients should be aware that they may pass this condition on to their children and should receive genetic counseling.

Warts and Molluscum Contagiosum

Warts

Warts are some of the most common growths on the human body. They are caused by infection with the human papillomavirus (HPV). There are over seventy different types of HPV; some are more likely than others to cause certain types of warts. These lesions are slow growing and if left alone will eventually disappear on their own. Unfortunately, they are often very unsightly and cause patients a considerable degree of embarrassment.

Why some people are affected by warts is not completely clear. There seems to be an association with immune system functioning. Children and adolescents are more likely to develop warts but adults may get them as well. Warts are acquired by contact with infected persons. This virus is very widespread, however, and most patients are not able to specifically identify where or when they were infected.

The typical wart is a rough, scaly flesh-colored to slightly gray bump. Warts tend to affect the hands and fingers, particularly around the nails. These are known as verruca vulgaris (common warts). Flat warts (verruca plana) are small, sometimes mildly pink, flat lesions that accumulate on the face and forehead. They may be difficult to see. Filiform warts are very spiny lesions that also arise on the central face and forehead. They often affect the nose and lips. Plantar warts are found on the feet. These may be very large and are often painful. They affect the heels, balls of the feet, and toes. Genital warts (condyloma accuminatum) are found in the groin and on the genitalia (see the section on sexually transmitted diseases). Warts may also affect the mucous membranes of the mouth where they appear as flesh-colored to pink growths. Since these conditions are so common, the diagnosis is usually quite easy. In some instances, however, as when sexual abuse of a child is suspected, determining the type of HPV causing the wart may become important. Specialized testing is available for such warts but is usually quite expensive.

Treatment of warts is frequently difficult. About two-thirds will disappear on their own in two years. During that time, however, they are capable of spreading the virus to other areas of the skin and causing more lesions. Since no known antibiotics will kill HPV, removal of warts involves destroying the tissue containing the virus. Unfortunately, the skin surrounding a wart may also be infected by HPV but not show a wart. Even if the lesion is removed it is therefore common for a new wart to arise in the same area. Treatment should be done as gently as possible; if done too aggressively a scar may result.

Over-the-counter agents for removing warts usually contain salicylic acid and may be effective for some lesions. They must be used faithfully to have a chance at a cure. These compounds tend to have a high failure rate. The most popular method of therapy for warts is liquid nitrogen. This is usually sprayed on or applied with a cotton-tipped applicator. This is typically done several times to each wart and the area allowed to slowly thaw. After several hours, the skin begins to blister. When the blister ruptures and the skin begins to reheal, hopefully the wart will be gone. In larger lesions, the blister may become bloody and heal with a dark area. At the next visit this area of dead tissue is then cut away, revealing infected tissue below. Another freezing is done and the cycle is repeated until the wart has been completely removed. Obviously, this is time consuming and may be expensive. If the liquid nitrogen is applied too vigorously, large unsightly and uncomfortable blisters develop. The major drawback to liquid nitrogen therapy is the pain, particularly if very sensitive areas are being treated. Children are not fond of this therapy and even adults may decide to just live with the problem after the first treatment. It is safe and fairly effective, however. Persons with darker skin may have some unsightly loss of pigment; this may take some time to resolve. Raising a blister may also be done with canthrone. This is less painful and useful for children. It is applied as mentioned below for molluscum contagiosum. Other chemicals have been used with some success. Application of salicylic acid and trichloroacetic acid may destroy some lesions. Creams containing 5-fluorouracil (Efudex®) also remove some warts but can be uncomfortable. Topical podophyllin, as used for venereal warts, is useful in selected patients. Imiquimod cream (Aldara®) has not been tested for use on routine warts. Some warts will respond to application of tretinoin (Retin-A®). This is particularly useful for flat warts and is applied in the same manner as for acne. For particularly stubborn warts, the injection of bleomycin (Blenoxane®) may be helpful. This treatment method is tricky and has to be done accurately or a substantial amount of healthy tissue will be destroyed. It tends to be painful and must be given with caution on the fingers.

Laser treatment of warts has gained popularity in recent years. Carbon dioxide lasers will destroy the wart-containing tissue but there is always the possibility that they may recur. The treated tissues have to be numbed with local anesthetic. Some dermatologists have begun to use lasers designed to destroy the underlying blood vessels such as the Candela® laser. This treatment is not nearly as uncomfortable and has a moderately good rate of success. Unfortunately, it is expensive.

A treatment option long been known to be effective is the power of suggestion.

As unusual as it may sound, there are a number of dermatologists who have treated patients, usually children, with suggestion therapy. In this method, the warts are painted with a colored solution or one that glows in the dark and then the child is told that over the next few days the warts will magically disappear. Shining a fine, bright light such as that produced by the red light of a pointer laser onto the lesions is another method. It is not clear how this works, but the power of suggestion possibly boosts the patient's immune system to eliminate the warts. This method may be used by parents but may be less effective.

Another method of treatment for children is giving high doses of cimetidine (Tagamet®). This drug has an effect on the immune system and presumably allows the body to rid itself of the warts. It is painless and well tolerated; the only drawback is the cost. The drug is usually given as a suspension at 40 mg/kg per day in divided doses. This is well above the usual dose for ulcer disease or gastritis. Cimetidine treatment has not been as effective in adult patients with warts, but may be worth a try. Injecting interferon (Intron-A®) into a wart is effective in some patients but is usually reserved for those with very stubborn lesions. This therapy is expensive, painful, and causes flulike side effects. Persons with poorly functioning immune systems such as those who have had organ transplants may develop hundreds of warts. Not only is this disfiguring but these warts have an increased risk of becoming cancerous. Most traditional therapies have not been successful in these patients. Isotretinoin (Accutane®) has been beneficial in some patients in at least controlling the problem. It is given in the same doses as for cystic acne.

Finally, for warts not responding to any other therapies, the option of surgery still exists. Excising a wart is usually effective but a recurrence from infected surrounding skin is possible.

Molluscum Contagiosum

This is a very common viral disease. It is totally benign and is limited to the skin. After exposure it takes two to seven weeks for the lesions to appear. Molluscum contagiosum occurs worldwide. The disease is spread by skin-to-skin contact. The two groups most affected are children and young adults. In children, the virus is spread on the playground, at day care, in school, and so on. In young adults, most cases are spread by sexual contact. Why some persons and not others are affected is not clear but it may have to do with the immune system. Some persons, such as those with AIDS, are more susceptible. Children develop molluscum on the face, neck, trunk, and extremities. Young adults tend to get them in the groin and on the genitalia. These lesions range in size up to the width of a pencil lead. They are flesh colored and usually have a small indentation. Persons with eczema or atopic dermatitis are prone to get these lesions and they may arise in the areas of inflamed skin. Most patients only have a few, but persons such as those with AIDS may get hundreds. If molluscum have been scratched or traumatized, they commonly become infected and then may appear like a pimple or boil.

Molluscum contagiosum will subside on its own. These lesions have the ability to infect other skin surfaces (autoinfection), however, and so as long as one is present there is the possibility that others will develop as well. The easiest way to remove these lesions is with a sharp instrument which can be used to flick them off the skin. This is not painless and may be fairly bloody. As a result, it is not popular for genital lesions or in children. It is very quick and effective, however. The most common treatment is liquid nitrogen. It is applied much as for warts and after the blister begins to heal, the molluscum hopefully has been permanently destroyed. This is also a painful procedure and is not 100 percent effective. A popular removal method, because it is relatively painless, is the application of canthrone. This is a vesiculating agent, meaning that it will cause a blister. The liquid is applied and then washed off in four hours (or earlier if stinging begins). Some dermatologists cover the individual spots to keep the medicine in place. Canthrone is very effective but some mild itching and stinging may occur at the sites of placement. It should be remembered that this medication causes a blister on *any* skin it contacts. Consequently, care should be taken while the medicine is on the skin. Two less well-known therapies are anthralin (Drithocreme®) and griseofulvin (Gris-PEG®). Anthralin may be applied to the individual spots for several hours per day. In some patients this will cause the molluscum to gradually shrink. Anthralin use is not without its own problems (see the section on psoriasis) and is not as effective as other methods of destruction. Griseofulvin is most commonly used for fungal infections. For some reason, it is effective in treating molluscum. Its greatest use is in patients with many lesions who have an underlying disease making them more susceptible to molluscum. It is given in the same doses as for fungal infections.

Miscellaneous Conditions

This section of the book includes conditions that are uncommon or do not fit under other sections. Not all these diseases are necessarily rare, but they may rarely be diagnosed.

Acanthosis Nigricans

Acanthosis nigricans is a fairly common condition. It is seen in several different settings; most commonly in persons who are modestly to profoundly overweight. Others include persons with diabetes, those who have an underlying cancer, or those with the type that runs in families. These last three are rare. Certain medications such as nicotinic acid, birth control pills, and corticosteroids may also provoke this condition.

Acanthosis nigricans begins around the time of puberty and is found most often in young adults. It starts as a darkening and thickening of the skin along the sides of the neck and in the armpits. The skin is not rough but rather velvety soft and has deep grooves. The groin, breasts, and mucous membranes may also be involved, but this is less common. The skin has a somewhat "dirty" look to it as though the discoloration could be washed off. There are no symptoms but some patients complain that there is a slight odor.

Treatment is difficult. If there is an underlying medical condition or the patient is taking a provoking medication, correcting these may help. In the majority of cases, however, acanthosis nigricans is associated with obesity and getting patients to lose weight is difficult. Applying alpha hydroxy acid–containing moisturizers may be useful. The most popular is Lac-Hydrin 12% Cream®. This must be applied three or four times per day. There is no danger in using this cream so often, but it is a prescription drug and such therapy may become somewhat expensive. Some dermatologists will also prescribe a light application of tretinoin cream (Retin-A®) at bedtime. There is no amount of scrubbing, rubbing, or soap usage which can relieve this discoloration. Since it is not due to dirt, the skin cannot be "cleaned."

Acrodermatitis Chronica Atrophicans

The same bacteria responsible for Lyme disease (*Borrelia burgdorferi*) in the United States also causes acrodermatitis chronic atrophicans (ACA) in Europe. It is unclear why the same organism can cause such different diseases on two separate continents, but it may have to do with the tick that transmits the infection. In Europe the tick *Ixodes ricinus* is largely responsible for spreading ACA, whereas in the United States Lyme disease is spread by different ticks. In ACA the skin becomes very thin and often ulcerates. The blood vessels beneath the skin are very visible and the muscles tend to stand out. The treatment is similar to that for Lyme disease and consists of penicillin (usually given intravenously) or oral administration of erythromycin (PCE®) or tetracycline (Sumycin®).

Amyloidosis

Amyloidosis is actually a collection of different conditions, all of which have in common the presence of a substance in the skin called "amyloid." This substance is thought to be derived from proteins in the blood as well as degenerating skin cells.

Primary amyloidosis usually occurs in persons who have a type of leukemia. The skin is very fragile and bruises easily. The tongue enlarges and small nodules of the skin may appear. This form of amyloidosis is rare. Treatment of the underlying blood disease is the best means of battling this condition. Nodular amyloidosis is also rare and usually involves the lower legs. On the skin are large nodules that may ulcerate and form thickened plaques. Treatment is very difficult and usually involves systemic chemotherapy-type drugs.

The two most common forms of amyloidosis are macular amyloidosis and lichen amyloidosis. Macular amyloidosis usually appears as very itchy patches on the upper back that are somewhat dark. Middle-aged women of Latin, Middle Eastern, or Asian descent are most often affected.

Lichen amyloidosis usually occurs on the lower legs as small bumps which are extremely itchy. These may become so numerous that they seem to grow together. They usually are flesh colored and have a slightly shiny appearance. Both of these conditions arise for unknown reasons and are very difficult to treat. Anti-itching creams such as Sarna® lotion and Aveeno Anti-Itch® cream may be useful, as is topical doxepin cream (Zonalon®). Topical corticosteroids are also employed but often are not strong enough to stop the itching. Class I preparations are probably the most helpful. In the past, superficial x-ray treatments called Grenz rays were used for these conditions but this therapy is much less available now.

Cellulite

The appearance of postpuberty bumpiness and lumpiness of the skin over the buttocks and thighs is termed *cellulite*. It arises due to the layering of fat and more often affects women, who have a greater number of fat layers. It doesn't occur prior to puberty and tends to disappear with age. In most persons, cellulite has no symptoms but in some persons it may be slightly tender, particularly when sitting for prolonged periods without changing position.

There have been numerous treatments for this condition; for most there is no significant evidence that they work. Numerous creams and lotions are available, all claiming that they can make cellulite disappear. They may make the skin appear smoother but not remove cellulite altogether. There is some evidence that applying tretinoin (Retin-A®, Renova®) is helpful in lessening the problem. Unfortunately, applying these creams on such a wide area is both expensive and time consuming.

Liposuction usually makes cellulite less obvious by removing some of the fat cells. It does not typically make it disappear, however. The most recent innovation in this battle is that of endodermologie. This technique was developed in France and is now very popular in the United States. The patient dons a tight-fitting sheer garment, much like a body stocking, and a machine is passed over the affected areas. This machine picks up the skin and applies a rolling action to it to break up the lumps of fat. A single session usually takes about half an hour and more than a dozen such treatments are required to obtain the desired result. This therapy is commonly performed after liposuction to give the skin a nicer contour. While this is a new therapy, it appears to be reasonably safe. It is expensive and not widely available, but likely will be in the near future.

Dandruff

This is not a disease per se, but rather is the normal scaling of skin from the scalp. In some persons, this scaling may be very heavy and have a greasy composition. In this case, the patient probably has seborrheic dermatitis, which is a different condition (see section on seborrheic dermatitis). Dandruff is the clumping together of normally shedding skin cells and some persons, for unclear reasons, are more prone to develop this than others. Fortunately, the same treatments for seborrheic dermatitis and scalp psoriasis are usually effective for dandruff. Shampoos containing tar, ketoconazole (Nizoral®), corticosteroids, zinc pyrithione, and salicylic acid usually control the problem.

Delusions of Parasitosis

This condition is actually a mental illness and a manifestation of an underlying psychosis. It is uncommon but spectacular in appearance. Affected patients are usually older, tend to be well educated, and are extremely fastidious. They claim to be infested with insects or bugs, often both on the skin and internally. They typically carry around a small bottle or jar with debris which they claim are insects that they have removed from their skin. An examination of this material rarely shows any bugs. These patients usually have some skin irritation which they are making worse by picking. Most patients use their fingernails but some use forks, needles, and other instruments to dig at these imaginary insects. Interestingly, most of these patients are otherwise normal and able to live routine, uneventful lives. Such patients should be thoroughly evaluated to make sure that they do not have some underlying infestation which is easily treated. Otherwise, therapy is difficult. Explaining that there are no attacking insects is useless. These patients will rarely accept such an explanation and may become angry at the suggestion that they do not have a real disease. Psychiatric therapy is useful but most patients will reject a referral to a psychiatrist. The oral antipsychotic drug pimozide (Orap®) is the most useful drug for this condition but has some side effects that make it difficult to take for extended periods. The drug alprazolam (Xanax®) is also helpful.

Ehler's Danlos Syndrome

This syndrome is actually a collection of different syndromes, all of which are thought to be inherited as a genetic deficiency; in this situation, one of the substances of the skin, the elastic tissue, is defective. There are at least twelve different types, with varying symptoms. The most common changes are very stretchable skin, easy formation of large scars, fragile blood vessels, and excessively extendable joints. Aside from genetic counseling and avoidance of trauma to the skin, there is no treatment. Gene therapy may someday be useful for these patients, but this is currently only experimental.

Erythema Nodosum

In erythema nodosum (EN), the skin changes result from the body reacting to a process elsewhere. This disease may result from different infections (streptococcal infections, leprosy, fungal infections, tuberculosis, and so on), drug ingestion (birth control pills, anti-inflammatory medications, sulfa drugs), sarcoidosis, and some types of cancer. In some patients, the cause is not known. The use of oral contraceptives and other hormonal agents by young women is the most frequent cause in the United States.

Most patients are young, between twenty and thirty years of age; more women than men are affected. The lesions are red lumps which are dime to quarter sized and usually tender. They are almost always found on the shins. Sometimes they affect the thighs and upper legs but involvement above the waist is rare. At most about a dozen spots will form. Systemic symptoms such as fever, chills, and muscle aches may also appear. Over half of all patients will have joint pains. The skin lesions persist for up to six weeks and then fade, leaving a dark spot on the skin but no permanent scarring. Recurrent outbreaks are possible, particularly in patients for which the initial cause is unknown.

Diagnosis is usually done with a skin biopsy. Since the disease processes are in the fat, large, deep biopsies may be needed to help make the diagnosis. Other laboratory evaluations such as chest x-rays, skin tests, blood work, and cultures may be useful in determining the underlying cause of EN.

Since EN resolves on its own, some dermatologists choose not to treat it. Since some patients are uncomfortable, however, most physicians opt for therapy. Treatment of any underlying infections and malignancies and removal of any inciting drugs is required. Intramuscular injections of corticosteroids (Kenalog®) or oral prednisone (Deltasone®) are helpful, but the disease may recur when the medicines are stopped. Oral administration of potassium iodide has been used with success.

Erythroderma (Exfoliative Dermatitis)

This condition consists of very red and irritable skin which involves most, if not all of the body. It may be due to several different causes but the most common are atopic dermatitis (eczema), psoriasis, drug reactions, underlying cancer, and some types of autoimmune blistering diseases such as pemphigus vulgaris and pemphigus foliaceus. Unfortunately, in up to half of the cases an underlying cause is not determined. The skin is red and usually very scaly. Hair loss, chills, fever, and malnutrition are common. Since large amounts of skin are being shed, protein loss is a significant problem. Itching is common and may be severe. The skin often oozes and develops a bacterial infection. Erythroderma is considered one of the few dermatologic emergencies, since it may be fatal. Most patients are hospitalized and their underlying disease treated. The specific therapy depends on the underlying cause of the erythroderma. Calming the skin with soothing baths containing oatmeal (Aveeno®) or oils (Keri®) usually helps the symptoms and gives the patient some relief. Since most patients are dehydrated, intravenous fluids are usually given along with antibiotics. This condition has a high mortality rate but is treatable if caught early.

Erythema Annulare Centrifugum

This condition is also called a migratory erythema, since it seems to move slowly across the skin's surface. The cause of erythema annulare centrifugum (EAC) is un-known, but it probably results from some minor infection in other parts of the body, such as a fungal infection. EAC begins as small red bumps that slowly enlarge to silver dollar- or palm-sized circles. A small amount of scale may be seen at the outer edge. There are no symptoms aside from some occasional mild itching. The central part of the rash clears, revealing normal skin. All age groups and both sexes are affected. Oral antihistamines and topical steroids have been used for EAC with minimal success. Some dermatologists prefer to treat patients for an unseen fungal infection using fluconazole (Diflucan®) or itraconazole (Sporanox®). The disease usually disappears on its own after weeks or months but often recurs.

Erythema Dyschromicum Perstans

Erythema dyschromicum perstans is also called ashy dermatosis since it gives the skin a slate gray or ashy color. It is most common in Hispanics and may be very dis-figuring. It begins as small red patches on the upper chest, back, and neck. These gradually expand and begin to turn dark. Eventually, all of the skin in these areas becomes involved. Treatment is difficult and no specific therapy has proven effec-tive. Oral corticosteroids (prednisone [Deltasone®]) or injections of triamcinolone (Kenalog®) may be helpful.

Erythema Toxicum Neonatorum

This condition is restricted to infants in the first few days of life and disappears after a week or so. Small pustules and red spots are seen over the entire body. There are no symptoms and the affected children are otherwise healthy. It is not clear what causes this condition but treatment is not necessary.

Erythromelanosis Follicularis Faciei et Colli

Although this condition has an unusual and burdensome name, it is more common than might be thought. The skin on the cheeks, jaw, and sides of the neck are af-fected. It is red to pink and makes the patient appear as though she is blushing. This reddish discoloration becomes very noticeable when patients are exercising or exerting themselves. Small, raised bumps around the hair follicles are present. There are no symptoms; adolescents and young adults are most often affected. Treatment is difficult. Topical tretinoin (Retin-A®, Renova®) may be helpful but has to be used for an extended period. Lactic acid–containing creams such as Lac Hydrin® may also be useful. Fortunately, this condition tends to fade with time but may take months or years to go away.

Frostbite

Frostbite occurs when the skin temperature falls below freezing and ice crystals form in the tissues. It usually affects the ears, fingers, toes, nose, and cheeks. The skin becomes white or bluish. Outdoor enthusiasts such as snowmobilers and skiers tend to be most affected. Alcoholics and the homeless may also develop frostbite. The amount of damage depends on the length of time the skin is exposed and other conditions such as snow, wind, nicotine consumption, and so on. The deeper the tissue freezing, the greater the damage done. After the skin is rewarmed, blisters will form and thick black scabs (eschars) develop. If the freeze has been severe enough, amputation of the tissues is necessary. While frostbite is developing there may be little or no pain; however, after the skin thaws the pain may be very great.

The treatment of frostbite unfortunately has been surrounded by old wive's tales; these procedures may harm the skin more than help it. Such practices as rubbing snow on the affected sites may dmaage the skin and should never be done. Rewarming the skin is necessary but it is important to carefully do it. Slow rewarming actually does more harm than good. A rapid rewarming should be done by soaking in water which is a little over 100°F. As this process is finished, the skin may become very painful and powerful pain medications may be required. Any blisters that form should be left alone, since they provide protection for the underlying skin. Antibiotic ointments should be applied to wounds as they heal. Whirlpool baths containing an antiseptic are also helpful. Persons who have received frostbite may be very sensitive to cold in the future and their hands may tend to sweat a lot. Wearing sufficient protective clothing is the best means of prevention.

Hidradenitis

Hidradenitis is a condition that affects the sweat glands and hair follicles. It is uncommon but is a very unpleasant disease. The armpits and groin are most often affected. The deeper parts of the skin develop painful pink to red swellings that scar and begin to leak puslike fluids. Large blackheads (comedones) may be present.

Smell is a major problem and most patients bathe several times per day to stay clean. It is worse in warm weather.

Treatment is difficult. Antibiotics such as tetracycline (Sumycin®), minocycline (Minocin®), and cephalexin (Keflex®) may be useful but won't cure the problem. Corticosteroids by mouth or injection are more helpful but cannot be used on a long-term basis. Isotretinoin (Accutane®) is the drug of choice for this condition. It may put hidradenitis into remission, and at least makes it better while the drug is being taken. If the problem is not too widespread, it is possible to surgically remove the sweat glands, and if not solve the problem, at least make it better. Unfortunately, this leaves significant scarring. If all the glands are not removed, the hidradenitis may reappear. Other treatment options include taking dapsone or the anabolic steroid stanozolol (Winstrol®).

Intertrigo

Intertrigo arises when two skin surfaces come into contact with each other for a prolonged time. This is most common in obese persons, particularly women. Friction, sweating, and heat eventually cause the skin to begin to turn red and break down. Infection by bacteria and fungus inevitably occurs. Intertrigo may be found beneath the breasts, under large rolls of excessive skin on the abdomen, in the armpits, and in the groin. A foul odor may be present as infection worsens.

The most effective treatment is weight loss. That failing the condition may be managed with antibacterial soap such as Hibiclens®, Betadine®, and Betasept®. Keeping the areas of skin as dry and friction free as possible will help control intertrigo. Thoroughly drying the area with a cotton towel and blow dryer (set on "cool") is necessary. Applying an absorbent powder such as Zeasorb® or Zeasorb AF® will reduce moisture. If bacterial infection is present, it must be treated. Antibiotics effective against staphylococci and streptococci, such as cephalexin (Keflex®) and erythromycin are the most often used. If a *Candida* infection is present, as is typically the case, the use of antifungal antibiotics such as ketoconazole (Nizoral®), fluconazole (Diflucan®), and itraconazole (Sporanox®) will be necessary. Topical antifungal creams and lotions may be helpful if the problem is not too widespread.

Keratosis Pilaris

This condition is more common in persons with a background of asthma, allergies, and eczema. The rash most often appears on the backs of the upper arms but may also be seen on the thighs, hands, and face. The skin develops small, raised, rough spines. There is a faint pink to orange or brown color as well. Mild itching may be present. For most patients this is an annoyance rather than a serious problem. It tends to run in families and may improve in warm sunny weather. Keratosis pilaris is more often present in adolescents and young adults. Treatment consists of topical lactic acid (Lac Hydrin Cream®, Amlactin Cream®) or urea-containing creams (Table 3) during the day and tretinoin (Retin-A®, Renova®) at bedtime. This regimen will almost always give some relief but it may not completely clear the skin. It is also time consuming and expensive. Scrubbing the skin to remove the spines is not likely to be helpful and may make the problem worse.

Leishmaniasis

Leishmaniasis is a parasitic infection caused by an organism called *Leishmania.* There are several different kinds of disease, depending on the *Leishmania* organism infecting the patient. It is most common in India, the Middle East, South America, and Central America. Most infections seen in the United States are in persons who have lived or vacationed in these areas. The disease is spread by the bite of the sandfly. The organisms are introduced into the skin and begin to grow. A red pustule and nodule develop; these ultimately ulcerate. They are usually slightly painful. Other types of infection occur with this organism but are not commonly seen in this country. Making the diagnosis usually requires a skin biopsy and a special type of culture. Treatment may be difficult, depending on how susceptible the *Leishmania* organisms are to different antibiotics. Useful antibiotics include dapsone, rifampin (Rifadin®), levamisole (Lamprene®), and ketoconazole (Nizoral®). Some dermatologists have used the application of liquid nitrogen (cryotherapy) to kill the organisms.

Langerhans Cell Histiocytoses

This is the newest name for a group of diseases that are characterized by the proliferation of a cell found in the skin called the Langerhans cell. Langerhans cell histiocytoses (LCHs) are uncommon and somewhat similar to forms of lymphoma. The prognosis depends both on the age of the patient and the amount of skin that is involved. A form affecting infants and young children looks like a very bad case of cradle cap or seborrheic dermatitis, but the child soon begins to run fevers and lose his or her appetite; he or she will die unless the disease is recognized and treated. When other forms of LCHs affect the skin they may look like red bumps and rashes or ulcerations. Sometimes the underlying bones are affected. The older the child, the better the overall prognosis. Treatment usually consists of chemotherapy-type drugs.

Leprosy

Leprosy is one of the oldest known diseases and is caused by infection with the bacteria *Mycobacterium leprae*. It is still present today, although rarely seen in this country. Most of the cases of leprosy in the United States are in immigrants from Asia, Mexico, and Central America. The only known animal to be infected by leprosy is the nine-banded armadillo; persons having contact with or eating infected animals have contracted the disease. Leprosy has several different forms, depending on the immune status of the patient. It is spread by personal contact with an infected patient, often a member of the household. In areas where this disease is common, many persons have come into contact with the bacteria but have been able to kill it and avoid an infection. The skin may have red to pink patches or nodules. Since the bacteria invade the nerves of the skin, affected patches may lose feeling and be numb. Treatment depends on the stage of the disease. Dapsone, rifampin, clofazimine, and isoniazid (Rifamate®) are the most common drugs used to treat leprosy. Often, treatment must be given for many months. A hospital dedicated to the treatment of leprosy and research into the disease has existed for many years in Carville, Louisiana, and is run by the United States Public Health Service.

Lichen Striatus

Lichen striatus is a condition seen most often in older children and adolescents. It begins as a few flesh-colored to pink or brown bumps on the lower legs or arms. Slight itching may occur. As the disease progresses, it forms a line several inches in length. The cause is unknown. Treatment with topical corticosteroids or tretinoin (Retin-A®, Renova®) may be of some help but after several months the lesion will subside and fade away on its own.

Livedo Reticularis

This condition is caused by abnormally reactive blood vessels in the skin. In most patients, it occurs for no known reason and is called idiopathic. It is usually present in women, on the lower legs. The skin develops a netlike or spider-web appearance and is slightly blue or red, depending on the temperature. It is most apparent during colder weather. There are no symptoms except for mild tingling; the condition is mostly a problem of appearance. If it is present long enough it may become permanent. This condition is unsightly but not dangerous. The other form of livedo reticularis is secondary, meaning that it arises from another condition elsewhere in the body. The list of diseases associated with it is very long and includes lupus erythematosus, scleroderma, rheumatoid arthritis, infections, and some types of cancer. It may lead to ulceration of the skin. There is no well defined treatment for livedo reticularis. Treating any underlying condition may help the skin as well. Pentoxifylline (Trental®) has been used to treat idiopathic livedo reticularis.

Mucinoses

One of the substances formed in the skin is mucin. While it has some subtle differences from that formed in the nose and other mucous membranes, it is essentially similar. Under certain circumstances, the skin may begin to form more mucin than necessary. In persons whose thyroid fails to produce enough hormone (hypothyroidism), the skin may begin to develop excess mucin. This is present in the face, giving it a puffy look (myxedema), and commonly on the lower legs as flesh-colored to slightly brown nodules and knots that form under the skin (pretibial myxedema). Some, but usually not all, of these changes will subside when the patient begins to take thyroid hormone replacement medication. Probably the most common type of mucin involvement of the skin is that of a myxoid or synovial cyst. These occur at the ends and on the sides of the fingers and toes. They are red to flesh colored and usually painful. They have a somewhat clear or shiny look to them. Myxoid cysts arise after some trauma to the area and tend to occur in women after age forty. These cysts are benign, but don't usually go away on their own; they are somewhat disabling. If they arise close enough to a nail it may be deformed. Treatment is often successful but must be done carefully since these collections of mucin come from the finger joint. Cutting or excising the cyst from the skin is successful, as is burning it with an electric needle (electrofulgeration). Giving the patient a sterile needle and asking her to puncture the cyst every several days and express the mucin is also useful. Obviously, this must be done in sterile surroundings or an infection of the skin will result.

Perioral Dermatitis

This is a common condition which usually affects young women. It looks much like acne since it consists of small, red bumps, some of which may become pustules.

They arise around the central face and particularly around the mouth. A type of perioral dermatitis called periocular dermatitis is identical but affects the skin around the eyes. The cause of perioral dermatitis is unclear, but it may be related to sunlight exposure, skin mite infections, bacteria and some fungi, contact with cinnamon oil, fluoride-containing toothpastes, and the use of very potent (Class I or II) topical corticosteroids. Stress and food additives have also been blamed. A great number of affected patients use Colgate® toothpaste. The rash is usually slightly itchy and may sting when in the sun. Some mild scaling may take place.

A number of good treatments for perioral (and periocular) dermatitis are available but it may be stubborn and difficult to get rid of. Most therapies are similar to those for acne. Oral antibiotics such as tetracycline, doxycycline (Monodox®), minocycline (Minocin®), and trimethoprim/sulfamethoxasole (Bactrim®) are useful as is topical tretinoin (Retin-A®). The same topical antibiotics used in acne are also helpful. Switching to Arm and Hammer Baking Soda Toothpaste® is suggested and gum chewing and eating hard candy should be avoided. If a topical corticosteroid has been used, stopping it "cold turkey" may make the disease significantly flare. Some dermatologists choose to gradually wean the patient off more potent creams by using progressively weaker ones over a few weeks or months. Fortunately, use of oral antibiotics at the same time may help blunt any worsening of the perioral dermatitis. In very stubborn cases it may be necessary to consider oral isotretinoin.

Perleche

Perleche is an inflammatory reaction that occurs in the corners of the mouth. It is usually present in older patients whose dentures do not fit well or anyone whose skin overlaps at the edges of the mouth. Adolescents with braces, babies with very chubby cheeks, drooling children, and those who suck their thumbs may also be affected. The skin is damp and thickened. It is mildly red and tends to crack and split. Perleche is usually somewhat uncomfortable, but most patients complain about the way it looks.

The cause is an abnormal amount of occlusive skin at the corners of the mouth. The skin become wet and infection occurs with bacteria or *Candida.* Treating the infection is not difficult but does nothing for the problems causing the perleche. Getting new dentures or having braces removed usually helps. Sometimes surgery to realign the facial skin must be done. Corticosteroid creams with antifungal drugs (Vytone®, Mycolog II®) are very useful. Oral antifungal agents such as fluconazole (Diflucan®) and ketoconazole (Nizoral®) are also helpful if the problem is extensive.

Poikiloderma

This term refers to a collection of three findings on the skin—increased or decreased pigmentation, thinning, and a red color from tiny dilated blood vessels. The increased pigmentation appears brown or dark and the decreased pigmentation is off white to cream colored. There are no symptoms. A number of different conditions will cause poikiloderma. The most common arises on the neck and upper shoulders in women with a long history of sun exposure. This is called poikiloderma of Civatte. The tendency to develop this condition is probably inherited. It is caused and worsened by sun exposure. There is no specific treatment; aggressive sunscreen use with topical tretinoin (Retin-A®, Renova®) may improve the condition.

Porokeratosis

Porokeratosis is a collection of several different conditions in which the skin forms small to large patches with raised borders and mild scaling. The most common is called disseminated superficial actinic porokeratosis, or DSAP. It is an inherited condition and is more common in women. Affected patients begin to develop lesions in adulthood. These occur on sun-exposed areas, particularly the legs and arms. They are flesh colored to faint brown and have a raised border around the edge. Mild scaling may be seen. They have no symptoms but are very obvious and unsightly. Continued sun exposure makes them grow and causes new lesions to develop. DSAP may be treated with topical tretinoin (Retin-A®, Renova®) and alpha hydroxy acids (Lac Hydrin®, Amlactin®) but these are usually only partially effective. Applying 5-fluorouracil (Efudex®) cream twice daily to DSAP lesions has also proven effective but is uncomfortable. Vaporizing the lesions with a very superficial carbon dioxide laser has been shown to be effective. Electrodessication and treatment with liquid nitrogen is also helpful but may lead to scarring. If there are enough lesions, the use of oral isotretinoin may be considered.

Purpura

The word *purpura* refers to bleeding in the skin. Most spots are at least the size of a pencil eraser or larger, have no symptoms, and occur after some kind of trauma. They heal much like a bruise with a yellow green color. The most common type is senile or Bateman's purpura. This is caused by a thinning of the skin, a normal consequence of aging. It is most often seen on the arms but may also occur on the chest, legs, and neck. A similar situation occurs in persons who have been on high doses of oral corticosteroids or who have been using a very potent topical corticosteroid on a selected site. Treatment of senile purpura is possible but time consuming and expensive. Topical or oral vitamin C (1,000 mg per day) may be of some help. This supposedly strengthens the collagen around the blood vessels and makes them less likely to open and bleed after trauma. Topical tretinoin (Retin-A®, Renova®) also may help, but it may make the skin slightly more sensitive to the sun. Applying tretinoin cream over the arms and chest is not only time consuming but expensive. Lac-Hydrin® may be useful and is easy to apply. It should be used three to four times per day. Other alpha hydroxy acid creams may be similarly useful. Since it is likely that persons who have not had a great deal of sun exposure over the years will have less trouble with Bateman's purpura, the regular use of a good sunscreen is advisable.

There are a number of other causes of purpura, including medications (particularly anticoagulant medications such as coumadin [Warfarin®]), blood-clotting abnormalities, decreased platelet counts, and certain types of cancerlike conditions.

Radiodermatitis

Forty to fifty years ago, the use of radiation to treat different skin conditions was quite common. Since the medications used for dermatologic diseases were not nearly as good as they are today, a new and effective treatment was welcomed and widely used. Acne, excessive facial hair, and granuloma annulare were some of the conditions successfully treated with radiation. Unfortunately, the long-term consequences of such therapy were not then known and many patients later developed radiation skin disease known as radiodermatitis. Additionally, because of the newness of this therapy, some patients were given inappropriate amounts of radiation. Radiation treatment for skin conditions is no longer used as it was. Very superficial Grenz-ray therapy is occasionally still employed for conditions such as hand dermatitis or psoriasis and may be very effective. Radiation treatment for skin cancers in persons who cannot or should not be treated surgically is a very good option and one which is still used. Other malignancies affecting the skin that respond to radiotherapy include lymphomas and different types of skin cancer.

Radiation's effects on the skin are divided into two categories—acute, or those occurring over a period of days to weeks, and chronic, occurring years later. Acute radiodermatitis does not necessarily appear in every instance since there are different types of radiation therapies, some of which affect the skin more than others. Acute effects resemble a sunburn. They begin several days to weeks after the radiation treatments have begun. The skin may be painful and can develop swelling and blisters. If the problems have been minor, healing takes one to three months. If acute radiodermatitis has been severe, skin changes may indefinitely persist. Taking care of such skin usually centers around treating it gently. A bland soap such as Dove® or Basis® should be used with lukewarm water. Other soaps and cleansers should be avoided, along with unnecessary perfumes and toiletries. Some dermatologists recommend the use of a mild corticosteroid ointment or cream to affected areas. This may help with redness and provide some relief from discomfort. If blisters occur, these should be left alone and allowed to heal by themselves if possible. Some patients require oral or topical antibiotics to prevent an infection. Bland moisturizers such as petroleum jelly (Vaseline®) or Aveeno® may be used to keep the skin well lubricated. Skin which has received radiation treatment should be protected from any subsequent sun exposure by daily use of sunscreen.

Chronic radiation changes may begin shortly after the radiation treatments are performed but usually occur several years later. The skin becomes thinned, wrinkled, and scaly. Since radiation destroys most hair follicles, the area is usually hairless. Dilated small blood vessels (telangiectasias) and decreased or increased pigmentation may also be seen. If the skin is very badly damaged an ulcer may form. One worry with chronic radiation dermatitis is a skin cancer will develop. Such skin must not only be taken care of but also watched closely for any evidence of a developing skin cancer. Moisturizers as for acute radiation dermatitis should be used. Any suspicious places must be biopsied to check for malignancy. Precancerous changes such as actinic keratoses may be treated with 5-fluorouracil cream (Efudex®). Theoretically, tretinoin (Retin-A®, Renova®) may be helpful but it would have to be applied very carefully so as not to irritate the skin. Again, protection from the sun is absolutely mandatory and sunscreen should be applied daily.

Reiter's Disease

Reiter's disease is a condition much like psoriasis. It consists of arthritis, inflammation of the urethra (urethritis), inflammation of the eye (conjunctivitis), and psoriasislike skin changes. It occurs almost exclusively in young to middle-aged men; there is an inherited susceptibility to it. The disease usually begins with mild fever, weakness, and weight loss. The arthritis usually involves a few large joints such as the knees or ankles. The skin develops very thick, crusty areas, particularly on the palms, soles, and penis. Hand and finger involvement may be so extensive as to be disabling. Reiter's disease occurs after infection of the bowel with *Shigella* and *Salmonella* or infection of the urethra with *Chlamydia*. In some respects, this condition may be considered a sexually transmitted disease. Many Reiter's disease patients today are HIV positive. Therapy for this condition should involve an ophthalmologist to evaluate the eye disease and a rheumatologist to help manage the arthritis. Antibiotics have been used to eliminate the bowel infection and urethritis. Unfortunately, the skin and joint disease tend to progress and are usually treated much like a severe case of psoriasis. Methotrexate (Rheumatrex®) and acitretin (Soriatane®) are the most popular drugs for this condition.

Rocky Mountain Spotted Fever

The name given to this disease is no longer accurate. Most cases occur in areas east of the Mississippi River and not in the Rocky Mountains. This condition is caused by an infection with a member of the *Rickettsia* family of bacteria called *Rickettsia rickettsia*. Other members of this family cause typhus, ehrlichiosis, and trench fever. The bacteria of Rocky Mountain spotted fever (RMSF) are spread by the bite of the wood tick in the west and the dog tick in the east. Most cases occur in the summer when ticks are more active. The infection begins after three to twelve days with a sudden fever, chills, headache, and flulike symptoms. A rash begins initially on the hands and feet and spreads *toward the center of the body*. This pattern of spread is important since it is very characteristic of RMSF. The rash is pink to orange and composed of small spots. After several days, the spots begin to look like a small bruise. Rarely, RMSF occurs without a rash. Infected patients usually appear quite ill and the disease may be fatal. Since many of the symptoms are very similar to those of influenza, the features of the rash are important. Diagnosis may be confirmed with blood testing. Treatment is usually well tolerated, inexpensive, and widely available. The common antibiotic tetracycline is very effective in killing this bacteria and may be given either intravenously or by mouth. This antibiotic may stain undeveloped teeth in children so another antibiotic, chloramphenicol (Chloromycetin®) is sometimes chosen for these patients. Patients are usually hospitalized to closely monitor their progress and give them intravenous fluids.

Sarcoidosis

Sarcoidosis is considered a granulomatous disease. This means that in the affected tissues, the inflammation forms a particular pattern known as a granuloma. In sarcoidosis, the granulomas affect several different organs, including the skin. It is not clear what causes this disease. For many years, it was suspected that sarcoidosis was associated with tuberculosis. Exposure to some dusts and metals may contribute to the disease; it is clear that the immune system is involved. This condition is seen mostly in adults. Some ethnic groups, such as blacks and Scandinavians are more commonly affected.

Skin involvement in sarcoidosis occurs in about 25 percent of patients. The most classic lesion is called lupus pernio and occurs on the nose, ears, and lips. It appears as a shiny, slightly purple to red patch with mild scaling. The most common skin lesions in this disease are sarcoidal plaques. These arise over almost all skin surfaces. They are usually circular and up to two inches in diameter. They have a raised edge and are skin colored to slightly red. Some areas are dark if they have been present for a long time. Sarcoidosis in the skin may also appear as deep nodules and hair loss (alopecia).

Sarcoidosis also affects internal organs, most commonly the lungs. Patients may have cough and shortness of breath. X-rays of the chest will often disclose swollen lymph nodes around the central lungs (perihilar adenopathy). The eyes are also involved. Uveitis is most common and consists of inflammation of the interior of the eye. Pain, redness, discomfort from bright lights, glaucoma, and ultimately blindness may result. Joint pain with redness and swelling may occur, particularly early in the disease. The larger joints such as the knees, ankles, and wrists are affected. Swollen lymph nodes in the neck and underarms may also be present.

Persons with sarcoidosis are occasionally anemic and have low white blood cell counts. Increased serum calcium is found in many persons and presents a potentially life-threatening condition. An enzyme regulating blood pressure called angiotensin-converting enzyme (ACE) is elevated in many patients with this disease. While increased amounts of this enzyme are not diagnostic of sarcoidosis, they are a reason to suspect it. Periodic evaluation of ACE blood levels helps to monitor the disease's progression.

Treatment is principally with corticosteroids. Prednisone will not only help the skin disease but also lower the blood calcium and shrink granulomas in the lungs, kidneys, and other internal organs. In persons with skin disease alone, injection of corticosteroids (triamcinolone) into a few lesions is helpful. Potent topical corticosteroid preparations are helpful in small areas if applied several times daily. Application under occlusion by plastic film may assist in this treatment. Antimalarial drugs such as chloroquine and hydroxycholorquine are effective. Since these medications occasionally affect the eyes, frequent examinations by an ophthalmologist are required. Methotrexate, azathioprine (Immuran®), and chlorambucil (Leukeran®) are also helpful. Other rarely used medications for sarcoidosis include allopurinol (Zyloprim®), levamisole (Ergamisol®), and colchicine (Colbenemid®).

Swimmer's Itch and Sea-Bather's Eruption

Both of these conditions are somewhat similar but are differently acquired. Swimmer's itch occurs in freshwater lakes, usually in the northern regions of the United States. Most outbreaks occur during warm weather. It appears as red bumps and welts which begin several hours after leaving the water. The skin disease starts to subside after about three days and is gone in a week or so. It is caused by infestation of the skin by tiny flat worms known as schistosomes. These are unable to penetrate past the skin and die there after several days. The rash appears only on exposed skin; covered areas are spared. Sea-bather's eruption occurs in salt water. It is not clear what causes this condition but jellyfish cysts and small insects are suspected. It is usually acquired while swimming in the Atlantic or Gulf Coast regions of Florida between March and September. The rash looks very similar to swimmer's itch and occurs on about the same time schedule, but affects the area covered by the swimsuit and spares the uncovered skin. When children are affected they may run a slight fever. Showering shortly after coming out of the ocean may help prevent sea-bather's eruption if a person is known to be swimming in an infested area.

Treatment for both conditions is similar. Topical corticosteroids are effective in making the condition much less uncomfortable. An injection of corticosteroid or a short course of oral prednisone will also reduce the itching. Oral antihistamines such as diphenhydramine (Benadryl®) or hydroxyzine (Atarax®) are useful. Applying a thick coating of grease or the use of barrier creams on the skin may help prevent swimmer's itch.

Transient Acantholytic Dermatosis (Grover's Disease)

Grover's disease is relatively common and typically seen in middle-aged to older white males on the trunk, neck, and arms. It itches and is common in warmer weather. The spots are red to skin colored. They typically have a small amount of crusting, but very tiny blisters may be present if the skin has been scratched. It arises from sun exposure, the presence of a fever, or increased sweating. There is no cure for Grover's disease but it can be controlled. If only a few spots are present, the use of topical corticosteroids should control the itching. Topical anti-itch creams such as Sarna® lotion or Aveeno Anti-Itch® cream are also useful. Avoidance of heat and sweating will often cause the condition to subside on its own. If the disease is widespread, treatment with isotretinoin, acitretin, and PUVA may be helpful.

Typhus

There are actually two different types of typhus—endemic and epidemic typhus. Endemic typhus is not well known but is actually the more common form of the disease in the United States and elsewhere. It is caused by infection with the bacteria *Rickettsia typhi* and is spread by the bite of the rat flea. As a result, most infections begin near areas where rats are abundant such as garbage dumps, granaries, and seaports. Endemic typhus begins with symptoms that are very much like the flu and similar, if not identical, to Rocky Mountain spotted fever (RMSF). Headache, fever, chills, and nausea occur followed by a red rash. The pattern of spread, however, is very different from that seen in RMSF and is used to distinguish between the two infections. The rash begins on the chest and back. It may spread to the arms and hands but does so to a very limited extent. In some patients, no rash occurs at all. Treatment is with tetracycline and chloramphenicol (Chlormycetin®) as for RMSF.

Epidemic typhus is what most persons consider to be typhus. This infection occurs when large groups of people are crowded together, such as in refugee or concentration camps. Epidemic typhus is caused by *Rickettsia prowazekii* and is spread by the common human body louse. Under conditions of crowding and poor hygiene, infected lice transmit the infection to humans. The symptoms are similar to those of endemic typhus, but the skin rash is less obvious. Treatment is the same and will result in prompt recovery if given in time.

Xanthoma

Xanthomas are small bumps on the skin which arise when a patient's blood fats (cholesterol and triglycerides) are abnormally high. There are several different types of xanthoma. The most common is called xanthelasma. These lesions begin as flesh-colored to yellow-orange plaques on the eyelids. They have no symptoms and unless removed will remain stationary. About half of these patients have abnormal blood fats. Xanthelasmas are not dangerous but are unsightly and some persons choose to have them removed for that reason. Eruptive xanthomas are commonly seen in persons who are diabetic, in kidney failure, or who are obese. These xanthomas appear as small red to flesh-colored bumps; they may occur on any skin surface. They arise over a short period of time (hence the name eruptive) and have no symptoms. Other types of xanthomas include tuberous xanthomas, which are large red to orange lumps on the elbows and knees, and tendon xanthomas which arise over the tendons of the hands and feet. Xanthomas may also occur in persons with underlying liver disease, lymphomas, and enzyme deficiencies. The best treatment is getting the patient's cholesterol and trigylceride levels under control by diet or medication or a combination of the two. This may cause the lesions in eruptive xanthomas to disappear completely and helps shrink the other xanthomas or prevent them from forming. Xanthelasmas do not respond very well to dietary changes and usually have to be surgically excised. Fortunately, the eyelids heal well with little scarring. These lesions may also be taken off with a carbon dioxide laser or burned off using bichloroacetic or trichloroacetic acid.

MEDICATIONS USED IN DERMATOLOGY

This section of the book will help the reader better understand some of their prescribed medications. This list is not inclusive; for example, not all side effects are listed. Pregnant women or nursing mothers should always clear the use of any medication with a physician.

The cost of these medications is estimated from ★ (very inexpensive) to ★★★★ (very expensive).

Antiacne Medications

Azelaic acid (Azelex®)   This new product is used for mild to moderate acne. It kills bacteria as well as helping the skin cells of the follicles normally mature and slough. Azelex® is applied to affected skin, often at bedtime.

PRECAUTIONS   Azelaic acid may lighten the color of treated skin. If this happens, the drug should be stopped immediately. Mild irritation and inflammation are also occasionally seen.

DRUG INTERACTIONS   Essentially none.

DOSAGE   A thin layer of the cream may be applied once or twice daily.

HOW SUPPLIED   30 gm tubes

COST   ★★★

Benzoyl Peroxide (Benzac®, Benzagel®, Brevoxyl®, Desquam®, PanOxyl®, Triaz®)   Benzoyl peroxide is a chemical in wide use in dermatology, particularly for mild to moderate acne. It is known to kill bacteria on the skin associated with acne and to help break up the contents of comedones (blackheads) so that they may easily resolve. Benzoyl peroxide also causes a slight scaling or exfoliation of the skin. Most preparations are 2.5–10% in strength. Formulations stronger than 2.5% are not more effective but may be more irritating. Benzoyl peroxide is available as washes, creams, gels, bar soaps, and shaving gel.

PRECAUTIONS   Benzoyl peroxide may be irritating to the skin. Redness, scaling, and irritation may result if it is used too long or in too strong a concentration.

DRUG INTERACTIONS   Benzoyl peroxide may inactivate tretinoin if applied at the same time. It may also bleach hair, skin (a significant problem for black patients), bedding, and clothing.

DOSAGE Apply a thin layer of the gels or creams to affected areas once or twice daily. The washes may be used as often as desired. Benzoyl peroxide usually loses its effectiveness after several hours and may be washed off if desired.

COST ★★-★★★

Brand Name	Formulation	Trade Size
Benzac® AC 2.5%, 5%, and 10%	Gel	60 gm and 90 gm tubes
Benzac AC® 2.5%, 5%, and 10%	Wash	8 oz. bottle
Benzac W® 2.5%, 5%, and 10%	Gel	60 gm and 90 gm tubes
Benzac W® 5% and 10%	Wash	8 oz. bottle
Benzac® 5% and 10%	Gel	60 gm tube
5 Benzagel®	Gel	1.5 oz. and 3.0 oz. tubes
10 Benzagel®	Gel	1.5 oz. and 3.0 oz. tubes
Brevoxyl®-4	Gel	1.5 oz. and 3.0 oz. tubes
Brevoxyl®-8	Gel	1.5 oz. and 3.0 oz. tubes
Brevoxyl® Cleansing Lotion	Liquid cleanser	10.5 oz. bottle
Desquam®-E 2.5%, 5%, 10%	Gel	1.5 oz. tube
Desquam®-X 5%, 10%	Gel	1.5 oz. and 3.0 oz. tubes
Desquam®-X 5%, 10%	Wash	5 oz. bottle
Desquam®-X 10%	Bar soap	3.75 oz. bar
Panoxyl® 5%, 10%	Cream	2 oz. and 4 oz. tubes
Panoxyl® AQ 2.5%, 5%, 10%	Gel	2 oz. and 4 oz. tubes
Triaz® 6% and 10%	Gel	1.5 oz. tube
Triaz® Cleanser	Liquid cleanser	3.0 oz. bottle

Benzoyl Peroxide Shaving Gel (Benzashave® 5% & 10%) Benzoyl peroxide shaving gel is used for mild to moderate acne. Some preparations have also been helpful for pseudofolliculitis barbae.

PRECAUTIONS Similar to benzoyl peroxide in washes and creams.

DRUG INTERACTIONS Essentially none.

DOSAGE Apply to damp beard area and use as other shave gels.

HOW SUPPLIED 4 oz. spray cans

COST ★★★

Clindamycin, topical (Cleocin T®) A potent antibiotic used for acne control. It is very effective for mild to moderate disease and is a very popular product, particularly the lotion (useful in persons with dry skin). Clindamycin, like other topical antibiotics, is believed to work by killing bacteria which contribute to acne.

PRECAUTIONS When given orally and intravenously, may cause a severe type of infectious diarrhea called pseudomembranous colitis. This is a potential risk with the topical medication but huge quantities of the lotion or gel would have to be used almost constantly for a person to absorb enough of the antibiotic to cause this infection. The gel and solution forms of Cleocin T are alcohol based and may irritate already inflamed skin.

DRUG INTERACTIONS   Essentially none when used in the topical form. Clindamycin should not be applied along with tretinoin.

DOSAGE   The skin may be dry or slightly damp when the drug is applied. It may be used twice daily if desired. Makeup may be applied over it.

HOW SUPPLIED   Cleocin® T Gel–30 gm and 60 gm tubes
Cleocin® T Solution–30 ml and 60 ml bottles
Cleocin® T Lotion–60 ml bottle

COST   ★★★ (generics may be much less)

Erythromycin and Benzoyl Peroxide (Benzamycin®)   This is a combination cream used for patients with acne or acne rosacea. It may also be helpful with perioral dermatitis. It is usually applied at bedtime.

PRECAUTIONS   May cause dermatitis from an allergy to the drug or cream (contact dermatitis). Dryness and scaling of the skin may occur. Clothing or bedding may become bleached.

DRUG INTERACTIONS   Essentially none.

DOSAGE   This medication may be applied once or twice daily.

HOW SUPPLIED   23.3 gm and 46.6 gm tubes

COST   ★★★

Erythromycin, topical (ATS®, Emgel®, Erycette®, Erygel®, Erymax®, Erythra-Derm®, T-Stat®, Theramycin Z®)   Of the topical antibiotics, erythromycin is the most popular. It is reasonably effective for mild to moderate acne. It is believed to work by killing acne-causing bacteria on the skin. This drug is available as alcohol-based solutions and gels. Most are packaged in dispenser bottles but some also come as single-use cotton pads (pledgets). Topical erythromycin usually has lost its effectiveness after several hours and may be washed off if desired.

PRECAUTIONS   Topical erythromycin should be avoided by persons allergic to the antibiotic or the formulations in which it is mixed.

DRUG INTERACTIONS   None. Should not be applied along with tretinoin.

DOSAGE   The skin may be dry or slightly damp when the drug is applied. It may be used twice daily if desired. Makeup may be applied after application.

COST   ★★–★★★ (generics may be much less)

Brand Name	Formulation	Trade Size
ATS®	Solution	60 ml bottle
ATS®	Gel	30 gm tube
Emgel®	Gel	27 gm and 50 gm tubes
Erycette®	Solution	Boxes of #60 pads
Erygel®	Gel	30 gm and 60 gm tubes

Erymax®	Solution	2 oz. and 4 oz. bottles
Erythra-Derm®	Solution	60 ml bottle
T-Stat®	Solution	60 ml bottle, jar of #60 pads
Theramycin Z®	Solution	60 ml bottle

Metronidazole, topical (Metrogel®, Metrocream®)   When given in pill form, is useful in controlling acne rosacea and, in some instances, acne vulgaris. For acne vulgaris, topical preparations are available. Both Metrogel® and Metrocream® are only approved for use in acne rosacea but have been used successfully for mild to moderate acne vulgaris.

PRECAUTIONS   Some patients may have their rosacea and acne worsened by topical metronidazole but this is rare. Allergy to the gel and cream has also been noted.

DRUG INTERACTIONS   Essentially none when used in the topical form.

DOSAGE   The skin may be dry or slightly damp when the drug is applied. It may be used twice daily if desired.

HOW SUPPLIED   Metrogel®–1 oz. and 45 gm tubes
Metrocream®–45 gm tube

COST   ★★★

Sodium Sulfacetamide (Klaron®, Sulfacet-R®)   An antibiotic used for treating acne. This product may be used in the morning but many patients prefer to apply it at bedtime and wash it off the next day. Sulfacet-R® contains sulfur and has a packet with color tints to make the product blend into the skin better.

PRECAUTIONS   Persons who have an allergy to sulfur drugs should not use this product.

DRUG INTERACTIONS   Essentially none.

DOSAGE   A thin layer of the lotion should be applied to affected areas. This may be done up to three times per day.

HOW SUPPLIED   Klaron® Lotion–2 oz. bottle
Sulfacet-R® Lotion–25 gm bottle

COST   ★★★

Tetracycline, topical (Topicycline®)   The topical use of tetracycline is less popular than it once was, probably because there are better drugs to use for mild to moderate acne. This drug is thought to kill the bacteria associated with acne.

PRECAUTIONS   Tetracycline is mixed in alcohol and may irritate already inflamed skin. Some persons may be sensitive to the sun while this drug is on their skin.

DRUG INTERACTIONS   Essentially none when used in the topical form.

DOSAGE   The skin may be dry or slightly damp when the drug is applied. It may be used twice daily if desired.

HOW SUPPLIED   70 ml bottle

COST   ★★ (generics may be less)

Antibiotics

Azithromycin (Zithromax®)   This antibiotic is closely related to erythromycin. It is used primarily for skin infections such as cellulitis and infected cysts or boils. In the future, azithromycin may be used for unusual infections such as leprosy or those caused by mycobacteria. The big advantage to this drug is that it is given only once daily for only five days.

PRECAUTIONS   Stomach upset and mild nausea and diarrhea are the most common side effects. Azithromycin is not known to cause the same heart irregularities as erythromycin when taken with terfenadine or other antihistamines, but this may be a possibility. This antibiotic needs to be taken on an empty stomach to enhance absorption.

DRUG INTERACTIONS   Blood levels of theophylline may be increased when taking azithromycin. Antacids prevent adequate absorption of the drug.

DOSAGE   In adults, azithromycin is given as 500 mg (two capsules) on the first day of treatment and then one capsule per day for the following four days. In children the dose is 2.25–5.5 mg per pound per day for five days.

HOW SUPPLIED   250 mg capsules and tablets
600 mg tablets
Liquid suspension—100 mg per teaspoon and 200 mg per teaspoon

COST   ★★★★

Cefadroxil (Duricef®)   Cefadroxil is an antibiotic of the cephalosporin class. It is similar to cephalexin and is often used to treat the same diseases.

PRECAUTIONS   Some persons allergic to penicillin are also allergic to cefadroxil. This medication may cause mild stomach upset and diarrhea in some patients. An infection of the intestines, pseudomembranous colitis, may also rarely occur if cefadroxil is taken for a long time.

DRUG INTERACTIONS   Essentially none, but probably should not be taken with other antibiotics.

DOSAGE   Adults: 1,000 mg per day in a single dose or in divided doses
Children: 30 mg/kg per day in divided doses

HOW SUPPLIED   500 mg and 1,000 mg (1 gm) tablets.
125 mg, 250 mg, and 500 mg suspension

COST   ★★★ (generics are much less)

Cephalexin (Keflex®, Keftab®, Keflet®)   Cephalexin is an antibiotic of the cephalosporin class. These are very closely related to penicillin and are often used to treat the same diseases. This drug is effective against staphylococci and streptococci. Skin infections such as furuncles (boils) and cellulitis are often treated with it. Some patients with stubborn acne may also respond to cephalexin.

PRECAUTIONS   Some persons allergic to penicillin are also allergic to cephalexin. May cause mild stomach upset and diarrhea in some patients.

DRUG INTERACTIONS Essentially none, but probably should not be taken with other antibiotics.

DOSAGE Adults: 250–500 mg three or four times daily
Children: 25–50 mg/kg per day over three or four doses

HOW SUPPLIED 250 mg and 500 mg tablets
125 mg and 250 mg suspension

COST ★★★★ (generics are much less)

Dapsone A sulfa drug used for certain infections such as leprosy. It also has anti-inflammatory properties and is used for vasculitis, lupus erythematosus, dermatitis herpetiformis, bullous pemphigoid, and other skin diseases. Since this drug has significant side effects, it is generally reserved for more serious conditions.

PRECAUTIONS Causes red blood cells to break down more easily and, as a result, causes a mild degree of anemia. In persons who lack a certain blood enzyme (glucose-6-dehydrogenase; G-6-PD) this breakdown may be severe and even fatal. Persons who take the drug must be tested to make sure they have this enzyme. Mild to moderate fatigue affects almost everyone taking dapsone. Taking this drug long term (months to years) may involve the nerves supplying the body's muscles (neuropathy). Headache, mild stomach upset, and a skin rash may also affect some patients.

DRUG INTERACTIONS Other sulfa drugs and rifampin should be taken with caution when a patient is also taking dapsone.

DOSAGE The dose depends on the disease being treated, but usually is between 50 mg and 300 mg per day.

HOW SUPPLIED 25 mg and 100 mg tablets

COST ★★

Dicloxacillin (Dycill®, Dynapen®, Pathocil®) A penicillin drug that is popular in dermatology, since few staphylococci and streptococci are resistant to it. Most often used for deeper skin infections such as cellulitis and infected cysts or boils. Usually very effective and well tolerated. The drug is best taken on an empty stomach. Acid-containing fruit juices or carbonated beverages may inactivate dicloxacillin and should not be consumed with this medication. Persons allergic to penicillin are also usually allergic to dicloxacillin

PRECAUTIONS Some stomach upset with diarrhea may be seen. Vaginal yeast infections may occur. Theoretically, this antibiotic may decrease the effectiveness of oral contraceptives.

DRUG INTERACTIONS This drug should be taken with caution when a patient is also taking certain types of high blood pressure medications, other antibiotics, and blood thinners.

DOSAGE Adults: 250–500 mg every six hours
Children: 6–12 mg per pound divided into four doses

HOW SUPPLIED 250 mg and 500 mg capsules

COST ★★

Doxycycline (Doryx®, Monodox®, Vibramycin®)   This antibiotic is used mostly for acne vulgaris and acne rosacea. However, it may also be given for other unusual infections. Doxycycline can be taken with food.

PRECAUTIONS   These are essentially identical to minocycline.

DRUG INTERACTIONS   Poorly absorbed when taken with antacids. Theoretically, doxycycline may decrease the effectiveness of birth control pills.

DOSAGE   50 mg or 100 mg twice daily.

HOW SUPPLIED   50 mg and 100 mg capsules

COST   ★★★ (generics are usually less)

Erythromycin, oral (E-Mycin®, Ery C® Ery-Tab®, E.E.S.®, Ery-Ped Suspension®, Erythrocin®, PCE®)   Erythromycin is widely used in dermatology. It is most commonly given for skin infections such as impetigo and cellulitis. It is also very useful for eczema and atopic dermatitis since these patients often have some degree of skin infection. Acne also responds to erythromycin. Since it is an older antibiotic, some bacteria have become resistant and many dermatologists prefer to use other, more powerful medications. Generic preparations are inexpensive. Erythromycin may be taken on an empty or full stomach, although many patients prefer to take it with food to decrease the likelihood of stomach upset.

PRECAUTIONS   Erythromycin is well tolerated by most patients although there are some persons who develop stomach upset with nausea and vomiting. Diarrhea is another side effect. Some preparations such as Ery C® and PCE® are designed to lessen these side effects and are better tolerated. Persons taking theophylline and digoxin may have increased blood levels if erythromycin is added. This may become a serious situation and is potentially fatal. Allergic reactions to this antibiotic also occur but are uncommon. Terfenadine may cause heart rhythm abnormalities if taken with erythromycin.

DRUG INTERACTIONS   Cyclosporine, carbamazepine, dilantin, disopyramide, lovastatin, ergotamine, triazolam, midazolam, oral anticoagulants, and dihydroergotamine may cause problems when taken with erythromycin.

DOSAGE   Adult acne: 250–500 mg once or twice daily

Other infections: 500 mg four times daily

Children's infections: 30–50 mg/kg per day in divided doses

HOW SUPPLIED   E-Mycin®—250 mg tablets

E-Mycin® 333—333 mg tablets

Ery-C®—250 mg capsules

Ery-Ped® 200 Suspension—100 ml and 200 ml bottles

Ery-Ped® 400 Suspension—60 ml, 100 ml, and 200 ml bottles

Ery-Ped® Drops—50 ml bottle

Ery-Tab®—333 mg and 500 mg tablets

E.E.S.® 200 Liquid—100 ml bottle

E.E.S.® 400 Liquid—100 ml bottle

E.E.S.® Granules—100 ml and 200 ml bottles

E.E.S.® 400 Filmtabs—400 mg tablets

Erythrocin—250 mg and 500 mg tablets

PCE® 333–333 mg tablets
PCE® 500–500 mg tablets
COST　★★★ for brand names, ★–★★ for generics

Minocycline (Dynacin®, Minocin®, Vectrin®)　This antibiotic is used mostly for acne vulgaris and acne rosacea but may be useful for other infections. The major advantage to this drug is that it can be taken with food (thus minimizing stomach upset).

PRECAUTIONS　Similar to tetracyclines. Increased sun sensitivity, stomach upset, diarrhea, headache, blurred vision, inflammation of the esophagus, and decreased mental alertness are possible. Since this drug may cause tooth and bone discoloration, it should not to be given to pregnant women or children under twelve and only with caution to patients under sixteen years.

DRUG INTERACTIONS　Poorly absorbed when taken with antacids. Theoretically, minocycline may decrease the effectiveness of birth control pills.

DOSAGE　50 mg or 100 mg twice daily.

HOW SUPPLIED　50 mg and 100 mg capsules

COST　★★★ (generics are usually less)

Tetracycline (Achromycin®, Sumycin®)　Tetracycline is an antibiotic used for infections such as syphilis, gonorrhea, and Rocky Mountain spotted fever, but its greatest use is to treat acne. This is one of the oldest antibiotics and some bacteria may be resistant to it.

PRECAUTIONS　The greatest problem with this drug is that it causes staining of the bones and teeth in children and infants. Therefore, it should not be given during pregnancy or to children under the age of sixteen. It will also make some patients more susceptible to the sun and cause an exaggerated sunburn. Stomach upset with nausea, vomiting, and diarrhea happens occasionally when the drug is taken on an empty stomach. While this is the best since it allows the drug to be better absorbed, it may be preferable in some persons to take the drug with food. In persons who take the drug for a long time, such as with acne therapy, increased blood levels of liver enzymes may occur; some dermatologists monitor blood work as part of their acne treatment.

DRUG INTERACTIONS　Oral anticoagulant drugs may become more potent if given with tetracycline. There is a theoretical decrease in the effectiveness of birth control pills if tetracycline is given with these medications.

DOSAGE　Acne: 250–500 mg two to four times daily
Infections: Usually 500 mg four times daily

HOW SUPPLIED　250 mg and 500 mg capsules

COST　★–★★

Trimethoprim-Sulfamethoxazole (Bactrim®, Cotrim®, Septra)　Trimethoprim-sulfamethoxazole (TMP-SMZ) is a combination of sulfa drugs very popular for treating infections of the bladder and ear. In dermatology, it is primarily given for acne and pneumocystis infections in AIDS patients.

PRECAUTIONS   TMP-SMZ is well known as a cause of toxic epidermal necrolysis, Stevens-Johnson syndrome, and certain types of anemia. For some reason it causes a rash in a large percentage of HIV-infected patients. It can also cause a mild rash in persons allergic to sulfa drugs.

DRUG INTERACTIONS   May interact with some diuretics used for blood pressure control, anticoagulants, dilantin, and methotrexate.

DOSAGE   The typical dose for acne is one DS (double-strength) or two regular tablets daily.

HOW SUPPLIED   Bactrim®–regular strength and DS tablets
Bactrim® suspension–16 oz. bottle
Cotrim®–regular strength and DS tablets
Cotrim® suspension–16 oz. bottle
Septra®–regular strength and DS tablets
Septra® suspension–100 ml and 16 oz. bottles

COST   ★–★★

Antifungal Medications

Ciclopirox Olamine (Loprox®)   An antifungal agent that is prepared in a cream and lotion. It is useful for skin infections (including tinea versicolor) but not nail involvement.

PRECAUTIONS   Some patients develop a mild allergy to the medication.

DRUG INTERACTIONS   Essentially none.

DOSAGE   Apply to skin infection once or twice daily.

HOW SUPPLIED   Cream–15 gm, 30 gm, and 90 gm tubes
Lotion–30 ml and 60 ml bottles

COST   ★★★

Clotrimazole (Lotrimin®)   Clotrimazole is one of the older topical antifungal medications. It is effective against most skin fungus infections including tinea versicolor. This drug is available over the counter and in generic preparations.

PRECAUTIONS   Some patients develop a mild allergy to the medication.

DRUG INTERACTIONS   Essentially none.

DOSAGE   Apply to skin once or twice daily.

HOW SUPPLIED   Cream–15 gm, 30 gm, 45 gm, and 90 gm tubes
Lotion–30 ml bottles
Solution–10 ml and 30 ml bottles

COST   ★★–★★★

Clotrimazole/Betamethasone (Lotrisone®)   This cream is a combination of clotrimazole and betamethasone, a potent topical corticosteroid. It is intended for use in situations where it is not clear if a patient's rash will respond to topical corticosteroids or is a fungal infection. The betamethasone likely takes care of most inflamed rashes with the clotrimazole doing little or nothing. Most dermatologists do not use and do not like it, since it usually causes more problems than it solves.

PRECAUTIONS   Some patients develop a mild allergy to either medication but this is uncommon.

DRUG INTERACTIONS   Essentially none.

DOSAGE   Apply to skin once or twice daily.

HOW SUPPLIED   15 gm and 45 gm tubes

COST   ★★★

Econazole (Spectazole®)   Econazole is a topical antifungal cream. It is useful for skin infections from fungus including *Candida* and tinea versicolor. It is not effective for nail infections.

PRECAUTIONS   Some patients may develop a mild allergy to the medication.

DRUG INTERACTIONS   Essentially none.

DOSAGE   Apply once or twice daily.

HOW SUPPLIED   15 gm, 30 gm, and 85 gm tubes

COST   ★★★

Griseofulvin (Fulvicin P/G, Grifulvin V, Gris-PEG, Grisactin®)   One of the oldest medications used for fungal infections of the skin and nails. It will not treat more serious fungal infections or those caused by yeasts such as *Candida.* Unfortunately, many fungus strains are resistant to griseofulvin and treating nail infections may take twelve months or longer. As a result, the use of this drug has dropped substantially since itraconazole and terbenafine have become available. It is still popular for fungal infections in children, but suspensions of itraconazole and fluconazole are now available. Griseofulvin comes in two different formulations—microsize and ultramicrosize. These relate to the medicine's capacity to be absorbed.

PRECAUTIONS   Griseofulvin may make persons susceptible to sunburn and can worsen lupus erythematosus. Stomach upset and headache are fairly common. Blood counts and liver enzymes may be affected by this drug and frequent blood monitoring is suggested for most patients if they will be taking griseofulvin for a long time.

DRUG INTERACTIONS   The effects of alcohol may be increased by griseofulvin. Barbiturates and some blood thinners may also be affected.

DOSAGE   Adults: 375-750 mg per day depending on the infection treated
Children: 5 mg per pound per day for microsize and 3.3 mg per pound with ultramicrosize formulations

HOW SUPPLIED   Fulvicin PG®—125 mg, 165 mg, 250 mg, 333 mg tablets
Grifulvin V®—250 mg and 500 mg tablets
Grifulvin V®—125 mg per teaspoon suspension
Gris-PEG®—125 mg and 250 mg tablets
Grisactin®—250 mg and 500 mg capsules
Grisactin Ultra®—250 mg and 333 mg tablets

COST   ★★★

Itraconazole (Sporanox®)   One of the imidazole type of antifungal antibiotics. It is a relatively new drug and one that has revolutionized the treatment of fungal infections of the skin, particularly of the nails. It is very useful in persons who have malfunctioning immune systems and have developed unusual fungal infections.

PRECAUTIONS   Some patients taking itraconazole develop an irritation of the liver and an increase in the blood levels of some liver enzymes. This can be screened for with blood tests. The liver inflammation almost always stops after discontinuing the drug. Some mild nausea and diarrhea may also occasionally occur.

DRUG INTERACTIONS   It is dangerous to take astemizole or terfenadine while on itraconazole since this combination may cause heart rate abnormalities. Some other drugs such as cyclosporin, digoxin, and oral antidiabetes agents may have their blood levels increased by taking itraconazole.

DOSAGE   There are numerous dosing schedules for nail fungus including two pills twice daily for seven days per month. This is done for three consecutive months. Daily dosing for three months is also done. Taking a single capsule daily for two weeks should treat fungus of the skin but longer courses are usually necessary for athlete's foot.

HOW SUPPLIED   100 mg capsules

COST   ★★★★

Ketoconazole (Nizoral® Cream and Shampoo)   The cream form of ketoconazole is useful for mild fungal infections of the skin. It can be used for nail fungus but is rarely effective. The shampoo form is most often used for severe dandruff, seborrheic dermatitis, and psoriasis of the scalp. It may also be used for tinea versicolor.

PRECAUTIONS   Some persons are allergic to these products and may break out in a mild rash. Otherwise, the drug is well tolerated.

DRUG INTERACTIONS   Essentially none.

DOSAGE   The cream may be applied once or twice daily. The shampoo can be used each day but some patients prefer to use it every other day or several times per week. The shampoo lather should be left on the scalp for five minutes before rinsing out. When used for tinea versicolor, the shampoo should be brought to a lather on the skin and left on for five to ten minutes before rinsing off.

HOW SUPPLIED   Cream—15 gm, 30 gm, and 60 gm tubes
        Shampoo—4 oz. bottle

COST   ★★★★

Ketoconazole (Nizoral® Tablets)   Ketoconazole was a major breakthrough in oral antifungal treatment. This drug is effective against many more fungal infections than griseofulvin. It is useful for *Candida* infections, the dermatophytes which cause skin and nail disease, and deep fungal infections affecting persons with poor immunity.

PRECAUTIONS   The concern with ketoconazole is liver damage. This occurs in about 1 in 10,000 patients, typically those who are overweight. Mild stomach upset and occasional rash are seen in persons taking the drug. Ketoconazole is also believed to diminish levels of male hormones (testosterone), but only in persons taking the drug for a long time or taking large doses. Ketoconazole is known to cause birth defects in animals and should be avoided during pregnancy.

DRUG INTERACTIONS   This is a considerable problem with this medication. The drugs that absolutely cannot be taken along with ketoconazole include phenytoin, terfenadine, cyclosporine, cisapride, and theophylline. Drugs such as antacids and stomach acid blockers such as cimetidine and ranitidine will prevent ketoconazole from being absorbed. Physicians should be made aware of all medications a patient is taking before prescribing ketoconazole.

DOSAGE   One to two tablets per day for several weeks are given for skin infections. Some dermatologists give ketoconazole prophylactically every few months to prevent tinea versicolor from returning. Nail infections usually have to be treated for three to six months. Blood work to monitor the effects on the liver are recommended in persons on the drug for prolonged periods.

HOW SUPPLIED   200 mg tablets

COST   ★★★★

Naftifine (Naftin®)   A topical antifungal drug believed to be more potent than other creams and lotions used for similar infections. There is evidence that the gel is effective in treating nail infections if used enough.

PRECAUTIONS   Some patients may develop mild skin irritation from using this drug.

DRUG INTERACTIONS   Essentially none.

DOSAGE   Apply to affected skin once or twice daily.

HOW SUPPLIED   Cream—15 gm, 30 gm, and 60 gm tubes
Gel—20 gm, 40 gm, and 60 gm tubes

COST   ★★★★

Oxiconazole (Oxistat®)   A topical antifungal cream and lotion. It is useful for skin infections from fungus including *Candida* and tinea versicolor. It has been used in some patients with nail infections (particularly the lotion) but is much less effective than oral medications.

PRECAUTIONS   Some patients may develop a mild allergy to the medication.

DRUG INTERACTIONS   Essentially none.

DOSAGE   Apply to affected skin once or twice daily.

HOW SUPPLIED   Cream—15 gm, 30 gm, and 60 gm tubes
Lotion—60 ml bottle

COST   ★★★

Sulconazole (Exelderm®)   An antifungal agent. Most often used for ringworm and jock itch but also effective against tinea versicolor. The solution may be used for treating nails but more effective medications are usually employed.

PRECAUTIONS   Some patients may develop mild skin irritation from using this drug.

DRUG INTERACTIONS   Essentially none.

DOSAGE   Apply to affected skin once or twice daily.

How Supplied   Cream—15 gm, 30 gm, and 60 gm tubes
Solution—30 ml bottle
Cost   ★★★★

Terbenifine (Lamisil®)   This drug is a little different from other oral antifungal antibiotics. It has been available as a cream in the United States for several years, but only recently was approved in pill form. It is effective for certain types of nail fungus. The same general precautions regarding blood work apply to terbenifine as to itraconazole. This drug is used almost solely for fungal infections of the fingernails and toenails. The 1% cream is used for infections of the groin, feet, and trunk.
Precautions   Aside from occasional stomach upset, the tablets are very well tolerated. The cream may occasionally cause a mild rash.
Drug Interactions   Essentially none.
Dosage   The tablets are given once daily for six weeks for fingernail infections and for twelve weeks for toenail infections. The cream cures over 75 percent of skin infections treated twice daily for several weeks. Like most creams, terbenifine does not have much effect in the treatment of nail disease.
How Supplied   250 mg tablets
1% cream—15 gm and 30 gm tubes
Cost   ★★★★

Antihistamines

Astemizole (Hismanal®)   A nonsedating antihistamine used for hives (urticaria) and other itching conditions.
Precautions   May worsen stomach ulcer conditions and glaucoma. The same cardiac effects that occur with terfenadine and taking ketoconazole or itraconazole may also arise if astemizole is taken with these drugs. Astemizole should not be taken with erythromycin, since liver damage may occur.
Drug Interactions   As with some other nonsedating antihistamines, there may be an interaction with itraconazole, cimetidine, ranitidine or theophylline.
Dosage   One pill daily.
How Supplied   10 mg tablets
Cost   ★★★★

Ceterizine (Zyrtec®)   A nonsedating antihistamine that blocks histamine receptors. It is used for seasonal allergies, urticaria, and itching.
Precautions   Rare drowsiness, headache, or nervousness.
Drug Interactions   Essentially none. Best taken on an empty stomach.
Dosage   5–10 mg daily, or 1–2 teaspoons daily.
How Supplied   5 mg and 10 mg tablets
10 mg per teaspoon suspension
Cost   ★★★★

Cimetidine (Tagamet®)   Technically an antihistamine; this has been used for gastritis and stomach ulcer disease. Recently, it has been found to interact with the body's immune system and is now used for hives (urticaria) and warts, particularly in children. It is well tolerated, but must be used in higher doses than for stomach disease.

PRECAUTIONS   Mild diarrhea and headache are the most common side effects. Some women experience some mildly uncomfortable breast swelling with the use of this medication. On rare occasions, a patient's blood counts may drop after taking cimetidine.

DRUG INTERACTIONS   Interferes with the metabolism of certain drugs such as anticoagulants, dilantin, propranolol, nifedipine, certain antidepressants, lidocaine, theophylline, and metronidazole.

DOSAGE   The typical dose for warts is 40 mg/kg per day in divided doses. For adults this may mean taking quite a number of pills. Doses for treating hives tend to be smaller.

HOW SUPPLIED   200 mg, 300 mg, 400 mg, and 800 mg tablets
300 mg per teaspoon suspension

COST   ★★★ (generics are less expensive)

Diphenhydramine (Benadryl®)   This is one of the older antihistamines. It is most often used for itching skin conditions such as eczema, hives (urticaria), and insect bites. It is available over the counter and in various generic forms. The use of diphenhydramine in a cream is not recommended since it usually is ineffective and may cause inflammation.

PRECAUTIONS   The greatest side effect of this drug is drowsiness; persons who are driving or need to be alert should avoid it. Some people experience jitteriness or nervousness.

DRUG INTERACTIONS   Other drugs such as narcotics and alcohol are also depressants and should not be taken with diphenhydramine.

DOSAGE   A typical dose is 25–50 mg two to four times per day for adults. Children should be given a teaspoon (5 ml) several times daily as needed.

HOW SUPPLIED   25 mg tablets
25 mg softgel capsules
12.5 mg chewable tablets
12.5 mg per teaspoon liquid

COST   ★★★ (generics are less)

Doxepin (Adapin®, Sinequan®)   Doxepin is actually an antidepressant with very prominent antihistamine actions. It is used in low doses to control the itch of certain skin conditions, notably eczema or urticaria. A topical cream is also available. Some persons respond very well to doxepin, whereas others do not. The greatest side effect is drowsiness. Almost all patients who take doxepin become drowsy and many dermatologists recommend it for use only at bedtime. Most patients are not able to take it during the day. The liquid form is useful for very severe cases of atopic dermatitis in children. This drug must be kept away from children since overdoses of doxepin are often fatal.

PRECAUTIONS   Persons taking doxepin should drive or operate machinery only with great caution. Dry mouth, urinary retention, confusion, and worsening of glaucoma are possible if the dose is high enough.

DRUG INTERACTIONS   Sedatives such as barbiturates and alcohol may be dangerous when taken with doxepin. Some high blood pressure medications, other antidepressants, and thyroid replacement drugs should be taken with caution.

DOSAGE   A typical dose for an adult is 25 mg every eight hours or so. Some patients receive the 10 mg capsules and begin taking a single capsule. The dose is then increased as tolerated using the 10 mg capsules. Pediatric doses should be arranged with a dermatologist familiar with the use of the drug in children.

HOW SUPPLIED   10 mg, 25 mg, 50 mg, 75 mg, 100 mg, and 150 mg capsules
10 mg/ml solution—120 ml bottle

COST   ★★★ (generics are less)

Hydroxyzine (Atarax®)   An antihistamine used for the relief of itching. It is considered more effective than diphenhydramine. This drug is most commonly used for skin diseases such as eczema, urticaria (hives), and drug reactions. Hydroxyzine may cause considerable drowsiness and should not be taken if persons have to drive or operate machinery. Some patients prefer to take this drug at bedtime to relieve itching and promote restful sleep.

PRECAUTIONS   As with other antihistamines, taking too much of this drug may cause anxiety and nervousness.

DRUG INTERACTIONS   Narcotics and alcohol are also depressants and should not be taken with hydroxyzine.

DOSAGE   A typical dose is 25–50 mg two to four times per day for adults. Children should be given a teaspoon (5 ml) several times daily as needed.

HOW SUPPLIED   10 mg, 25 mg, 50 mg, and 100 mg tablets
10 mg syrup

COST   ★★★ (generics are less)

Loratidine (Claritin®)   A nonsedating antihistamine used for allergies, urticaria, and itching. Claritin-D® contains a decongestant, pseudoephedrine. Besides the lack of sleepiness, the big advantage to loratidine is that it only has to be taken once per day.

PRECAUTIONS   Occasional drowsiness, dry mouth, and headache.

DRUG INTERACTIONS   As with some other nonsedating antihistamines, there may be an interaction with ketoconazole, erythromycin, cimetidine, ranitidine, or theophylline.

DOSAGE   One tablet daily.

HOW SUPPLIED   10 mg tablets

COST   ★★★★

Terfenadine (Seldane®) This drug was the original nonsedating antihistamine. It is used primarily for seasonal allergies but may also be helpful with hives (urticaria) and some types of itching. The use of terfenadine has diminished since it was learned that this drug may cause irregular heart rhythms, particularly in persons taking erythromycin, clarithromycin, ketoconazole, or itraconazole. Seldane-D® contains pseudoephedrine as a decongestant.

PRECAUTIONS   Some mild drowsiness occurs in some persons, as may some mild stomach upset.

DRUG INTERACTIONS   Terfenadine should not be taken with erythromycin, clarithromycin, ketoconazole, or itraconazole. This medication is best taken on an empty stomach.

DOSAGE   One tablet twice daily.

HOW SUPPLIED   60 mg tablets

COST   ★★★★

Antiscabies Medications

Crotamiton (Eurax®) Crotamiton is an older preparation used for treating scabies infestations and itching skin. It may stain bedding and clothing. It is not as effective as some of the newer medications.

PRECAUTIONS   Crotamiton may cause some irritation and inflammation of treated skin.

DRUG INTERACTIONS   Essentially none.

DOSAGE   A layer of the cream or lotion should be massaged into the skin from the chin to the toes after taking a bath or shower. Toe and finger web spaces should be treated. A second application should be done in twenty-four hours and a cleansing bath taken at forty-eight hours. Bedding and clothes should be washed and cleaned after the first application.

HOW SUPPLIED   Cream—2 oz. tubes
Lotion—2 oz. bottles

COST   ★★★

Ivermectin (Stromectol®) Ivermectin has been used in veterinary medicine to control worm infestations. It was recently shown to be effective in treating scabies and is now given orally. A one-time treatment is typical, but a repeat dose several days later is sometimes required.

PRECAUTIONS   This drug should not be taken by pregnant women since it causes birth defects in animals. Ivermectin should be taken with water. Occasional patients may complain of stomach upset, mild itching, or minor rash.

DRUG INTERACTIONS   No known interactions.

DOSAGE   Dosage is based on patient's weight. Adults usually take two tablets in a single dose.

HOW SUPPLIED   6 mg tablets

COST   ★★★★

Lindane (Kwell® Cream, Lotion, and Shampoo)   This chemical is one of the older drugs used to treat scabies and head lice. It can be used as well for other mite and louse infestations. In recent years, some insects have developed a resistance to lindane. Lindane is available as a generic preparation, making it much cheaper and still effective in most instances. Some dermatologists recommend a second treatment with the cream, lotion, or shampoo the next day to increase the chances of killing the mites.

PRECAUTIONS   Lindane absorbed through the skin may cause seizures and other neurological problems in some patients. The problem is more common in children; some dermatologists do not recommend using lindane in patients under twelve years of age. The cream or lotion should not be left on the skin for more than twelve hours and no more than an ounce should be used to cover the skin of a child. It is important that lindane not be ingested and children should be prevented from sucking their fingers or licking off the lotion.

DRUG INTERACTIONS   Essentially none.

DOSAGE   Lindane cream or lotion is massaged into the skin from the scalp to the soles of the feet. A nighttime application is most popular. Application between the fingers and toes is important. The medication is then washed off eight to twelve hours later. If desired, this treatment may be repeated the following night.

  The shampoo is used in a somewhat different manner. The hair should be shampooed with an ordinary shampoo and then completely dried. The lindane shampoo should be massaged thoroughly into the dry hair and allowed to remain for a few minutes. Water should then be added to the hair and a lather raised. Rinse the shampoo out and remove the nits with a nit comb or tweezers.

HOW SUPPLIED   Cream—60 gm tube
Lotion—2 oz. and 16 oz. bottles
Shampoo—2 oz. and 16 oz. bottles

COST   ★★-★★★ (generic preparations are less costly)

Permethrin (Elimite Cream®)   Permethrin is the preferred drug for treating scabies infections and other conditions caused by insect mites. It is very effective and usually only one treatment is necessary. Some dermatologists recommend that the drug be applied a second time to ensure that all the insects have been killed. Permethrin is also considered a safer method of treatment, particularly for children.

PRECAUTIONS   The cream should get into the eyes since it will irritate them. Eczema and dry skin may be slightly worsened by permethrin. A mild rash may develop in some patients.

DRUG INTERACTIONS   Essentially none.

DOSAGE   Permethrin cream is massaged into the skin from the scalp to the soles of the feet. A nighttime application is the most popular. Getting between the fingers and toes is important. The cream is then washed off eight to fourteen hours later. If desired, this treatment may be repeated the following night.

HOW SUPPLIED   60 gm tubes

COST   ★★★

Antiviral Antibiotics

Acyclovir (Zovirax®)   Originally used for treating herpes simplex infections. In recent years, it has been used as well for chickenpox (varicella) and herpes zoster (shingles). It is usually well tolerated and may be given intravenously if needed. Patients with poorly functioning kidneys must have the dose reduced. The ointment is used for fever blisters (herpes labialis) and genital herpes, but does not work as well as when the drug is given by mouth. Acyclovir should be used as soon as the symptoms begin even if there is no evidence of skin lesions. Some strains of herpes virus have become resistant to acyclovir.

PRECAUTIONS   This medication should be given to persons with kidney disease only under well-supervised conditions.

DRUG INTERACTIONS   Probenecid increases the amount of acyclovir in the bloodstream.

DOSAGE   Genital herpes: 200 mg five times per day for five days; apply ointment six times per day for seven days
Genital herpes prevention: 400 mg twice daily
Herpes labialis: 200 mg five times per day for five days; apply ointment six times per day for seven days
Chickenpox: 800 mg four times per day for five days in adults
Chickenpox: 20 mg/kg four times per day for five days in children
Shingles: 800 mg five times per day for seven to ten days

HOW SUPPLIED   200 mg and 800 mg tablets
200 mg per teaspoon suspension
Ointment—3 gm and 15 gm tubes

COST   ★★★ (generics are less)

Famciclovir (Famvir®)   Similar to acyclovir and works against the same viruses. Used for treating shingles (herpes zoster) or recurrent genital herpes outbreaks. It is easier to take than acyclovir but is more expensive.

PRECAUTIONS   The same precautions as for acyclovir apply to famciclovir. Headache and mild nausea are the most common side effects.

DRUG INTERACTIONS   Similar to acyclovir.

DOSAGE   Genital herpes: 125 mg twice daily for five days
Shingles: 500 mg three times daily for seven days

HOW SUPPLIED   125 mg and 500 gm tablets

COST   ★★★★

Imiquimod (Aldara®)   Imiquimod cream works by an unknown method in the treatment of genital warts (condyloma acuminata). It is thought to cause the skin to produce more alpha interferon causing the wart to disappear.

PRECAUTIONS   May cause mild redness and irritation of the skin.

DRUG INTERACTIONS   Unknown.

DOSAGE   Apply three times weekly to warts for six to ten hours (overnight). The cream is then washed off with mild soap and water. This course is followed as long as the warts remain and the patient tolerates the treatment.

How Supplied   250 mg in single-use cream packets

Cost   ★★★★

Penciclovir (Denavir®)   An antiherpes cream for use in persons with cold sores (herpes labialis). It is free of any serious side effects but must be applied every two hours while the patient is awake.

Precautions   Contact of the medication with the eyes may cause irritation.

Drug Interactions   Unknown.

Dosage   Applied every two hours while awake.

How Supplied   2 gm tube

Cost   ★★★★

Podofilox (Condylox®)   A derivative of podophyllin used to treat genital (venereal) warts. It works by killing the tissue containing the wart virus. Until this preparation became available, there was no treatment for home use with these warts. Effective in certain patients, but therapy is expensive.

Precautions   This drug causes irritation and burning of the skin in a large number of patients who use it. Women tend to be affected more than men. Usually, this discomfort is not so bad that the therapy can't be continued. Podofilox should not be used by women who are pregnant or thinking of conceiving.

Drug Interactions   Essentially none.

Dosage   Apply to wart tissue twice daily for three consecutive days and then withhold for four days. This weekly cycle should be repeated for four weeks and if no significant benefit is noted, the drug should be stopped.

How Supplied   3.5 ml solution bottle

Cost   ★★★★

Valacyclovir (Valtrex®)   A "prodrug" of acyclovir, meaning that it is converted into acyclovir in the body. As such, the same precautions for giving acyclovir apply to valacyclovir. The main advantage to this drug is that there is less resistance than with acyclovir and it does not have to be given as often.

Precautions   May lower blood counts in persons with damaged immune systems. As such, it should not be given to transplant patients or those with HIV disease. Patients with kidney disease should be given reduced doses. Headache and mild stomach upset are the most common side effects.

Drug Interactions   Cimetidine and probenecid prevent the excretion of valacyclovir and will raise the blood levels.

Dosage   Genital herpes: two 500 mg tablets twice daily for five days
Shingles: two 500 mg tablets three times daily for seven days

How Supplied   500 mg tablets

Cost   ★★★★

Immune System–Suppressing Medications

Azathioprine (Immuran®)   A drug used to suppress the immune system. It is most useful for conditions such as lupus erythematosus, dermatomyositis, psoriasis, and lichen planus.

PRECAUTIONS   The most worrisome side effect of taking this drug is decreased blood counts. These must be watched carefully with blood work. Stomach upset with diarrhea is also possible. Since azathioprine can cause severe birth defects, it is mandatory that women not take this medication while pregnant or thinking about conceiving.

DRUG INTERACTIONS   Azathioprine should be taken with great care in patients using other immune-suppressing medications. Other drugs which should be avoided include allopurinol, certain high blood pressure medications, and warfarin.

DOSAGE   The usual beginning dose is 50–100 mg per day. This may be increased to 200 mg per day. Doses above this level continue to suppress the immune system without benefiting the treated disease.

HOW SUPPLIED   50 mg tablets

COST   ★★★ (generics are less)

Cyclophosphamide (Cytoxan®)   Used to treat cancer, but has been found effective for some conditions of the skin such as lupus erythematosus, vasculitis, pemphigus vulgaris, and lichen planus. Also useful for inflammatory conditions of the blood vessels (vasculitis). Usually well tolerated and may be taken by mouth.

PRECAUTIONS   May decrease blood counts; these have to be watched carefully with intermittent blood work. When higher doses are used, particularly if they are given intravenously, bleeding into the bladder (hemorrhagic cystitis) may develop. As a result, it is suggested that the patient consume large quantities of water when using this drug. Routine evaluation of the urine (urinalysis) is done by some physicians. Stomach upset, nausea, mild hair loss, and mouth ulcers may occur. This drug will badly deform unborn children and must not be taken during pregnancy. Patients who take cyclophosphamide have an increased susceptibility to infection.

DRUG INTERACTIONS   Patients who take phenobarbitol may find that the effectiveness of cyclophosphamide is reduced.

DOSAGE   The usual adult dose is between 25 mg and 100 mg per day. This may be given in divided doses and is best taken with food.

HOW SUPPLIED   25 mg and 50 mg tablets

COST   ★★★ (generics are less)

Cyclosporine (Sandimmune®, Neoral®)   This drug was initially developed to prevent the body from rejecting transplanted organs. It suppresses the body's immune system and is known to make several skin diseases much better. Psoriasis, atopic dermatitis, alopecia areata, and lichen planus all respond readily to this drug. The doses used are less than in organ transplantation. Cyclosporine is best reserved for serious conditions that have not responded to more traditional therapy. It is also preferable for the prescribing dermatologist to have some experience in the use of this drug. Cyclosporine has been used topically but with varying degrees of success. There is no commercially available topical cyclosporine preparation so most have to be made from different "recipes."

PRECAUTIONS   The most worrisome side effect of cyclosporine use is its effects on the kidneys. Treated patients should regularly have blood work to evaluate their kidney function. Increased blood pressure, increased hair growth, enlargement of the gums, and headache may also occur. This drug is absolutely not to be taken during pregnancy since birth defects may occur. As with all immune system–suppressing drugs, patients who take cyclosporine are more susceptible to infection from bacteria, viruses, and fungi.

DRUG INTERACTIONS   A long list of drugs interact adversely with cyclosporine. Most, such as fluconazole, itraconazole, and erythromycin, increase the drug's blood levels. Nafcillin, carbamazepine, phenobarbitol, and phenytoin, on the other hand, decrease cyclosporine blood levels. Cyclosporine increases blood levels of potassium and should be used carefully with other drugs that do the same.

DOSAGE   The dosage is based on the patients weight. The typical dose is 1–3 mg/kg per day. The oral solution is best mixed with room temperature orange or apple juice in a glass container and taken with food.

HOW SUPPLIED   Neoral®–25 mg capsules
Neoral®–100 mg capsules
Neoral®–solution 100 mg/ml
Sandimmune®–25 mg, 50 mg, and 100 mg capsules
Sandimmune®–100 mg suspension

COST   ★★★★

Methotrexate (Rhematrex®)   Most often used in dermatology for treating psoriasis and psoriatic arthritis. It may also be used for cutaneous T cell lymphoma. Methotrexate is a chemotherapy drug and may have some serious side effects. The doses used in dermatology are usually much smaller than those for cancer therapy. Methotrexate is a very cost-efficient means of treating skin disease but has to be done very carefully and the patients closely watched.

PRECAUTIONS   May damage the lungs, causing breathing difficulty. The most worrisome effects of this drug, however, are those involving the liver. When given for too long or in too high doses, the liver may be damaged. Regular monitoring of liver function is required when using this medication. Decreased blood cell counts may also occur. Patients who take methotrexate may have mild to moderate stomach upset with diarrhea. It is best to take this drug on an empty stomach, but some persons must take it with food to avoid stomach upset. Mouth ulcers may occur while taking methotrexate.

DRUG INTERACTIONS   Toxic blood levels of methotrexate may occur when aspirin and nonsteroidal anti-inflammatory drugs (NSAIDs) are taken with it. Examples of NSAIDs include ibuprofen, naproxen, and phenylbutazone. Other drugs to be avoided include phenytoin, sulfa drugs, acitretin, antibiotics, theophylline, and folic acid. It is best for the physician dispensing methotrexate to be familiar with all the medications a patient is taking or is likely to take during his or her treatment. Since methotrexate is capable of causing severe birth defects, it is mandatory that women not take this medication while pregnant or if thinking about conceiving.

DOSAGE   There are several different ways to take methotrexate. The usual dose is between 5 and 30 mg per week. Most dermatologists give the dose all at once but others have patients take it in three doses over twenty-four hours (every twelve hours). The liquid is usually used for injecting but may be taken by mouth and is less expensive. Giving an intramuscular injection once a week is useful for persons who for one reason or another cannot take the pills.

HOW SUPPLIED   2.5 mg tablets
25 mg/ml liquid

COST   ★★★

Vitamin A Derivatives (Retinoids)

Acitretin (Soriatane®)   Acitretin is very similar to isotretinoin. It is used for severe and disabling psoriasis and a few other rare skin conditions.

PRECAUTIONS   These are essentially the same as for isotretinoin. Pregnancy must be avoided while taking the drug but also for three years after stopping it, since it takes that long for the drug to leave the body. For this reason, many dermatologists will not prescribe acitretin to women who are still capable of having children.

DRUG INTERACTIONS   These are the same as for isotretinoin. Milk seems to decrease the amount of the drug absorbed.

DOSAGE   The dose is based on the patient's weight and is usually given as 0.5–1.0 mg/kg per day. It is best to take the drug with food.

HOW SUPPLIED   10 mg and 25 mg capsules

COST   ★★★★

Adalapene (Differin®)   This gel has only recently been released on the market and is used for psoriasis and acne. Adalapene is very similar to tretinoin and is used in essentially the same way.

PRECAUTIONS   Adalapene gel may initially worsen acne for a brief period. Mild inflammation of the skin and an increased sensitivity to the sun may also occur similar to tretinoin. Because this is a retinoid, its use in pregnant or nursing women is discouraged.

DRUG INTERACTIONS   Believed to be the same as for tretinoin.

DOSAGE   Apply to affected areas of skin at bedtime and wash off in the morning.

How Supplied   Gel—15 gm and 45 gm tubes
Cost   ★★★★

Isotretinoin (Accutane®)   For all practical purposes, isotretinoin is essentially tretinoin (Retin-A®) in pill form. It is intended for persons with severe scarring or disfiguring acne. It works extremely well and is curative in most patients. The major disadvantage of isotretinoin use is the cost (the drug is extremely expensive) and the need for strict avoidance of pregnancy.

Precautions   Since isotretinoin raises blood fats (cholesterol and triglycerides), this drug should be given with caution to diabetics and other patients who may have increased blood fats. Blood work is also done to monitor how the liver handles the drug. Almost all patients develop chapped lips, dry eyes (making contact lens wearing difficult), and dry skin. Mild headaches, muscle pains, and joint aches are sometimes seen early in treatment. Mild hair thinning is seen in some persons but hair grows back when the drug is stopped. Isotretinoin badly deforms unborn children and must not be taken by pregnant women. Rarely, isotretinoin may cause an unusual increase in the pressure within the brain called pseudotumor cerebri. This is associated with severe headache and visual disturbances. If this occurs, the drug should be stopped and the patient should seek treatment at an emergency room. Under some unusual circumstances isotretinoin is taken for prolonged periods (years) and problems such as calcium deposits in joints and tendons may be seen.

Drug Interactions   Isotretinoin should not be taken with drugs that raise blood fats or are similar to vitamin A.

Dosage   The drug is given according to the patient's weight. The typical dose is 0.75–1.25 mg/kg per day. Treatment typically takes five or six months.

How Supplied   10, 20, and 40 mg capsules
Cost   ★★★★

Tazarotene (Tazorac®)   Tazarotene works similarly to tretinoin and isotretinoin. It is indicated currently only for psoriasis but likely will someday be used for acne and other conditions. It is very expensive.

Precautions   Like any topical medication, tazarotene may irritate the skin with stinging and burning. Worsening of psoriasis has also been described but is uncommon. Because this drug is a retinoid, it should not be used during pregnancy or while breast-feeding.

Drug Interactions   Essentially none.

Dosage   Apply a thin layer to psoriasis plaques once daily at bedtime.

How Supplied   0.05% and 0.1% strengths in 30 gm and 100 gm tubes
Cost   ★★★★

Tretinoin, topical (Retin-A®, Renova®, Retin-A Micro®)   Tretinoin is one of the most written about and used medications of the last decade. It was originally prescribed as a gel for treatment of acne. While very effective, it was too irritating for many patients and fell out of favor. Creams were then introduced; the medication was better tolerated and it has become a mainstay in treating acne. When it was discovered that tretinoin was capable of reversing some of the signs of aging skin, the drug became very popular and currently is one of the most used medications on the market. Since the drug is used topically (an oral form does exist but is only used for certain types of leukemia) it is usually well tolerated. Some persons do have a mild degree of irritation when treatment is begun, but this usually fades with continued use. Currently, tretinoin is used for mild to moderate acne (not the cystic form), solar lentigos (age spots), fine wrinkling of the face and forehead, and preventing or treating precancers on the skin. The gel formulations are best for oily skin. The Micro Gel® brand is designed to allow more medication to be applied to the skin. Some generic preparations have recently become available and are significantly less expensive, but since the cream bases vary there is some question as to how well they work. Most dermatologists prefer to use brand-name medications.

PRECAUTIONS   Some persons become slightly sensitive to the sun after using tretinoin. Irritation at the corners of the nose, eyes, and mouth occasionally occurs. If tretinoin is applied and then the skin exposed to light, the medication may be inactivated and incapable of providing any benefit. It is best to apply the cream, gel, or solution at bedtime and wash it off in the morning. Because tretinoin is a retinoid, its use in pregnant or nursing women is discouraged.

DRUG INTERACTIONS   Essentially none. Applying tretinoin with other creams and lotions, such as benzoyl peroxide, may cause the drug to lose its effect.

DOSAGE   A thin layer of the medication should be applied to the affected skin at bedtime and washed off in the morning.

HOW SUPPLIED   Renova® Cream—40 gm and 60 gm tubes
Retin-A® Cream 0.025%—20 gm and 45 gm tubes
Retin-A® Cream 0.05%—20 gm and 45 gm tubes
Retin-A® Cream 0.1%—20 gm and 45 gm tubes
Retin-A® Gel 0.01%—15 gm and 45 gm tubes
Retin-A® Gel 0.25%—15 gm and 45 gm tubes
Retin-A® Liquid 0.05%—28 ml bottle
Retin-A® Micro—20 gm and 45 gm tubes

COST   ★★★–★★★★

Miscellaneous

Aluminum Chloride (Drysol®, Xerac AC®)   Aluminum chloride slows down the production of perspiration by sweat glands. It is a common ingredient in many antiperspirants. Stronger concentrations are available in two products, Drysol® (20%) and Xerac AC® (6.25%). This liquid may be harmful to certain fabrics and metals.

PRECAUTIONS   May irritate the skin. It should not be applied to already inflamed skin. A mild burning sensation occasionally results from its use.

DRUG INTERACTIONS   Essentially none.

DOSAGE   Apply to skin at bedtime.
HOW SUPPLIED   Drysol®—37.5 ml bottle
   Drysol®—35ml and 60 ml Dab-O-Matic bottles
   Xerac AC®—35ml and 60 ml Dab-O-Matic bottles
COST   ★★★

Ammonium Lactate (Lac-Hydrin® 12% Cream and Lotion, Amlactin® 12% Lotion)
Ammonium lactate is an alpha hydroxy lotion. It is very useful for dry skin, xerosis, psoriasis, and ichthyosis. It stings if it comes into contact with open skin so in patients with cracked skin this lotion will be uncomfortable.
PRECAUTIONS   Contact of the medication with the eyes may cause irritation.
DRUG INTERACTIONS   Unknown.
DOSAGE   These medications may be applied to intact skin as often as desired.
HOW SUPPLIED   Amlactin®—8 oz. and 14 oz. bottles
   Lac-Hydrin® Cream—140 gm tube
   Lac-Hydrin® Lotion—225 gm and 400 gm bottles
COST   ★★★

Anthralin (Drithocreme®, Dritho-Scalp®, Micanol®)   Anthralin is an older but still very useful product for treating psoriasis. Not all persons with psoriasis are good candidates for this drug, but in certain patients it works very well. It is considered safe for long-term use.
PRECAUTIONS   This is a fairly strong medication and should not be applied to sensitive areas such as the face, underarms, and groin. Anthralin stains bedding and clothing and when washed off may leave a residue with staining. This drug may irritate the skin and cause redness and burning. Some staining of gray or blond hair may occur when Drithoscalp® is used.
DRUG INTERACTIONS   Essentially none.
DOSAGE   The cream is applied to the skin or scalp and washed off after a certain time. Usually, a low concentration of anthralin is started and only allowed to remain on the skin for thirty minutes to an hour. After the skin has become accustomed to this drug, stronger preparations are used and applied for longer periods.
HOW SUPPLIED   Drithocreme® 0.1% 50 gm tube
   Drithocreme®—0.25% 50 gm tube
   Drithocreme®—0.5% 50 gm tube
   Drithocreme®—1.0% 50 gm tube
   Drithoscalp®—0.25% 50 gm tube
   Drithoscalp®—0.5% 50 gm tube
COST   ★★★ (generics are less)

Beta-carotene (Solatene®)   Beta-carotene is a form of vitamin A found in fruits and vegetables. It absorbs light in the visible range (not UVA, UVB, or UVC). It is used for treating light-sensitive skin conditions such as lupus erythematosus, porphyria, and polymorphous light eruption.

PRECAUTIONS   Beta-carotene may turn the skin slightly yellow to orange.

DRUG INTERACTIONS   Essentially none.

DOSAGE   Children (one to eight years): 30–60 mg per day

Adolescents: (nine to sixteen years) 90–120 mg per day

Adults: 120–180 mg per day (may be increased to 250 mg per day)

HOW SUPPLIED   30 mg capsules

COST   ★★

Calcipotriene (Dovonex®)   A synthetic vitamin D drug that is most often used for psoriasis. It is safe if used in reasonable amounts and effective for many patients. The main drawback to the use of calcipotriene is that it is expensive. Other skin disorders such as eczema have been treated with this drug with some success. The solution is used to treat scalp psoriasis.

PRECAUTIONS   Calcipotriene causes a higher-than-normal incidence of mild skin irritation when used as directed.

DRUG INTERACTIONS   Essentially none.

DOSAGE   Apply to affected skin once or twice daily.

HOW SUPPLIED   Cream—30 gm, 60 gm, and 100 gm tubes

Ointment—30 gm, 60 gm, and 100 gm tubes

COST   ★★★★

Chloroquine (Aralen®)   An antimalarial antibiotic used for the same skin diseases as hydroxychloroquine. The same precautions are to be followed as well. It is unclear why some skin conditions seem to respond better to one drug than the other.

PRECAUTIONS   The major worry with the use of chloroquine is that of eye damage with long-term use. This is unlikely for most patients since they won't remain on the drug for very long. Chloroquine tastes extremely bitter so breaking the tablets in half is not recommended.

DRUG INTERACTIONS   Similar to hydroxychloroquine.

DOSAGE   As with hydroxychloroquine, the dose depends on the disease being treated. Most patients receive no more than one tablet daily and some take only one or two per week.

HOW SUPPLIED   500 mg tablets

COST   ★★★

Doxepin (Zonalon®)   The antihistamine doxepin has been formulated in a cream for use on itching skin. It seems to work well but is expensive. The major side effect of doxepin cream is drowsiness (about 20 percent of patients). It should be used with caution by persons who drive or operate machinery.

PRECAUTIONS   Persons susceptible to glaucoma and urinary retention should be careful of using topical doxepin.

Medications Used in Dermatology   ~   359

DRUG INTERACTIONS   Certain types of antidepressants should not be taken if large amounts of doxepin cream are going to be used.

DOSAGE   Doxepin cream may be applied daily every three to four hours.

HOW SUPPLIED   30 gm and 45 gm tubes

COST   ★★★★

Finasteride (Propecia®)   This drug inhibits the function of an enzyme, 5-alpha reductase, in hair follicles, causing them to be less likely to be lost with male pattern baldness (androgenetic alopecia).

PRECAUTIONS   Finasteride causes deformities of male fetuses in women who take this drug while pregnant, so it should not be used in pregnant or nursing women. Broken or crushed pills also should not be handled by pregnant patients, since small amounts of the medication may be absorbed through the skin. A small percentage of men (less than 2 percent) experience a loss of libido or difficulty achieving or maintaining an erection.

DRUG INTERACTIONS   None known.

DOSAGE   One pill daily.

HOW SUPPLIED   1 mg pills

COST   ★★★★

Fluorouracil (Efudex®, Fluoroplex®)   A chemotherapy drug used to treat colon cancer. Patients who received this drug often had an inflammation and then disappearance of their actinic keratoses. For that reason, the drug was put into a cream. It has also been used on stubborn warts, porokeratosis, and other skin growths, but seems to work best for actinic keratoses. Depending on how often the cream is applied, it causes an irritation in just about everyone. The treated skin lesions become red and sore but the surrounding skin is also red and inflamed. If this drug is applied regularly, especially to the face, the discomfort may be significant. In addition, since the skin tends to turn bright red, the treated patient may look as if scalding water had been thrown in his or her face.

PRECAUTIONS   Since fluorouracil causes increased sensitivity to the sun, applying sunscreen at the same time is suggested.

DRUG INTERACTIONS   None.

DOSAGE   There are several different regimens for applying this drug. The most common is application (with sunscreen) twice daily for two to six weeks, depending on how inflamed the skin becomes. The drug is then stopped and the skin allowed to heal. Several weeks later, after healing, new skin replaces the actinic keratoses and the patient looks much better. One or 2% cream may be used on facial skin, with the 5% cream reserved for treating the arms and hands. A more popular method is twice-daily application for two consecutive days per week for several months; with this regimen, patients have much less redness and irritation.

HOW SUPPLIED   Efudex® Cream 5%—30 gm tube

Efudex® Solution 5%–10 ml bottle
Efudex® Solution 2%–10 ml bottle
Fluoroplex® Cream 1%–30 gm tube
Fluoroplex® Solution 1%–30 ml bottle

COST ★★★ (generics cost much less)

Hydroquinone (Eldoquin®, Eldopaque®, Melanex®, Melpaque®, Nuquin®, Solaquin®, Viquin®) Hydroquinones are used as "bleaching creams" to rid the skin of excess pigment or darkening. They have traditionally been used for "liver spots" or melasma and are quite effective. They need to be used with sunscreens since they may make the patient more susceptible to the sun. Many formulations contain sunscreens. Creams with lower concentrations of hydroquinones are available over the counter but do not work as well.

PRECAUTIONS Dermatitis from an allergy to the drug or cream (contact dermatitis) and excessive bleaching of the skin may occur. Some patients become more sun sensitive after using the cream.

DRUG INTERACTIONS None.

DOSAGE Applied once or twice daily, usually at bedtime or during the day with a sunscreen.

HOW SUPPLIED Eldoquin Forte® 4% Cream–1 oz. tube
Eldopaque Forte® 4% cream–1 oz. tube
Melanex® Solution–1 oz. bottle
Melpaque® HP 4% Cream–1 oz. tube
Melquin® HP 4% Cream–0.5 oz. and 1 oz. tube
Melquin®-3 Topical Solution®–1 oz. bottles.
Nuquin® HP 4% Cream–0.5oz., 1oz., and 2 oz. tubes
Nuquin® HP 4% Gel–1 oz. tube
Solaquin Forte® 4% Cream–1 oz. tube
Solaquin Forte® 4% Gel–1 oz. tube
Viquin Forte® 4% Cream–1 oz. tube

COST ★★★

Hydroxychloroquine (Plaquenil®) Hydroxychloroquine is most often used in rheumatologic diseases such as arthritis and lupus erythematosus. It is occasionally used in sarcoidosis, dermatomyositis, porphyria cutanea tarda, and granuloma annulare. Overall, this drug is well tolerated, although some patients experience stomach upset or increased sun sensitivity.

PRECAUTIONS The most worrisome aspect of this drug is its effects on the eyes. The drug may be deposited in the corneas and the retina may be affected as well. Persons who take hydroxychloroquine in high doses or for extended periods should be followed by an ophthalmologist. Some persons develop a rash or a mild bleaching of the hair. Hydroxychloroquine should not be taken by alcoholics or those with liver disease.

DRUG INTERACTIONS   Drugs which may damage the liver should not be taken with hydroxychloroquine.

DOSAGE   The dose of drug depends on the disease being treated. For adults the standard dose is 400 mg per day for lupus erythematosus. Lower doses are also used, depending on the patient's condition. For some persons with porphyria cutanea tarda, treatment with one pill several times per week is effective.

HOW SUPPLIED   200 mg tablets

COST   ★★★ (generics are less)

Iodoquinol (Vytone®)   This medication is very popular for inflammatory skin conditions. Iodoquinol is a topical antibiotic effective against some bacteria and fungi. Vytone® is popular for diaper rash, leg ulcers, and some rashes occurring on the face. This cream contains 1% hydrocortisone; this helps with inflammation and irritation but is not strong enough to cause serious long-term side effects.

PRECAUTIONS   This cream may cause mild irritation in persons allergic to it.

DRUG INTERACTIONS   None.

DOSAGE   A small amount of the cream may be applied several times daily.

HOW SUPPLIED   1 oz. tube

COST   ★★

Methoxsalen (Oxsoralen-Ultra® Capsules, Oxsoralen® Lotion)   Methoxsalen is the most popular psoralen compound for use in PUVA treatment. This therapy is useful for psoriasis, lichen planus, and cutaneous T cell lymphoma. This drug should only be used in conjunction with a dermatologist experienced with it. Persons who have taken this drug and then been exposed to extensive sunlight or tanning beds have developed serious and life-threatening sunburns. The lotion form is applied to individual areas on the skin (usually with vitiligo) and avoids the problems with giving the drug by mouth.

PRECAUTIONS   Methoxsalen makes the skin sensitive to ultraviolet light; as a result, persons who take this medication or apply the lotion have to be responsible about sun exposure. Persons with diseases worsened by sunlight such as lupus erythematosus and porphyria, are usually not candidates for PUVA treatment. After taking the drug and having the light therapy, patients must be careful about sun exposure for the following twenty-four hours. Special sunglasses are needed to protect the eyes during that time period as well. Some increased likelihood of skin cancers and precancerous changes are seen in persons who receive PUVA for extended periods.

Mild nausea is the most common side effect from this drug. Taking methoxsalen with milk or food usually helps. This medication may rarely affect the liver and blood counts, so blood work is routinely done. There is also a potential for development or worsening of cataracts, so many dermatologists suggest that treated patients be periodically evaluated by an ophthalmologist.

DRUG INTERACTIONS   Other drugs causing sensitivity to light (tetracyclines, griseofulvin, certain diuretics, and so on) should be taken with great caution or, preferably, avoided altogether.

DOSAGE This drug is given based on the patient's weight. It is taken 90 to 120 minutes before light therapy, preferably in a single dose.

HOW SUPPLIED 10 mg capsule
1 oz. lotion bottle

COST ★★★

Minoxidil (Rogaine®) A potent high blood pressure medication that caused hair growth in persons who took it by mouth. A topical solution was prepared and found to be useful in hair regrowth or preventing hair loss in men and women with male pattern baldness (androgenetic alopecia). It is now available without a prescription and some generic preparations have come on the market. Minoxidil works reasonably well in about one-half to two-thirds of patients but must be used regularly. It must also be used for about six months before a patient can accurately determine whether it will be effective. There is some evidence that the drug loses its effectiveness after several years. Nevertheless, minoxidil is a safe and well-tolerated method for combating male pattern baldness. Alopecia areata may also respond to this medication.

PRECAUTIONS A rare patient may have a slight rash after using minoxidil. There is a rare but possible risk in patients with heart disease and blood pressure problems. If a substantial amount of the drug is absorbed through the skin, heart failure may occur. Persons with such a medical history should check with their doctors before using minoxidil.

DRUG INTERACTIONS Theoretically, the use of other antihypertension medications with minoxidil may cause too great a drop in blood pressure. Guanethidine should not be used with this drug.

DOSAGE One ml of the medication should be applied to the scalp twice daily. Some dermatologists give their patients tretinoin gel for use with the minoxidil since it helps absorption of the drug.

HOW SUPPLIED 60 ml bottle

COST ★★★ (generics are less)

Mupirocin (Bactroban®) This antibacterial ointment is used for wounds or slight skin infections such as impetigo. Only certain types of staphylococci and streptococci are susceptible to this drug but it is very useful for preventing infection of skin surgery sites, scrapes, and cuts.

PRECAUTIONS A rare patient may develop an allergy to this ointment.

DRUG INTERACTIONS Essentially none.

DOSAGE The ointment should be applied several times daily or at each dressing change.

HOW SUPPLIED 15 gm and 30 gm tubes

COST ★★★

Pramoxine (Pramasone®, Zone A Forte®)   This drug is a topical anesthetic that is used to control itching and burning. It is mixed with 1% or 2.5% hydrocortisone; this also helps the itching and inflammation. These medications are very useful for sunburns, eczema, insect bites, and other itchy conditions. They are considered safe for extended use since they contain such low concentrations of hydrocortisone, but should be used with caution in infants and children.

PRECAUTIONS   Some patients develop a mild rash from using these products. They should not be used for a long time without medical supervision.

DRUG INTERACTIONS   None.

DOSAGE   Pramoxine may be applied several times daily as needed.

HOW SUPPLIED   Pramasone® Ointment 1%–1 oz. tube
Pramasone® Ointment 2.5%–1 oz. tube
Pramasone® Cream 1%–1 oz. and 2 oz. tubes
Pramasone® Cream 2.5%–1 oz. and 2 oz. tubes
Pramasone® Lotion 1%–1 oz. tube
Pramasone® Lotion 2.5%–1 oz. tube
Zone A® Cream 1%–1 oz. tube

COST   ★★★ (generics are less)

Prednisone/Prednisolone (Deltasone®, Orasone®, Prelone®)   Prednisone and prednisolone are two corticosteroids used a great deal in dermatology. They are very helpful but must be given with care. When given for short periods of time, they have few significant side effects. The problems with these drugs almost always occur when they are given in moderate to high doses for extended periods. Prednisone reduces inflammation and itching and is most often given for eczema, hives (urticaria), drug reactions, contact dermatitis, vasculitis, and blistering diseases. Use in children may be very helpful but needs to be done with caution. Some skin conditions such as psoriasis may worsen with prednisone, so it is important that it be given by persons with knowledge of skin diseases and experience in their use.

PRECAUTIONS   Prednisone causes side effects such as increased blood pressure, increased blood sugar (which may be a problem for persons with diabetes), retardation of growth in children, cataract formation, worsening of ulcer disease, increased risk of infection, psychiatric symptoms (depression, psychosis, and so on), thinning of the skin, suppressed pituitary and adrenal gland activity, muscle weakness, water retention, increased bruising, and weight gain. Most of these are seen when the drug has been taken for a long time.

DRUG INTERACTIONS   None.

DOSAGE   Dose depends on the disease being treated and its severity. Most dermatologists begin with a daily dose of between 20 and 60 mg given all at once or in divided doses. This may be reduced over several days or a week (a "tapered" dose). Children usually receive between 0.5 and 2.0 mg/kg per day. When the drug will be taken for a long time, the dose may be given every other day.

HOW SUPPLIED   Deltasone® (prednisone)–2.5 mg, 5 mg, 10 mg, 20 mg, and 50 mg tablets

Liquid Pred® (prednisone)–5 mg per teaspoon
Orasone® (prednisone)–2.5 mg, 5 mg, 10 mg, 20 mg, and 50 mg tablets
Prelone® Syrup (prednisolone)–5 mg per teaspoon
Prednisone Tablets–1mg, 2.5 mg, 5 mg, 10 mg, 20 mg, and 50 mg tablets
Prednisone Oral Suspension–5 mg per teaspoon

COST　★★

Salicylic Acid (Occlusal-HP®, Salacid Plaster®, Salactic Film®, Sal-Plant Gel®)　Salicylic acid for use on warts had been available only by prescription. It is now available over the counter. These products usually contain at least 15% salicyclic acid and patches or plasters contain around 40%. These are most helpful for small warts although larger lesions may respond as well if the drug is used long enough. Some of these products contain lactic acid to help the dead skin flake off and the salicylic acid penetrate better.

PRECAUTIONS　Salicylic acid may irritate normal surrounding skin. This medication is not intended for genital warts or those on the mucous membranes.

DRUG INTERACTIONS　None.

DOSAGE　A small amount of the liquid should be applied to the wart and allowed to dry. The area may be covered with a bandage. This should be repeated each day until the wart disappears. Gently removing the buildup once or twice weekly with a pumice stone or emery board is helpful.

HOW SUPPLIED　Duofilm® Liquid–0.5 oz. bottle
Duofilm® Patch for Kids–18 medicated patches
Duoplant® Gel–0.5 oz. bottle
Occlusal-HP®–10 ml bottle
Sal-Acid® Plaster–14 plasters per pack
Salactic® Film–0.5 oz. bottle
Sal-Plant® Gel–0.5 oz. bottle
Trans-plantar® pads
Viranol® Solution–8 gm bottle
Viranol® Gel–8 gm bottle
Viranol® Ultra Gel–8 gm bottle

COST　★★

Triamcinolone (Aristospan®, Kenalog®)　Triamcinolone is a corticosteroid and is available for use as a cream, ointment, spray, and lotion as well as an oral pill and injectable suspension. Tablets may be used as prednisone is taken but this is not common since triamcinolone by mouth usually causes more side effects than does prednisone. The greatest use for this drug is as an intramuscular injection (a shot); however, shots cannot be given too often or the patient will develop the same problems as persons taking prednisone.

PRECAUTIONS　Essentially the same as for prednisone or prednisolone.

DRUG INTERACTIONS　None.

DOSAGE   Triamcinolone can be injected into a treated lesion such as in psoriasis, alopecia areata, or a nail. Under these circumstances, the injected concentration is usually between 1 and 5 mg/ml. It may also be given as an intramuscular injection of between 20 and 60 mg. Children may be rarely given this medication. Shots usually last between ten days and three weeks; then their effects wear off.

HOW SUPPLIED   Aristocort® Forte–40 mg/ml
Aristocort® Intralesional–25 mg/ml
Aristospan®–5 mg per ml and 20 mg/ml
Cinalone®–40 mg/ml
Kenalog®–10 mg/ml
Kenalog®–40 mg/ml

COST   ★★★ (generics are less)

Trioxsalen (Trisoralen®)   Trioxsalen is similar to methoxsalen but is used more for treating vitiligo than psoriasis. The same precautions apply to this drug as to methoxsalen.

PRECAUTIONS   Identical to methoxsalen.

DRUG INTERACTIONS   Identical to methoxsalen.

DOSAGE   Two tablets are taken two to four hours before light therapy preferably as a single dose.

HOW SUPPLIED   5 mg tablet

COST   ★★★

Zinc pyrithione (DermaZinc®)   Zinc pyrithione is a weak antifungal drug found in some types of shampoos (Head & Shoulders®). It is very popular for psoriasis. It is available without a prescription. It appears to be safe but its effectiveness has not been tested. Another product, Skin Cap®, was recently found to include a powerful topical corticosteroid, clobetasol, and is now off the American market.

PRECAUTIONS   Contact with the eyes may cause irritation and stinging.

DRUG INTERACTIONS   Unknown.

DOSAGE   Apply to areas of psoriasis several times daily initially and then taper off until used only several times per week.

HOW SUPPLIED   4 oz. pump spray
Bar soap
Scalp solution
(These must be purchased through Dermalogix Products, Inc. at 1-800-753-0047)

COST   ★★★

SELF-DIAGNOSIS

Acnelike Lesions
Acne vulgaris
Acne rosacea
Chemical induced acne
Cosmetic induced acne
Iodine and bromine toxicity
Medication induced acne
Oil acne
Perioral dermatitis
Secondary syphilis
Steroid acne

Blisters (Large)
Bullous impetigo
Bullous pemphigoid
Contact dermatitis
Drug eruptions
Erythema multiforme
Friction blister
Insect bites
Pemphigus vulgaris and foliaceus
Porphyria
Thermal burn
Toxic epidermal necrolysis

Blisters (Small)
Dermatitis herpetiformis
Dyshidrotic eczema (pompholyx)
Fungal infection of the foot
    (athlete's foot)
Grover's disease
Hand, foot, and mouth disease
Herpes simplex
Herpes zoster (shingles)

Insect bites
Miliaria crystallina
Scabies
Varicella (chickenpox)

Bumps on the Face
Acne rosacea
Acne vulgaris
Adenoma sebaceum
Alopecia mucinosa
Basal cell carcinoma
Blue nevus
Comedone (blackhead)
Fixed drug eruption
Hemangioma
Hydrocystoma
Keloid
Lupus erythematosus
Miliaria
Moles
Molluscum contagiosum
Neurofibroma
Nevus sebaceus
Papular urticaria (insect bites)
Perioral dermatitis
Pilomatricoma
Polymorphous light eruption
Pyogenic granuloma
Sarcoidosis
Sebaceous hyperplasia
Seborrheic keratosis
Squamous cell carcinoma
Syringoma
Trichoepithelioma

Bumps on the Face continued
Wart
Xanthelasma

Hair Loss
Adrogenetic alopecia (male pattern baldness)
Alopecia areata
Dissecting cellulitis of the scalp
Drugs (including chemotherapy)
Endocrine disease (hormonal)
Follicular degeneration syndrome
Hair shaft abnormalities
Illness
Lichen planopilaris
Lupus erythematosus
Radiation exposure
Scalp dermatitis
Secondary syphilis
Telogen effluvium
Traction alopecia
Trichotillomania

Itching Without a Rash
Adrenal disease
Anemia (iron deficiency and others)
Blood disorders
Cancer (some types)
Diabetes
Drug reactions
Anabolic steroids
Antimalarials
Erythromycin estolate
Hormones (estrogen, progesterone, testosterone)
Narcotics
Phenothiazines
Tolbutamide
Vitamin B complexes
HIV disease and AIDS
Kidney failure and hemodialysis
Liver disease
Lymphoma and leukemia

Parasite infestations (i.e., scabies)
Psychiatric disease
Thyroid disease

Lumps and Bumps
Angiokeratoma
Cysts
Dermatofibroma
Dupuytren's contracture
Keloids/Folliculitis keloidalis
Miliaria
Molluscum
Mucocele
Leiomyoma
Lipoma
Lymphangioma
Metastases
Neurofibroma
Pyogenic granuloma
Sebaceous hyperplasia
Seborrheic keratosis (Dermatosis papulosa nigra)
Skin tags
Syringoma

Mouth Ulcers
Aphthous ulcers
Epidermolysis bullosa
Erythema multiforme
Hand, foot, and mouth disease
Herpangina
Herpes simplex
Lichen planus
Pemphigus
Pemphigoid, bullous and cicatricial
Squamous cell carcinoma
Syphilis

Pustules (Localized)
Erythema multiforme
Fungal infection (jock itch, tinea, etc.)
Furuncle (boil)

Hand, foot, and mouth disease
Herpes simplex
Subcorneal pustular dermatosis

Pustules (Widespread)

Acne
Candida infection (yeast)
Folliculitis
Fungal infections
Herpes zoster (shingles)
Impetigo
Insect bites
Intertrigo
Miliaria
Pustular psoriasis
Scabies
Steroid acne
Varicella (chickenpox)

Rashes That Form Lines

Contact dermatitis
Insect bites
Lichen planus
Lichen striatus
Linear epidermal nevus
Shingles (herpes zoster)
Warts

Rashes That Itch

Atopic dermatitis (eczema)
Bullous pemphigoid
Contact dermatitis
Dermatophytosis and Candidal
  infections (fungal infections)
Drug eruptions
Folliculitis
Impetigo
Insect bites
Lichen planus
Lichen simplex chronicus
Mastocytosis
Miliaria

Mycosis fungoides
Parasitic infestations
Scabies and other infestations
Seborrheic dermatitis
Sun sensitivity disorders
Transient acantholytic disease
  (Grover's disease)
Urticaria (hives)
Varicella (chickenpox)
Viral infections
Xerosis

Red and Inflamed Nodules

Atypical mycobacterial infection
Basal cell carcinoma
Erythema nodosum
Foreign body inflammation
Fungal infection
Furuncle/Carbuncle
Kaposi's sarcoma
Keratoacanthoma
Metastases
Polyarteritis nodosa
Pyogenic granuloma
Sarcoidosis
Sporotrichosis
Sweet's syndrome
Vasculitis
Xanthomas

Scaling Skin

Chemical contact (tretinoin, salicylic-
  acid, benzoyl peroxide, etc.)
Drug reactions
Erythroderma (exfoliative dermatitis)
Ichthyosis
Kawasaki's disease
Keratolysis exfoliativa
Scarlet fever
Sunburn and other sun sensitivity
  diseases
Staph scalded skin syndrome
Stevens-Johnson syndrome

Scaling Skin continued
Toxic epidermal necrolysis
Toxic shock syndrome
Viral infections

Spots (Brown)
Acanthosis nigricans
Addison's disease
Amyloidosis
Becker's nevus
Cafe au lait spots (birthmarks)
Drug intake
Fixed drug eruption
Freckles (ephilides)
Lentigo
Melasma
Mongolian spots
Nevus (mole)
Nevus of Ota and Ito
Post inflammatory hyper-
    pigmentation
Seborrheic keratosis
Sun sensitivity disorders

Spots (White)
Albinism
Chemical depigmentation
Halo nevus without a nevus
Idiopathic guttate hypomelanosis
Lichen sclerosus

Lupus erythematosus
Morphea or scleroderma
Pityriasis alba
Post inflammatory hypo-pigmentation
Radiation dermatitis
Tinea versicolor
Vitiligo

Ulcerations
Burns
Chancroid
Decubitus
Fungal infection
Hypertension ulcer
Pyoderma gangrenosum
Sickle cell ulcer
Stasis ulcers
Syphilis
Trauma

Widespread Red Bumps
Eruptive xanthomas
Folliculitis
Insect bites
Miliaria
Papular drug eruption
Pityriasis lichenoides et varioli-
    formis acuta (PLEVA)
Scabies

SKIN DISEASE ORGANIZATIONS

American Academy of Dermatology
980 North Meacham Road
Schaumburg, IL 60173-4965
847-330-0230
Fax 847-330-0050
www.aad.org

American Cancer Society
1599 Clifton Road, NE
Atlanta, GA 30329
1-800-227-2345
404-320-3333
Fax 404-325-2217

American Celiac Society (Dermatitis
    Herpetiformis)
58 Musano Court
West Orange, NJ 07052
201-325-8837

American College of Mohs Micrographic
    Surgery and Cutaneous Oncology
930 North Meacham Road
Schaumburg, IL 60173-6016
708-330-9830
Fax 708-330-0050

American Foundation for AIDS Research
733 3rd Avenue, 12th Floor
New York, NY 10017
212-682-7440
Fax 212-682-9812

American Lupus Society
3914 Del Amo Boulevard, Suite 922
Torrance, CA 90503
310-542-8891
1-800-331-1802
Charlean Wakefield

American Melanoma Foundation
USC/Norris Cancer Center
2025 Zonal Avenue
GH-10-442
Los Angeles, CA 90033-1034
213-226-6352
Fax 213-224-6925

American Porphyria Foundation
P.O. Box 22712
Houston, TX 77227
713-266-9617
Fax 713-871-1788
Desiree Lyon, Executive Director
www.enterprise.net/apf/

American Skin Association
150 East 58th Street, 33rd floor
New York, NY 10155-0002
212-753-8260
1-800-499-SKIN
Fax 212-688-6547
Joyce Weidler, Managing Director

American Society of Dermatopathology
3601 Fourth Street, Suites 4A-118
Lubbock, TX 79430
806-743-1106
Fax 806-743-1609

American Society for Dermatologic
  Surgery
930 North Meacham Road
Schaumburg, IL 60173-6016
708-330-9830
Fax 708-330-0050

Arthritis Foundation
P.O. Box 1900
Atlanta, GA 30326
404-872-7100
1-800-283-7800

American Behcet's Foundation, Inc.
P.O. Box 54063
Minneapolis, MN 55454-0063
1-800-723-4238
1-800-7BEHCETS

Canadian Psoriasis Foundation
1565 Carling Avenue
1306 Wellington Street, Suite 500F
Ottawa, Ontario CANADA K1Y-3B2
613-728-4000
(In Canada: 1-800-265-0926)

Congenital Nevus Support Group
2585 Treehouse Drive
Lake Ridge, VA 22192
703-492-0253
405-377-3403

Dermatology Foundation
1560 Sherman Avenue, Suite 302
Evanston, IL 60201-4802
708-328-2256
Sandra Rahn Goldman, Executive
  Director

Dermatopathology Foundation
P.O. Box 377
Canton, MA 02021
617-821-0648
Wendy Christison

Dystrophic Epidermolysis Bullosa
  Research Association of America, Inc.
  (D.E.B.R.A.)
40 Rector Street
New York, NY 10006
212-513-4090
Miriam Feder, Executive Director

Ehlers Danlos National Foundation
6399 Wilshire Boulevard, Suite 510
Los Angeles, CA 90048
213-651-3038
www.stgenesis.org/EDS/ednf.html

Ehlers Danlos Syndrome Foundation
P.O. Box 1212
Southgate, MI 48195
313-282-0180
Fax 313-282-2793
Nancy Rogowski, Executive Director

Fanconi's Anemia International Registry
c/o Arleen Auerbach, Ph.D.
Laboratory for Investigative Dermatology
The Rockefeller University
1230 York Avenue
New York, NY 10021-6399
212-327-8862

Foundation for Ichthyosis and Related
  Skin Types (F.I.R.S.T.)
P.O. Box 669
Ardmore, PA 19003-0669
1-800-545-3286
e-mail: 74722.1571@compuserve.com

Gluten Intolerance Group of North
    America (Dermatitis Herpetiformis)
P.O. Box 23503
Seattle, WA 98102-0353
206-325-6980

Histiocytosis Association of America, Inc.
609 New York Road
Glassboro, NJ 08028
609-881-4911

Human Papillomavirus Support Program
American Social Health Association
P.O. Box 13827
Research Triangle Park, NC 27709
1-800-227-8922

International Society for Dermatologic
    Surgery
930 North Meacham Road
Schaumburg, IL 60173-6016
708-330-9830
Fax 708-330-0050

International Society of Cosmetic Laser
    Surgeons, Inc.
415 Pier Avenue
Hermosa Beach, CA 90254
310-372-8802
Fax 310-318-6369

International Society of Hair Restoration
    Surgery
930 North Meacham Road
Schaumburg, IL 60173-6016
708-330-9830
Fax 708-330-0050

Lupus Foundation of America, Inc.
1300 Picard Drive, Suite 200
Rockville, MD 20850-4503
301-670-9292
1-800-558-0121
Fax 301-670-9486
John Huber, Executive Director
Barbara Butler, Board of Directors
www.lupus.org/lupus

Melanoma Foundation
750 Menlo Avenue, Suite 250
Menlo Park, CA 94025
Marsden S. Bloise, M.D., President

Muscular Dystrophy Association (MDA)
3300 East Sunrise Drive
Tucson, AZ 85718-3208
1-800-572-1717
www.mdusa.org

National Alopecia Areata Foundation
710 "C" Street, Suite 11
P.O. Box 150760
San Rafael, CA 94915-0760
415-456-4644
Fax 415-456-4274
e-mail: 74301.1642@compuserve.com
Vicki Kalabokes, Executive Director
http://weber.u.washington.edu/~dvic-
    tor/natl.html

National Arthritis and Musculoskeletal
    and Skin Diseases Information
    Clearinghouse
National Institutes of Health
1 AMS Circle
Bethesda, MD 20892-3675

National Association for Pseudoxanthoma
  Elasticum
1420 Ogden Street
Denver, CO 80218-1910
303 832-5055
Fax 806 743-1603
e-mail: derkhn@ttuhsc.edu
Al Ferrari, President

National Cancer Institute
Office of Communications
National Institute for Health
9000 Rockville Pike
Building 31, Room 10A31
Bethesda, MD 20892
301-496-6631
1-800-4-CANCER Cancer Information
  Service
Fax 301-402-4945
Paul Van Nevel, Associate Director

National Congenital Port Wine Stain
  Foundation
123 East 63rd Street
New York, NY 10021
516-867-5137
Fax 516-869-1278

National Eczema Association
1221 SW Yamhill, Suite 303
Portland, OR 90035
503-228-4430
Fax 503-228-4430
Irene Crosby, Board of Directors

National Eczema Society
Travistock House North
London WC1 9SR United Kingdom
01-38804097

National Epidermolysis Bullosa Registry
Clinical Coordinating Center
University of North Carolina—Chapel Hill
Department of Dermatology
Room 137—NCMH
Chapel Hill, NC 27514
919-966-3321
919-966-6383

National Foundation for Ectodermal
  Dysplasia
219 East Main Street, Box 114
Mascoutah, IL 62258
618-566-2020
FAX 618-566-4718
e-mail: NFED1@aol.com
Mary Kaye Richter, Executive Director
www.nfed.org

National Foundation for Vitiligo and
  Pigment Disorders
9032 South Normandy Drive
Centerville, OH 45459
513-885-5739

National Herpes Hotline
919-361-8485

National Herpes Resource Center
American Social Health Association
P.O. Box 13827
Research Triangle Park, NC 27709
919-361-8488

National Incontinentia Pigmenti
  Foundation
41 East 57th Street, 5th Floor
New York, NY 10022
212-207-4636
Fax   212-371-7345
e-mail: nipf@pipeline.com
Susanne Bross Emmerich, Executive
  Director
http://medhlp.netusa.net/www/nipf.htm

National Marfan Foundation
382 Main Street
Port Washington, NY 11050
516-883-8712
1-800-8-MARFAN
Fax 516-883-8712
e-mail: staff@marfan.org
Carolyn Levering, Executive Director
www.marfan.org

National Neurofibromatosis Foundation
95 Pine Street, 16th Floor
New York, NY 10005
1-800-323-7938
Fax 212 747-0004
e-mail: NNFF@aol.com
Peter R.W. Bellerman, President

National Organization for Albinism and
    Hypopigmentation
1530 Locust Street, Box 29
Philadelphia, PA 19102-4415
215-545-2322
1-800-473-2310
e-mail: noah@albinism.org
www.albinism.org/

National Pediculosis Association
P.O. Box 149
Newton, MA 02161
617-449-6487
Deborah Altschuler, Executive Director

National Pemphigus Vulgaris Foundation
P.O. Box 9606
Berkeley, CA 94709-0606
510-527-4970

National Porphyria Foundation
P.O. Box 22712
Houston, TX 77227
713-266-9617

National Psoriasis Foundation
6600 SW 92nd, Suite 300
Portland, OR 97223
503-244-7404
1-800-723-9166
Fax 503-245-0626
e-mail: 76135.2746@compuserve.com
Gail M. Zimmerman, Executive Director
www.psoriasis.org

National Registry for Ichthyosis and
    Related Disorders
Dermatology, Box 356524
University of Washington
Seattle, WA 98195-6524
Geoff Hamill, R.N., Registry Coordinator
e-mail: geoff@u.washington.edu
Philip Fleckman, M.D., Principal
    Investigator
e-mail: fleck@u.washington.edu
1-800-595-1265

National Rosacea Society
220 South Cook Street, Suite 201
Barrington, IL 60010
708-382-8971
Fax 708-382-5567
Suzanne Corr, Director

National Sjögren Syndrome Association
21630 North 19th Avenue
Phoenix, AZ 85027
602-516-0787
Fax 602-516-0111

National Tuberous Sclerosis Association
1-8000 Corporate Drive, Suite 120
Landover, MD 20785
Carolyn Wilson, Director
301-459-9888
1-800-225-6872

National Vitiligo Foundation, Inc.
Box 6337
305 South Broadway, Suite 403
Tyler, TX 75711
903-534-2925
Fax 903-534-8075
e-mail: 73071.33@compuserve.com
Allen C. Locklin, President
Cheryl McInnis, Executive Director
www.nvfi.com

National Vulvodynia Association
P.O. Box 4491
Silver Spring, MD 20914-4491
301-299-0775
www.ivf.com

Nevoid Basal Cell Carcinoma Syndrome
    Support Network
162 Clover Hill Street
Marlboro, MA 01752
508-485-4873
1-800-815-4447
Fax 213-244-6925
e-mail: Souldansur@aol.com
Susan A. Charron, Executive Director

North American Society of Phlebology
930 North Meacham Road
Schaumburg, IL 60173-6016
708-330-9830
Fax 708-330-0050

Pediatric AIDS Foundation
1311 Colorado Avenue
Santa Monica, CA 90404
310-395-9051
Fax 310-395-5149

Plastic Surgery Research Foundation
P.O. Box 2586
La Jolla, CA 92038
619-454-3212
Edith Brookstein, Director

PFB Project (Pseudofolliculitis Barbae)
1875 Connecticut Avenue, Suite 1140
Washington, DC 20009-5728
202-588-5300
Melvin A. Alexander, Director

Pseudoxanthoma Elasticum International
23 Mountain Street
Sharon, MA 02067-2234
617-784-8006
617-784-3817
Fax 617-749-6538
e-mail: Tshar@aol.com
Sharon Terry, President
www.med.harvard.edu/programs/PXE

Psoriasis Society of Canada
National Office
P.O. Box 25015
Halifax, NS B3M 4H4 Canada
902-443-8680
Fax 902-457-1664

San Francisco AIDS Foundation
P.O. Box 6182
San Francisco, CA 94101-6182
415-863-AIDS
Pat Christen, Director

Sarcoidosis Family Aid and Medical
    Research Foundation
460 Central Avenue
East Orange, NJ 07018
201-399-3644
1-800-203-6429
Geneva Ausley, President and Founder

Scleroderma Federation
Peabody Office Building
One Newbury Street
Peabody MA 01960
508-535-6600
1-800-422-1113
Fax 508-535-6696
Jacqueline Magoon, Director
www.scleroderma.org

Scleroderma Info Exchange, Inc.
150 Hines Farm Road
Cranston, RI 02921
401-943-3909
Nancy D. Hersy, Executive Director

Scleroderma Society
1725 York Avenue, Suite 29-F
New York, NY 10128
212-427-7040
Mark Flagan, Ph.D., President

Scleroderma Research Foundation
Pueblo Medical Commons
2320 Bath Street, Suite 307
Santa Barbara, CA 93105
805-563-9133
Fax 805-563-2402
Shael Johnson, Executive Director

Sjögren's Syndrome Foundation, Inc.
333 North Broadway, Suite 2000
Jericho, NY 11753
516-933-6365
www.sjogrens.com

Skin Cancer Foundation
245 Fifth Avenue, Suite 2402
New York, NY 10016
212-725-5176
Fax 212-725-5751
Mitzi Moulds, Executive Director

Society of Dermatology Physician
  Assistants
5705 NE 116th Street
Vancouver, WA 98686
360-574-6919
e-mail: jomonroe@pacifier.com
Joe Monroe, Director
www.halcyon.com/physasst

Sturge-Weber Foundation
P.O. Box 418
Mt. Freedom, NJ 07970-0418
1-800-627-5482
Fax 210-895-4846
Karen Ball, Executive Director
www.inforamp.net

United Scleroderma Foundation
P.O. Box 399
Watsonville, CA 95077-0399
408-728-2202
1-800-722-HOPE
Fax 408-728-3328
e-mail: outreach@scleroderma.com
Robert J. Riggs, Executive Director
www.scleroderma.com

VZV Research Foundation (Chicken Pox/
  Shingles [Varicella/zoster])
36 East 72nd Street
New York, NY 10021
212-472-3181

Xeroderma Pigmentosum Society
57 Sleight Plass Road
Poughkeepsie, NY 12603
914-473-4735
e-mail: jcqc92a@prodigy.com
Caren J. Mahar, Director

BIBLIOGRAPHY

Abeck, D. "Chancroid." *Current Problems in Dermatology* 24 (1996): 90–96.

Adams-Gandhi, L.B. "Diagnosis and management of dermatomyositis." *Comprehensive Therapy* 22 (1996): 156–64.

Al-Ghazal, S.K. "Merkel cell carcinoma of the skin." *British Journal of Plastic Surgery* 49 (1996): 491–96.

Allen, R.A. "Pityriasis rosea." *Cutis* 56 (1995): 198–202.

Aly, R. "Common superficial fungal infections in patients with AIDS." *Clinical Infectious Diseases* 22 (1996): S128–S132.

Andress, C.J. "Perleche: report of a case." *ASCD Journal of Dentistry for Children* 50 (1983): 228.

Arvin, A.M. "Varicella zoster virus: overview and clinical manifestations." Seminars in Dermatology 15 (1996): 4–7.

Assaf, R.R. "The superficial mycoses." *Dermatologic Clinics* 14 (1996): 57.

Azana, J.M. "Urticaria pigmentosa: a review of 67 pediatric cases." *Pediatric Dermatology* 11 (1994): 102–106.

Bailey, R.E. "Diagnosis and treatment of infectious mononucleosis." *American Family Physician* 49 (1994): 879–88.

Barrenetxea, G. "Pruritic urticarial papules and plaques of pregnancy." *International Journal of Gynecology and Obstetrics* 33 (1990): 69–72.

Barron, D.F. "Granuloma annulare: a clinical review." *Lippincotts Primary Care Practice* 1 (1997): 33–39.

Becker, B.A. "Pemphigus vulgaris and vegetans." *Dermatologic Clinics* 11 (1993): 429–53.

Beltrani, V.S. "Contact dermatitis." *Annals of Allergy, Asthma, and Immunology* 78 (1997): 160–73.

—————. "Urticaria and angioedema." *Dermatologic Clinics* 14 (1996): 171–98.

Berger, B.W. "Current aspects of Lyme disease and other Borrelia burgdorferi infections." *Clinics in Dermatology* 15 (1997): 247–55.

Bergfeld, W.F. "Androgenetic alopecia: an autosomal dominant disorder." *American Journal of Medicine* 98 (1995): 95S–98S.

Berman, J.D. "Human leishmanisis." *Clinical Infectious Diseases* 24 (1997): 684–703.

Boyd, A.S. "Lichen planus." *Journal of the American Academy of Dermatology* 25 (1991): 593.

—————. "Typhus disease group." *International Journal of Dermatology* 31 (1992): 823–32.

Breathnach, A.S. "Melanin hyperpigmentation of skin: melasma, topical treatment with azalaic acid and other therapies." *Cutis* 57 (1996): S36–S45.

Brehler, R. "Recent developments in the treatment of atopic eczema." *Journal of the American Academy of Dermatology* 36 (1997): 983.

Brown, M. "Insect repellents: an overview." *Journal of the American Academy of Dermatology* 36 (1997): 243–49.

Burkhart, C.G. "An assessment of topical and oral prescription and over-the-counter treatment for head lice." *Journal of the American Academy of Dermatology* 38 (1998): 979–82.

Casson, P. "Dysplastic and congenital nevi." *Clinics in Plastic Surgery* 20 (1993): 105–111.

Clark, C.P. "Alpha hydroxy acids in skin care." *Clinics in Plastic Surgery* 23 (1996): 49–56.

Cohen, D.J. "Porphyria cutanea tarda: a clinical review." *Comprehensive Therapy* 22 (1996): 175–78.

Cohen, L.M. "Lentigo maligna and lentigo maligna melanoma." *Journal of the American Academy of Dermatology* 33 (1995): 923–36.

Cohen, P.R. "Pityriasis rubra pilaris: a review of diagnosis of treatment." *Journal of the American Academy of Dermatology* 20 (1989): 801–807.

Colven, R.M. "Topical vitamin C in aging." *Clinics in Dermatology* 14 (1996): 227–34.

Conant, H.A. "Genital herpes: an integrated approach to management." *Journal of the American Academy of Dermatology* 35 (1996): 601–605.

Daniel, C.R. "Traditional management of onychomycosis." *Journal of the American Academy of Dermatology* 35 (1996): 521–25.

David, T.J. "Dietary regimens for atopic dermatitis in childhood." *Journal of the Royal Society of Medicine* 90, S30 (1997): 9–14.

Denning, D.W. "Fungal nail disease." *British Medical Journal* 311 (1995): 1277–81.

Dillon, M.J. "Vasculitis in children and adolescents." *Rheumatologic Disease Clinics in North America* 21 (1995): 1115–36.

du Peloux Manage, H. "Aquagenic pruritus." *Seminars in Dermatology* 14 (1995): 313–16.

Egeler, R.M. "Langerhans cell histiocytosis." *Journal of Pediatrics* 127 (1995): 1–11.

Elewski, B. "Tinea capitis." *Dermatologic Clinics* 14 (1996): 23–32.

Elgart, G.W. "Ant, bee, and wasp stings." *Dermatologic Clinics* 8 (1990): 229–36.

Epstein, E. "Hand dermatitis: practical management and current concepts." *Journal of the American Academy of Dermatology* 10 (1984): 395–424.

Estes, S.A. "Therapy of scabies." *Seminars in Dermatology* 12 (1993): 26–33.

Fabbri, P. "Erythema multiforme and drug intake." *Clinics in Dermatology* 11 (1993): 479–89.

Fazio, V.W. "The management of perianal diseases." *Advances in Surgery* 29 (1996): 59–78.

Feng, E. "Miliaria." *Cutis* 55 (1995): 213–16.

Fiedler, V.C. "Treatment of alopecia areata." *Dermatologic Clinics* 14 (1996): 733–37.

Fiumara, N.J. "The diagnosis and treatment of infectious syphilis." *Comprehensive Therapy* 21 (1995): 639–44.

Garwood, J.D. "Keratosis pilaris." *American Family Physician* 17 (1978): 151–52.

Ghadially, R. "Ichthyoses and hyperkeratotic disorders." *Dermatologic Clinics* 10 (1992): 597–607.

Ghersetich, I. "A pathogenic approach to the management of systemic sclerosis (scleroderma)." *International Journal of Dermatology* (1990)29: 616–622.

Gibson, L.E. "Cutaneous vasculitis." *Rheumatic Diseases Clinics of North America* 21 (1995): 1097–113.

Glogaur, R.G. "Chemical peels." *Dermatologic Clinics* 13 (1995): 263–76.

————. "Chemical peels. Trichloroacetic acid and phenol." *Dermatologic Clinics* (1995)13: 263–76.

Gloster, H.H. "Dermatofibrosarcoma protuberans." *Journal of the American Academy of Dermatology* 35 (1996): 355–74.

Goihman-Vahr, M. "Skin aging and photoaging: an outlook." *Clinics in Dermatology* 14 (1996): 153–60.

Gold, E. "Almost extinct diseases: measles, mumps, rubella, and pertussis." *Pediatrics in Review* 17 (1996): 120–27.

Goldberg, L.H. "Basal cell carcinoma." *Lancet* 347 (1996): 663–67.

Goldman, M.P. "Diagnosis and treatment of varicose veins: a review." *Journal of the American Academy of Dermatology* 31 (1994): 393–415.

Goodfield, M. "Optimal management of chronic leg ulcers in the elderly." *Drugs & Aging* 10 (1997): 341–48.

Gorlin, R.J. "Nevoid basal cell carcinoma syndrome." *Dermatologic Clinics* 13 (1995): 113–25.

Gottleib, S.L., et al. "Molluscum contagiosum." *International Journal of Dermatology* 33 (1994): 453–61.

Graham-Brown, R. "Soaps and detergents in the elderly." *Clinics in Dermatology* 14 (1996): 85–87.

Green, H.A. "Aging, sun damage and sunscreens." *Clinics in Plastic Surgery* 20 (1993): 1–8.

Griffin, E.I. "Hair transplantation. The fourth decade." *Dermatologic Clinics* 13 (1995): 363–87.

Gross, D.J. "A widespread hemorrhagic and crusted eruption of recent onset. Pityriasis lichenoides et varioliformis acuta. (PLEVA)." *Archives of Dermatology* 129 (1993): 365.

Guercio-Hauer, C. "Photodamage, photoaging, and photoprotection of the skin." *American Family Physician* 50 (1994): 327–34.

Guitart, J. "Intertrigo: a practical approach." *Comprehensive Therapy* 20 (1994): 402–409.

Guzzo, C. "Recent advances in the treatment of psoriasis." *Dermatologic Clinics* 15 (1997): 59–68.

Hagermarck, O. "Treatment of itch." *Seminars in Dermatology* 14 (1995): 320–25.

Haik, B.G. "Capillary hemangioma." *Survey of Ophthalmology* 38 (1994): 399–426.

Hannuksel, M. "Erythema multiforme." *Clinics in Dermatology* 4 (1986): 88–95.

Headington, J.T. "Cicatricial alopecia." *Dermatologic Clinics* 14 (1996): 773–82.

Helm, K.F. "Juvenile melanoma (Spitz nevus)." *Cutis* 58 (1996): 35–39.

Hochman, L.G. "Paronychia: more than just an abscess." *International Journal of Dermatology* 34 (1995): 385–86.

Hogan, D.J. "Perioral dermatitis." *Current Problems in Dermatology* 22 (1995): 98–104.

Hom, D.B. "Irradiated soft tissue and its management." *Otolaryngology Clinics of North America* 28 (1995): 1003–19.

Huff, J.C. "Erythema multiforme: a critical review of characteristics, diagnostic criteria, and causes." *Journal of the American Academy of Dermatology* 8 (1993): 763.

Hughes R.A. "Reiter's syndrome and reactive arthritis: a current view." *Seminars in Arthritis and Rheumatism* 24 (1994): 190–210.

Huilgol, S.C. "Management of the immunobullous disorders. II. Pemphigus." *Clinical and Experimental Dermatology* 20 (1995): 283–93.

Jackson, E.M. "Moisturizers." *American Journal of Contact Dermatitis* 7 (1996): 247–50.

Janniger, C.K. "Seborrheic dermatitis." *American Family Physician* 52 (1995): 149–60.

Jansen, T. "Pathogenesis and treatment of acne in children." *Pediatric Dermatology* 14 (1997): 17–21.

—————. Rosacea. "Classification and treatment." *Journal of the Royal College of Medicine* 90 (1997): 144–50.

Johnson, T.M. "Current therapy for cutaneous melanoma." *Journal of the American Academy of Dermatology* 32 (1995): 689–707.

Jones, R.O. "Lichen simplex chronicus." *Clinics in Podiatric Medicine & Surgery* (1996)13: 47–54.

Kennedy, D. "Lichen striatus." *Pediatric Dermatology* 13 (1996): 95–99.

Kilmer, S.L. "Laser treatment of tattoos." *Dermatologic Clinics* 15 (1997): 409–17.

King, L.E. "Treatment of brown recluse spider bites." *Journal of the American Academy of Dermatology* 14 (1986): 691.

Kirchner, J.T. "Erythema infectiosum and other parvovirus B 19 infections." *American Family Physician* 50 (1994): 335–41.

Korman, N.J. "Bullous pemphigoid." *Dermatologic Clinics* 11 (1993): 483–98.

Kurzl, R.G. "Paget's disease." *Seminars in Dermatology* 15 (1996): 60–66.

Laman, S.D. "Cutaneous manifestations of lupus erythematosus." *Rheumatic Diseases Clinics of North America* 20 (1994): 195–212.

Lawrence, N. "Liposuction." *Advances in Dermatology* 11 (1996): 19–49.

Lee, M.M. "Bowen's disease." *Clinics in Dermatology* 11 (1993): 43–46.

Le Poole, C. "Vitiligo." *Seminars in Cutaneous Medicine and Surgery* 16 (1997): 3–14.

Lesher, J.L. "Recent developments in antifungal therapy." *Dermatologic Clinics* 14 (1996): 163.

Leung, A.K. "Hair loss in children." *Journal of the Royal Society of Health* 113 (1993): 252–56.

Linhardt, P.W. "Prurigo nodularis." *Journal of Family Practice* 37 (1993): 495–98.

Lorincz, A.L. "Cutaneous T cell lymphoma." *Lancet* 347 (1996): 871–76.

Luz Ramos, M. "Acne keloidalis and tufted hair folliculitis." *Dermatology* 194(1997): 71–73.

Lynch, P.J. "Delusions of parasitosis." *Seminars in Dermatology* 12 (1993): 39–45.

McDonald, L.L. "Sexually transmitted diseases update." *Dermatologic Clinics* 15 (1997): 221–32.

McFarlane, R. "Dupuytren's disease." *Journal of Hand Therapy* 10 (1997): 8–13.

McNally, M.A. "Conditions peculiar to the tongue." *Dermatologic Clinics* 14 (1996): 257–72.

Mana, J., et al. "Cutaneous involvement in sarcoidosis." *Archives of Dermatology* 133 (1997): 882–88.

Masri-Fridling, G.D. "Dermatophytosis of the feet." *Dermatologic Clinics* 14 (1996): 33–40.

Matsuoka, L.Y. "Acanthosis nigricans." *Clinics in Dermatology* 11 (1993): 21–25.

————. "Acne and its related disorders." *Clinics in Plastic Surgery* 20 (1993): 35–41.

Meade, R.H. "Exanthem subitum (roseola infantum)." *Clinics in Dermatology* 7 (1989): 92–96.

Meffert, J.J. "Lichen sclerosus." *Journal of the American Academy of Dermatology* 32 (1995): 393–416.

Menage, H.D. "The red face: chronic actinic dermatitis." *Clinics in Dermatology* 11 (1993): 297–305.

Michael, S. "Lasers in dermatology." *Journal of the American Academy of Dermatology* 34 (1996): 1–25.

Midgley, G. "Nail infections." *Dermatologic Clinics* 14 (1996): 41–50.

Miller, P.K. "Focal mucinosis (myxoid cyst)." *Journal of Dermatologic Surgery and Oncology* 18 (1992): 716–19.

Mitchell, H. "Scleroderma and related conditions." *Medical Clinics of North America* 81 (1997): 129–49.

Mulvihill, C.A. "Swimmer's itch: a cercarial dermatitis." *Cutis* 46 (1990): 211–13.

Murad, H. "The use of glycolic acid as a peeling agent." *Dermatologic Clinics* 13 (1995): 285–367.

Mutasim, D.F. "Cicatricial pemphigoid." *Dermatologic Clinics* 11 (1993): 499–510.

Nedwich, J.A. "Summer and skin." *Australian Family Physician* 21 (1992): 35–41.

Orentreich, N. "Dermabrasion." *Dermatologic Clinics* 13 (1995): 2313–27.

O'Sullivan, S.T. "Aetiology and management of hypertrophic scars and keloids." *Annals of the Royal College of Surgeons of England* 78 (1996): 168–75.

Orlow, S.J. "Albinism: an update." *Seminars in Cutaneous Medicine and Surgery* 16 (1997): 24–29.

Parks, R.W. "Pathogenesis, clinical features, and management of hidradenitis suppurativa." *Annals of the Royal College of Surgeons of England* 79 (1997): 83–89.

Parsons, J.M. "Transient acantholytic dermatosis: a global perspective." *Journal of the American Academy of Dermatology* 35 (1996): 653–66.

Pearson, R.W. "Clinicopathologic types of epidermolysis bullosa and their nondermatological complications." *Archives of Dermatology* 124 (1988): 718–25.

Peters, W. "The chemical peel." *Annals of Plastic Surgery* 26 (1991): 564–71.

Piacquadia, D.J. "Topical corticosteroids in clinical practice." *Cutis* 57 (1996): 4–9.

Poland, J.M. "Current therapeutic management of recurrent herpes labialis." *General Dentistry* 42 (1994): 46–50.

Powell, F.C. "Glossodynia and other disorders of the tongue." *Dermatologic Clinics* 5 (1987): 687–693.

Prasad, S.M. "Molluscum contagiosum." *Pediatrics in Review* 17 (1996): 118–19.

Pulla, R.J. "Frostbite." *Journal of Foot & Ankle Surgery* 33 (1994): 53–63.

Ramsay, C.A. "Solar urticaria." *International Journal of Dermatology* 19 (1980): 233–36.

Ray, M.C. "Dermatologic manifestations of HIV infection and AIDS." *Infectious Diseases Clinics of North America* 8 (1994): 583–605.

Rees, T.D. "Recurrent aphthous stomatitis." *Dermatologic Clinics* 14 (1996): 243–56.

Roenigk, H. "Methotrexate in psoriasis: revised guidelines." *Journal of the American Academy of Dermatology* 19 (1988): 145–56.

Rogers, M. "Epidermal nevi and the epidermal nevus syndrome: a review of 233 cases." *Pediatric Dermatology* 9 (1992): 342–44.

Rothe, M.J. "Atopic dermatitis: an update." *Journal of the American Academy of Dermatology* 35 (1996): 1–13.

Roujeau, J.C. "Severe adverse cutaneous reactions to drugs." *New England Journal of Medicine* 331 (1994): 1272–85.

Russo, G.G. "Hyperlipidemia." *Current Problems in Dermatology* 22 (1995): 98–104.

Sadick, N.S. "Current aspects of bacterial infections of the skin." *Dermatologic Clinics* 15 (1997): 341–49.

Sahn, E.E. "Alopecia areata in childhood." *Seminars in Dermatology* 14 (1995): 9–14.

Scherwitz, C. "So-called cellulite." *Journal of Dermatologic Surgery and Oncology* 4 (1978): 230–34.

Schiller, P.L. "Angiokeratomas: an update." *Dermatology* 193 (1996): 275–82.

Schwartz, R.A. "Acanthosis nigricans." *Journal of the American Academy of Dermatology* 31 (1994): 1–19.

————. "Keratoacanthoma." *Journal of the American Academy of Dermatology* 30 (1994): 1–19.

————. "Kaposi's sarcoma: advances and perspectives." *Journal of the American Academy of Dermatology* 34 (1996): 804–14.

Sehgal, V.N. "Porokeratosis." *Journal of Dermatology* 23 (1996): 517–25.

Sherrard, J. "Modern diagnosis and management of gonorrhea." *British Journal of Hospital Medicine* 55 (1996): 394–98.

Ship, J.A. "Recurrent aphthous stomatitis. An update." *Oral Surgery, Oral Medicine, Oral Pathology, Oral Radiology, and Endodontics* 81 (1996): 141–47.

Shornick, J.K. "Herpes gestationis." *Dermatologic Clinics* 11 (1993): 527–33.

Shriner, D.L. "Impetigo." *Cutis* 56 (1995): 30–32.

Shulman, S.T. "Kawasaki disease." *Comprehensive Therapy* 23 (1997): 13–18.

Sibbald, R.G. "Skin and diabetes." E*ndocrinology & Metabolism Clinics of North America* 25 (1996): 463–72.

Siegfried, E.C. "Warts on children: an approach to therapy." *Pediatric Annals* 25 (1996): 79–90.

Silber, J.L. "Rocky Mountain Spotted Fever." *Clinics in Dermatology* 14 (1996): 245–58.

Silva-Lizama, E. "Tinea versicolor." *International Journal of Dermatology* 34 (1995): 611–17.

Singalavanija, S. "Diaper dermatitis." *Pediatrics in Review* 16 (1995): 142–47.

Smith, E.P. "Dermatitis herpetiformis and linear IgA bullous dermatosis." *Dermatologic Clinics* 11 (1993): 511–26.

Sober, A.J. "Precursors to skin cancer." *Cancer* 75 (1995): 645–50.

Sodaify, M. "Erythromelanosis follicularis faciei et colli." *International Journal of Dermatology* 33 (1994): 643–44.

Spach, D.H. "Tick-borne disease in the United States." *New England Journal of Medicine* 329 (1993): 936–47.

Spencer, J.M. "Indoor tanning: risks, benefits, and future trends." *Journal of the American Academy of Dermatology* 33 (1995): 288–98.

Steere, A.C. "Lyme disease." *New England Journal of Medicine* 321 (1989): 586–96.

Stegman, S.J. "Basal cell carcinoma and squamous cell carcinoma." *Medical Clinics of North America* 70 (1986): 95–107.

Sterling, J. "Treating the troublesome wart." *Practitioner* 239 (1995): 44–47.

Stevens, D.L. "The toxic shock syndromes." *Infectious Disease Clinics of North America* 10 (1996): 727–46.

Stitt, V.J. "Stevens-Johnson syndrome: a review of the literature." *Journal of the National Medical Association* 80 (1988): 104, 106–108.

Sugita, Y. "Leprosy." *Clinics in Dermatology* 13 (1995): 235–43.

Sykes, N.L. "Condyloma acuminatum." *International Journal of Dermatology* 34 (1995): 297–307.

Thiboutot, D.M. "An overview of acne and its treatment." *Cutis* 57 (1996): 8–12.

Thomas, I. "Hand, foot, and mouth disease." *Cutis* 52 (1993): 265–66.

Thomson, H. "Cutaneous hemangiomas and lymphangiomas." *Clinics in Plastic Surgery* 14 (1987): 341–56.

Tyring, S.K. "Reactive erythemas: erythema annulare centrifugum and erythema gyratum repens." *Clinics in Dermatology* 11 (1993): 135–139.

Van Poppel, G. "Vitamins and cancer." *Cancer Letters* 114 (1997): 195–202.

Van Praag, M.C. "Diagnosis and treatment of polymorphous light eruption." *International Journal of Dermatology* 33 (1994): 233–39.

Weightman, W. "Toxic epidermal necrolysis." *Australasian Journal of Dermatology* 37 (1996): 167–75.

Weiss, R.A. "Advances in sclerotherapy." *Dermatologic Clinics* 13 (1995): 431–45.

Wheeland, R.G. "Cosmetic use of lasers." *Dermatologic Clinics* 13 (1995): 447–59.

White, A.D. "Sunburn. Management and prevention." *Australian Family Physician* 17 (1988): 953–54.

Wilson, D.C. and L.E. King. "Spiders and spider bites." *Dermatologic Clinics* 8 (1990): 277.

——————. "Erythroderma and exfoliative dermatitis." *Clinics in Dermatology* 11 (1993): 67–72.

Winchester, R. "Psoriatic arthritis." *Dermatologic Clinics* 17 (1995): 779–92.

Wojnarowska, F. "Chronic bullous disease of childhood." *Seminars in Dermatology* 7 (1988): 58–65.

INDEX